1983

Selye's Guide
to
Stress
Research

Selye's Guide
to
Stress
Research

Volume I

Edited by

Hans Selye

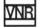 **VAN NOSTRAND REINHOLD COMPANY**
NEW YORK   CINCINNATI   ATLANTA   DALLAS   SAN FRANCISCO
LONDON   TORONTO   MELBOURNE

Van Nostrand Reinhold Company Regional Offices:
New York   Cincinnati   Atlanta   Dallas   San Francisco

Van Nostrand Reinhold Company International Offices:
London   Toronto   Melbourne

Library of Congress Catalog Card Number: 79-18512
ISBN: 0-442-27483-1

Manufactured in the United States of America

Published by Van Nostrand Reinhold Company
135 West 50th Street, New York, N.Y. 10020

Published simultaneously in Canada by Van Nostrand Reinhold Ltd.

15   14   13   12   11   10   9   8   7   6   5   4   3   2   1

Library of Congress Cataloging in Publication Data

Main entry under title:

Selye's guide to stress research.

    Includes index.
    I.   Stress (Physiology)   2.   Stress
(Psychology)   I.   Selye, Hans, 1907–
II.   Title: Guide to stress research.
QP82.2.S8S46   155.9   79-18512
ISBN 0-442-27483-1 Vol. 1

Preface

THE PURPOSE OF THIS VOLUME

When I was first approached by Mr. Ashak M. Rawji of Van Nostrand Reinhold to edit a guide to contemporary stress research (if possible as an annual series), I immediately realized both the enormous value and the extreme difficulty of such a task.

I was to select the most timely topics, and the best specialists to represent their respective fields. This was to be done regardless of whether the chosen material was highly technical or understandable to the educated layman. The work was to reflect but one thing: the current status of the stress concept. It would hardly have been possible to assess the relative importance of biochemical, neurological or psychosocial topics impartially, or even to decide who best could deal with the theoretical intricacies of neurohumoral transmission systems, and it would have bordered on the ridiculous to compare the relative importance and timeliness of these topics with the very practical problems facing the businessman, the athelete and the family counselor. The one common link among all these authors would be that they know a great deal about individual facets of stress, its mechanism and the techniques of facing its demands.

The only problem all living beings share is that of surviving as happily as possible in an ever-changing environment. Microbes, plants and most of the living organisms situated lower on the evolutionary scale achieve this by means of more or less automatic cellular responses or instincts, which have evolved in accordance with "the survival of the fittest." Only the higher organisms, and particularly man, have acquired a brain sufficiently complex to endow them with a sense of logic and ethics, through which they can learn to control, at least in part, their hereditary impulses.

For man, this process led to a variety of increasingly sophisticated codes of behavior which best suited particular individuals at a particular time, helping them to choose consciously how they should respond to the demands of life. Of course, the basic concept of what we now call stress goes back to prehistoric times; it must have occurred to primitive man occasionally when he was tired, tense, sick or unhappy and felt the need to adapt. He had no name for it and did not at first inquire into its causes and mechanisms. But later, he ascribed it to some superior being, usually an omniscient deity. The very fact of primitive man's own existence was, to him, sufficient proof that there must be a creator whose wisdom and power far exceed that of his creations. For this reason, all the most ancient codes of behavior or ethics were based on the apparently obvious conclusion that our main problem is to satisfy our creator and avert his displeasure.

Since it seemed self-evident that anything that happens must be purposeful, and since the creator was conceived as the source of every happening, man arrived at the concept of universal teleology, according to which the cause of every happening is the will of the creator. And since man cannot imagine anything totally unrelated to his experience, the creator was endowed with human feelings, such as love, hate and the wish to achieve dominance over his creations through reward and punishment.

So it was that a variety of religious and philosophical codes of ethics were developed to guide us in our wish to satisfy the all-powerful being under the most diverse circumstances of life.

Various forms of teleology are still common in contemporary thought because it is difficult to imagine anything that has no purpose; it takes a considerable power of abstraction to imagine something that just happens, and not to ask why.

Herein lies the essential difference between the concept of a law that tells you what to do and what not to do, and one that is purely descriptive and only states what is. In fact, perhaps the word "law" should not even have been applied to what we call the laws of Nature; perhaps they are better described as facts that can be discovered, clearly formulated, proved and taught. Their knowledge is most useful to man (who does have purposes and can better achieve them by behaving in conformity with natural principles than by acting exclusively on tradition or superstition), but they are instruments, not final aims.

As we shall see, I have tried to develop a code of behavior or a philosophy of life based on the facts of Nature. It is still incomplete, but at least it represents a first step toward a code of conduct independent of all creeds and authorities assumed a priori to be infallible. Even in its present immature form, it has helped many people to find their way toward what they themselves consider their ultimate aim or port of destination, by improving their mastery over the innumerable unpredictable dangers posed by the stress of life.

These apparently very theoretical, philosophical remarks seemed indispensable to me as a prelude to what I have to say concerning the stress concept in general, and the purpose and use of this anthology in particular.

What is stress? Nowadays, everyone seems to be talking about stress. You hear it not only in daily conversation but also through television, radio, the newspapers and the constantly increasing number of conferences, stress centers and university courses that are devoted to the topic. Yet remarkably few people define the concept the same way or even bother to attempt a clear-cut definition. The businessman thinks of it as frustration or emotional tension, the air traffic controller as a problem in concentration, the biochemist and endocrinologist as a purely chemical event, the athlete as muscular tension. This list could be extended to almost every human experience or activity, and, somewhat surprisingly, most people—be they chartered accountants, businessmen or surgeons— think of their own occupations as being the most stressful. Similarly, most of us believe that ours is "the age of stress," forgetting that the caveman's fear of being attacked by wild animals while he slept, or of dying from hunger, cold or exhaustion, must have been just as stressful as our fear of a world war, the crash of the stock exchange, overpopulation or the unpredictability of the future.

Somewhat ironically, there is a grain of truth in every formulation of stress because all demands upon our adaptability do evoke the stress phenomenon discussed in the present work. But we tend to forget that there would be no reason to use the single word "stress" to describe such diverse circumstances as those just enumerated were there not something common in all of them, just as we would have no reason to use a single word in connection with the production of light, heat, cold or sound, if we had been unable to formulate the concept of energy, which is required to bring about any of these effects. We formulated a definition of stress as "the nonspecific (that is, common) result of *any* demand upon the body," be it a mental or somatic demand for survival and the accomplishment of our aims.

It is the formulation of this definition, based on objective indicators such as bodily and chemical changes which appear after any demand, that has brought the subject (so popular now that it is often referred to as "stressology") out of the stage of vague cocktail party chitchat into the domain of science.

In 1936, when this definition was formulated, we knew of only three objective indicators that could be recognized no matter how stress was produced. They showed that there is a common element in the most varied demands for adaptation. These indicators were: the mobilization of the anterior pituitary-adrenal axis, the readily observable involution of the thymico-lymphatic system and the appearance of peptic ulcers. Now, if these indicators (as well as many others since described, which are totally nonspecific) appear, the phenomenon is stress *by definition,* irrespective of any other specific changes that may occur after exposure to one or the other "stressor" or stress-producing agent.

In selecting the contributors to this volume, I purposely requested the cooperation of generally recognized, eminent experts in their fields, who, I knew, see stress from different perspectives. This assures the readers that whatever they read in these pages will be based on first-rate expertise; at the same time they will see that even among the greatest stress specialists some fundamental problems are either ignored or misunderstood. I had suggested the contributors follow the general rules of this publishing company, but as you will see, even that is not what happened. Though some contributors wrote in very classical scientific style, others were much less observant of conventions, and one author even decided to ·write his chapter in the form of a personal letter to me. Yet, I let them speak in their own way because with authors of this caliber I felt that I should not use the customary editorial prerogatives; moreover, it is part of the benefit you can derive from a book of this kind to learn about the personalities who participate in this effort and the way they interpret the task assigned to them as expressed in the title. After all, to understand a science fully you must also understand the scientists who formulated it.

Here I shall make no specific reference to any chapter, but in studying the text readers will have no difficulty in recognizing the main sources of confusion that I shall now enumerate:

1. *Stress is nonspecific.* This does not mean that all stress situations are identical because stress is never seen in isolation. You cannot produce stress in pure form without using a stressor, and the latter necessarily always has specific effects. In the cold, you shiver; in the heat, you sweat—but these are specific actions of cold and heat respectively. What

is common among them is only those manifestations which we now consider characteristic of a demand in itself; of the demand to resist cold, heat or any other stressor that you may encounter.

2. *A stressor is whatever produces stress, with or without functioning hormonal or nervous systems.* This may be a somatic demand such as an athletic effort, the healing of a wound or resistance to infection or poisoning; but it may be purely psychogenic, such as putting up with an almost intolerable partner in private or business life. In all these situations, the stressor makes certain specific demands that are not common to anything but the condition under consideration; yet it also necessitates the mobilization of the general resistance phenomenon as such.

The first experiments on the stress reaction and the entire general adaptation syndrome (G.A.S.) were conducted mainly from the viewpoint of the hormonal system. Hence, we hastened in 1937 to perform experiments to prove that even in totally hypophysectomized and/or adrenalectomized rats, exposure to stress produces all the stereotyped nonspecific responses characteristic of demands as such, except those made by stimuli that are relayed through the pituitary-adrenocortical axis. The importance of corticotropin-releasing factor (CRF) or even adrenocorticotropic hormone (ACTH) is still debated, yet it is universally accepted that variations in CRF or ACTH production are the most reliable indicators showing that a state of stress exists.

3. *Much confusion exists concerning various views on corticoid and ACTH feedback and corticoid utilization.* This confusion needs clarification. There appears to be little doubt that, at least under normal conditions, excess corticoid administration can diminish corticoid production through the inhibition of ACTH secretion. Similarly, administration of excessive amounts of ACTH will act back on the pituitary, and decrease ACTH production itself and thus, secondarily, corticoid secretion. In both instances, ACTH production is diminished either directly by ACTH itself or by a longer loop going from the adrenal cortex to the pituitary and/or hypothalamus. The much-debated older idea, that while corticoids exert their action they are "utilized," and that this mechanism rather than increased blood levels of corticoids is the stimulus for the rise in ACTH production, has long been disproven. The corticoids act more or less as catalysts by their mere presence, and are not used up during this process to a much greater extent than normally. For example, it was shown that, in hypophysectomized rats, administration of a given amount of ACTH produces essentially the same enlargement of one adrenal whether the

contralateral gland is present or removed. Hence the stimulation of adrenal gland tissue does not appreciably elevate the catabolism of corticoids.

4. *The shift in pituitary activity during stress was the subject of much discussion.* In the early thirties we described the fact that in animals, as in man, the adrenal cortex enlarges during extreme and prolonged stress, whereas somatic growth, lactation and other phenomena—then known to be under pituitary control—diminish. This led us to the concept of a "shift" in pituitary activity. We assumed it to be due to the fact that during intense emergencies, in the interests of survival, increased life-maintaining corticoid production receives priority over other functions, and we speculated that this may be due to the diminished ability of pituitary cells to produce maximal amounts of ACTH while maintaining their other secretory actions.

Since then, the existence of such a shift in pituitary *activity* has been confirmed in many laboratory experiments and by current clinical observations on patients exposed continuously to a variety of intense stressors; but it has also been confirmed that such a shift may be due to diverse mechanisms that could not have been forseen in the early thirties. For example, the various trophic hormones of the pituitary are not produced by the same cells. Also, diminished peripheral activity is not necessarily the result of lowered production, but may be due to lowered receptivity of peripheral organs and a variety of other conditioning factors, such as species differences or significant variations depending upon the intensity and the duration of exposure. These possibilities have been clearly brought out by several contributors to this volume.

5. *A psychologic stressor can only act if it is appreciated as such.* Otherwise there is no stress; in fact, there is no demand. Under deep anesthesia, a person cannot be placed under stress of the most irritating boss, spouse or financial calamity, just as exposure to X-rays makes no demand if we are completely protected by a lead screen.

6. *The fact that all stress situations are apparently different does not nullify their nonspecificity.* That both the event and the response to it are always specific is self-evident and was emphasized in the earliest papers on this subject. This is explained by two circumstances: (A) the stressor is always accompanied by specific side effects; (B) both internal and external predisposing or immunizing factors modify the response. These last factors have long been recognized in stress research; we call them conditioning factors. They may be internal (e.g., heredity, previous exposure

to stress) or external (e.g., air pollution, traditions or education, seasonal variations).

7. *There is a distinction between good stress and bad stress.* Good stress we call eustress (eu = good, as in euphonia, euphoria), and bad stress we call distress, which is the detrimental variety.

Here again, we must remember that everything depends not upon what actually happens to us but upon how we appreciate the events. The news that a war was won may cause eustress for the victor and distress for the vanquished nation. A letter from the bank stating that you have $1000 in your account may cause you horrible distress if you are a multimillionaire, and as a result you may lose all your self-esteem and commit suicide; whereas a Battery bum who never had more than a few cents to his name would regard this as a most satisfying, eustressful event.

In ordinary conversation, I think it is perfectly acceptable to speak of stress when we mean distress because eustress is rarely what we complain about, and it simplifies matters to employ a brief terminology. We speak of Johnny's running a temperature when we mean he is running a high temperature because that is usually what causes us to worry. It is important for us to realize, however, that there are two types of stress, and that both are conducive to certain common objective manifestations.

8. *Stress is not a yes or no phenomenon.* We must recognize that stress can exist in various degrees. Different demands, and different intensities of the same demands, do not always cause equal stress reactions. Almost anything we feel or do represents a demand, but in each situation the role of stress may be more or less important.

9. *The stress diseases are also a matter of degree.* Some maladies are almost completely due to our appreciation of their stressful effect. High blood pressure, heart accidents, mental breakdowns, migraines and insomnia are usually listed in this category, although even here additional factors likewise play a role. Other maladies, such as a lethal bullet wound through the head or paralysis after complete transection of the spinal cord, are totally unrelated to stress—they make no demands because there is nothing you can do about them; it is only their consequences that may cause stress. Most likely, the vast majority of all maladies for which the patient seeks medical attention are predominantly due to stress—particularly to psychogenic stress, which is the basis of psychosomatic medicine.

10. *"Stress tests" are useful to the degree to which they can be individualized.* Most of the current questionnaires and physical or chemical

stress tests have been accepted as measuring stress on the basis of averages taken from large populations. To my mind, this is very much like computerized diagnoses or recommendations for therapy. These procedures may be quite valid in that they show how most persons would behave under certain circumstances; but they say nothing about the individual patient himself because no one is average. In contrast, stress tests based on statistically significant data about, say, the crew of an American battleship or school children or inhabitants of old folks' homes, give more pertinent and useful rules concerning regulations that should be instituted for the average member of such a group. Of course, it is not feasible to test everybody from every point of view, but the closer you can get to what in medicine we call a personal visit by your physician (as when doctors still made house calls), the more valuable the test. This is the basis of holistic medicine; you must consider the whole patient including his environment in order to come as close as possible to a correct diagnosis. Naturally, in practice it is impossible to do this for everyone, but with specialized tests one can give advice at various levels; for example, the executive or the blue collar workers in a particular company, or the students or staff of a school in a certain country at a particular time. This can be achieved by questionnaires. Of course, the more individualized the quiz, the more expensive and time-consuming the testing procedure will be; therefore, it is necessary to adjust wishes to the possibilities in any specified group.

At our Institute, we are now working on a personalized stress test which could be used by individuals or by increasingly large groups. Its main characteristic is that you compose and fill out your own questionnaire, putting down events that are likely to occur in your personal life, and then arrange these events in decreasing order of their stressor impact upon each individual. The results will then be useful for each person so examined, and can also be averaged, using the results for regulating the conditions to be imposed upon groups of increasing size. The same principles would apply to somatic, i.e., chemical or biophysical, indicators.

11. *A clear distinction must be made between treatment techniques (biofeedback, relaxation, physical exercise) and a philosophy of life.* Naturally, both are of considerable importance, but I believe that the greatest challenge to humanity at present is to find a philosophy of life, a code of behavior, which gives good guidance, not to avoid stress (for that is impossible), but to cope with it in order to achieve health, long life and happiness.

It would be repetitious to review in detail all our work in this domain, but the major points mentioned are to be found in six key publications of mine (1-6).

As I have said, in undertaking the task of editing this guide, I was fully aware of the difficulties it would pose. Aside from those already discussed, how could anyone select authors and present articles so as to give a true image of the stress concept as we see it this year? It does seem worthwhile, however, to try to come as close to perfection as possible. Most of our readers will realize how great the confusion is in our field, and how easily even the most eminent experts can fall into the simplest traps, which we are bound to encounter if we want to follow such a complex problem as the stress concept in its countless applications; but we can still remain on a steady course by remembering the basic definition of what we are talking about.

I am very glad that so many eminent colleagues in the most diverse branches of stressology have agreed to contribute to this group effort. Here you will find opinions expressed by sociologists, psychologists, organic chemists and teachers of stress-reduction techniques. The only feature these authors have in common is that they are all internationally recognized experts in their respective fields. So read their contributions with the respect and attention they deserve.

In the Epilogue, which I was asked to write, I shall try to outline my favorite subject, one that I consider to be the most important in stress research—namely, the means for the accomplishment of the objective of Stress without Distress.

HANS SELYE

References

1. Selye, H. A syndrome produced by diverse nocuous agents. *Nature 138:* 32, 1936.
2. Selye, H. The general adaptation syndrome and the diseases of adaptation. *J. Clin. Endocr. 6:* 117, 1946.
3. Selye, H. *The Stress of Life*. New York: McGraw-Hill, first ed., 1956; second ed., 1976.
4. Selye, H. *Stress Without Distress*. Philadelphia—New York: J. B. Lippincott, 1974.
5. Selye, H. *Stress in Health and Disease*. Reading, Massachusetts: Butterworths, 1976.
6. Selye, H. *The Stress of My Life: A Scientist's Memoirs*. New York: Van Nostrand Reinhold, 1979.

Contents

Selye's Guide
to
Stress
Research

1
What is A Stressful Life Event?

Barbara Snell Dohrenwend and Bruce P. Dohrenwend
The City College of the City University of New York and College of Physicians and Surgeons, Columbia University

An extensive body of clinical and epidemiologic research suggests that stressful life events are causally implicated in a variety of undesirable effects on functioning and health (e.g., Dohrenwend and Dohrenwend, 1974; Gunderson and Rahe, 1974; Wolff, Wolf, and Hare, 1950). The effects described range from lowering the grade-point averages of college freshmen (Harris, 1972) to sudden death (Engel, 1971). However, at the same time that these studies have discovered many possibly pathogenic effects of stressful life events, they have raised questions, as yet unanswered, about the process whereby these effects are produced. A number of critics have argued that further progress toward answering these questions depends on solving numerous methodological problems that are common in research on stressful life events (e.g., Brown, 1974, pp. 218–226; Dohrenwend and Dohrenwend, 1977; Dohrenwend and Dohrenwend, 1974; Hough, Fairbank, and Garcia, 1976; Hudgens, 1974). We will not repeat this catalogue of criticisms but will focus instead on a critical question that has been bypassed in much of this methodological discussion, namely: What is a stressful life event?

WHY WE NEED TO KNOW:

Before trying to answer this question, however, let us consider why it is necessary to do so. Our reasoning on this issue is based on a psychosocial

*This work was supported in part by Research Grant MH 10318 and by Research Scientist Award KO5-MH 14663 from the National Institute of Mental Health, U.S. Public Health Service. It was also supported by the Foundations' Fund for Research in Psychiatry.

model of the stress process. This model, which is shown in Figure 1.1, is designed to provide a comprehensive description rather than to represent any particular, possibly controversial theory about psychosocial stress (cf. Scott and Howard, 1970).

Note first that the process described in this model starts with a proximate rather than distant cause of stress-induced pathology, with recent events in the life of an individual rather than with distant childhood experiences. Furthermore, this initial step in the model rests on a distinction emphasized by Selye (1956), and made by others as well (Dohrenwend, 1961), between a stressor, an event that initiates the stress process, and the immediate reaction to that event, the state of stress. The state of stress is usually inferred rather than observed, and for our purpose its nature does not need to be specified.

The next step in the model suggests that what follows after the stress state depends on the mediation of situational and personal factors that constitute the context in which this state occurs. Situational mediators are conditions in the environment that are external to, but impinge on, the individual. They include material supports or handicaps and social supports or handicaps. Some social theorists have argued that, instead of stressful life events, it is these relatively constant conditions, particularly deprivations associated with disadvantaged ethnic status and poverty, that are the primary cuases of stress-induced pathology (e.g., Langner and Michael, 1963; Gersten, Langner, Eisenberg, and Simcha-Fagan, 1977).

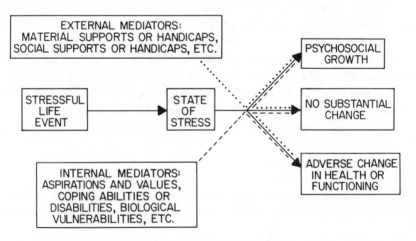

Figure 1.1. Model of life stress process.

The model does not prejudge this issue. Situational constraints may play a more important role than stressful life events in determining the nature of the outcome of the psychosocial stress process; the premise underlying the model is, however, that relatively constant situational factors are not sufficient, in the absence of one or more precipitating events, to explain the occurrence of stress-induced changes in an individual's functioning or health.

The final step in the model indicates that a state of stress interacts with situational and personal mediators to produce one of three general outcomes. A person who experiences stressful life events may as a result (1) undergo psychosocial growth, (2) resume his life without substantial permanent change, or (3) experience a change for the worse in his functioning or health.

This grossly simplified model of the psychosocial stress process states that if a stressful life event impinges on an individual and certain unfavorable states of internal and external mediating factors are present, then dysfunctional behavior or illness will result. The occurrence of dysfunctional behavior or illness does not, however, imply the existence of a stress process, since changes in behavior or health can arise from other causes. Consider, for example, Glass and Singer's (1972) observation that persons exposed to stressors under certain conditions subsequently did badly on a proofreading task. One would also predict that individuals with low scores on a test of reading ability, associated perhaps with a poor education, would perform badly as proofreaders without being exposed beforehand to a stressor. Nor does the presence of unfavorable mediating factors alone indicate that associated dysfunctional behavior or illness was induced by psychosocial stress. For example, if a person who is a poor member of a disadvantaged ethnic group develops pneumonia, it does not follow that psychosocial stress must have been involved. Poor nutrition, heavy alcohol consumption, and a hard winter in unheated housing might well be sufficient. In general, in the absence of evidence that a person has recently experienced one or more stressful life events, one cannot infer that his dysfunctional behavior or illness was induced by psychosocial stress. Therefore, to study the psychosocial stress process we need to know how to identify stressful life events.

Furthermore, we can ask certain interesting questions about the psychosocial stress process only if we can measure the severity of stressful life events. Such measurement would enable us to ask the simple question: How does the severity of the stressor relate to the outcome of the stress process? (Cf. Weick, 1970, pp. 288–292.) Another, more complex question that also depends on the measurement of the severity of stressful life events for an answer, is: What is the relative contribution of stressors of different severity as against variations in mediating factors to the outcome of the stress process? (Cf. Dohrenwend and Dohrenwend, 1978, p. 14; Glass and Singer, 1972, p. 51.)

CONCEPTUALIZATION AND MEASUREMENT OF STRESSFUL LIFE EVENTS IN STRESS RESEARCH

As a step toward arriving at a way of conceptualizing and measuring stressful life events, we will review the stress research literature to see what ideas it provides. We note first that a large portion of research on stress uses animals as subjects. Although these studies obviously do not investigate stressful life events directly, they are not necessarily irrelevant.

Studies of Animals

There are two possible reasons for using animal subjects in any kind of psychological research. One is to determine how behavior varies as a function of a species' position on the phylogenetic scale. The other is to do experimental studies that ethics rule out with human subjects. The literature indicates that the second is the overriding reason. On the one hand, the argument is that animal studies are useful insofar as they demonstrate cross-species similarity in the stress process and thereby strengthen generalizations from results obtained with animals to humans (e.g., Seligman, 1975, pp. 27–31). On the other hand, where species differences have been found, as in the conditions required to produce experimental neuroses by means of Pavlovian conditioning, researchers have emphasized the need to use higher, primate species so that they can "conduct experiments under the conditions closest to natural life situations, and analogous to those which are observed during conflict situations in man" (Lapin and Cherkovich, 1971, p. 266).

Many of the stress experiments with animals involve the introduction of stressors that appear analogous to life events in the paradigm shown in Figure 1.1. However, the conceptual definitions of stressors are left vague. In Selye's research, for example, a stressor is defined as any agent that produces stress. Perhaps the reason for the vagueness is that the operational definitions of stressors in research on animals seem so clear-cut; for example, the introduction of electroshock whose strength, all would agree, can adequately be measured in volts.

Nevertheless, if researchers who investigate the responses of animals to stressors generally intend their studies to serve as analogues to human expected stimulation, highly persistent stimulation, and fatigue-producing and boredom-producing settings, among others, have also been correspond. Unfortunately, this correspondence has seldom been considered at all and has nowhere been considered in a systematic way as far as we are aware. For example, Selye, who is certainly concerned about the implications of his studies of animals for the quality of human life, has barely suggested what life situations are relevant: "The businessman who is under constant pressure from his clients and employees alike, the air-traffic controller who knows that a moment of distraction may mean death to hundreds of people, the athlete who desperately wants to win a race, and the husband who helplessly watches his wife slowly and painfully dying of cancer, all suffer from stress" (1974, p. 26). Perhaps reasonably, the problem of conceptualizing stressful life events has been left to others by stress researchers who use animal subjects.

Studies of Human Subjects

Let us see, then, how this problem is handled by investigators who work with human subjects. For our purpose it will be useful to group stress studies of human subjects into three categories: analogue experiments, specific life event studies, and comprehensive life event studies.

Analogue Experiments. Analogue experiments with human subjects, like those with animal subjects, often use physical stressors such as electric shock or noise, which are easily manipulated and measured. In addition, as Appley and Trumbull illustrated in their attempt at a comprehensive description of experimentally applied stressors, stress studies using human subjects also involve stimuli described in cognitive or affective terms: ". . . situations characterized as new, intense, rapidly changing, sudden or unexpected, including (but not requiring) approach to the upper thresholds of tolerability. At the same time, stimulus deficit, absence of expected stimulation, highly persistent stimulation, and fatigue-producing and boredom-producing settings, among others, have also been described as stressful, as have stimuli leading to cognitive misperception, stimuli susceptible to hallucination, and stimuli calling for conflicting responses'' (1967, p. 5). Apparent contradictions in this set of conditions, such as new and changing conditions as against those that are boring, suggest that the choice of experimental stimuli has not been based on a systematic conception of stressors. Instead, it is probably fair to say that in analogue experiments the conditions that serve as stressors are usually chosen for their face validity, that is, because it seems obvious to the experimenter that they are stressful (cf. Appley and Trumbull, 1967, p. 6).

The question is, however: What do these analogues represent in life outside the experimenters' laboratories? In practice, this question has usually been ignored. When not ignored, it has been answered by referring to some abstract category such as "aversive stimuli" (Glass and Singer, 1972, p. 6) without specifying criteria for identifying the events that belong in the category. In general, then, analogue studies of human subjects provide little guidance as to how to conceptualize and measure stressful life events.

Specific Life Event Studies. Stress researchers working in natural life settings have studied the effects of a number of specific stressful life events, such as widowhood (e.g., Clayton, Desmarais, and Winokur, 1968; Clayton, 1975; Parkes, 1972), severe injury (e.g., Hamburg and Adams, 1967), and loss of job (Cobb and Kasl, 1977; Kasl, Gore, and Cobb, 1975). Some of these studies were not intended to lead to conclusions concerning life stress in general but were, instead, designed to increase comprehension of a particular event and its sequelae (e.g., Clayton, Desmarais, and Winokur, 1968; Cobb and Kasl, 1977).

Others, in contrast, aimed to derive principles from particular events that would apply to stressful life events in general. The domain to which these generalizations were to be applied has been described as including: "threatening, difficult experiences for many individuals. Some of these are inherent components of the life cycle; others reflect major features of urbanized, technologically complex societies" (Hamburg and Adams, 1967, p. 277); or, along with bereavement, "Less obvious forms of loss, and losses that take place some time before the onset of an illness [which] may be overlooked" (Parkes, 1972, p. 4). These descriptions of the general domain of life events make two useful points: first, that stressful life events are not limited to those that are inherent in the life cycle; and second, that their domain extends beyond a set of dramatic and obvious life events. For further help in specifying the domain of stressful life events, however, we must turn to comprehensive life event studies.

Comprehensive Life Event Studies. In these studies the subjects were sampled on some basis other than their participation in particular life events, with the aim of determining the effects of a wider range of events. Thus, for example, Hinkle drew samples of telephone company employees (1974), Theorell studied Stockholm residents who had had a recent myocardial infarction (1974), and Myers and his colleagues (1974) investigated a representative sample of the population of a mental health center catchment area.

This study design seems to force investigators to attend to the question of what constitutes the class of stressful life events, since lists of events to be inquired about must be constructed and must make sense to the persons being studied. For example, Holmes and Rahe, extrapolating from the types of events that they extracted from "life charts" recording case histories of patients admitted to treatment for medical problems, defined stressful life events as those "whose advent is either indicative of or requires a significant change in the ongoing life pattern of the individual" (1967, p. 217). Brown and Birley focused on "events which on common sense grounds are likely to produce emotional disturbance in many people . . . [and usually involve] either danger; significant changes in health, status or way of life; the promise of these; or important fulfillments or disappointments" (1968, p. 204). Similarly, Myers and his colleagues defined "crises" or "events" as "experiences involving role transformations, changes in status or environment, or impositions of pain" (1974, p. 399). And Antonovsky and Kats referred to "life crises" consisting of "objective situations which, on the face of it, would seem to be universally stressful" and involving "an experience which either imposed pain or necessitated a role transformation" (1967, p. 16).

These definitions indicate broad agreement at a highly abstract level concerning what is stressful about life events apart from their outcome. The agreement centers on the idea that stressful life events include those that involve change in the usual activities of most individuals who experience them. In addition, there appears to be further agreement on the part of most investigators on the need to distinguish events that are likely to be experienced as negative from those likely to be experienced as positive or neutral.

However, there is also a basic difference among life researchers about how to define the stressful characteristics of life events. The issue is whether the stressfulness of life events is idiographic or nomothetic in character.

This conceptual distinction was originally introduced to psychology by Gordon Allport, who noted, "In the field of medicine, diagnosis and therapy are idiographic procedures, but both rest intimately upon a knowledge of the common factors in disease determined by the nomothetic sciences of bacteriology and biochemistry" (1937, p. 22), and "The generalizations [made by psychologists] are not, or should not be, concerned only with the operations of an hypothetical 'average' mind. Their aim is rather to state explicitly the [idiographic] principles by virtue of which unique personalities are created by nature and understood by men" (1937, p. 61).

In the context of research on stressful life events, the nomothetic approach is implicit in the work of Holmes and his colleagues (Holmes and Masuda, 1974; Holmes and Rahe, 1967) and of Paykel and his colleagues (Paykel, Prusoff, and Uhlenhuth, 1971), in that both groups predicted the impact of stressful life events on individuals from average perceptions of these events. In contrast, Hinkle argued that "people react to their 'life situations' or social conditions in terms of the meaning of these situations to them" (1973, p. 46). In their review of stress research, Appley and Trumbull drew a conclusion consistent with Hinkle's position: "With the exception of extreme life-threatening situations, it is reasonable to say that no stimulus is a stressor to all individuals exposed to it" (1967, p. 7). Among researchers and theorists who have dealt explicitly with the problem of defining stressful life events, the idiographic conception is widely accepted (e.g., Hinkle, 1973, p. 46; McGrath, 1970, p. 17; Rahe, 1974, pp. 76–77; Theorell, 1974, p. 111; Vinokur and Selzer, 1975, p. 335).

Conclusions from Stress Research

Stress research, whether on human or animal subjects, whether in the form of analogue experiments or life event studies, does not answer the question of how to conceptualize and measure stressful life events. Instead, it becomes clear in reviewing this research that all of it requires an answer to the question. This answer is needed as an aid in specifying the correspondence implied in analogue studies and the generalizations to be made from specific life event studies. Comprehensive life events studies, while not providing a single answer to the question of conceptualization and measurement, do provide a starting point in that they delineate an issue that will have to be resolved: the issue of idiographic versus nomothetic conception and measurement of stressful life events.

IDIOGRAPHIC VERSUS NOMOTHETIC CONCEPTUALIZATION AND MEASUREMENT OF STRESSFUL LIFE EVENTS

The conceptualization and measurement of stressful life events must take two facts into account. First, it is not possible to measure the stressfulness of the event in terms of physical dimensions, such as the number of volts or decibels, as it is when electric shock or noise is the stressor. Second, stressful life events are not limited to extremely severe, life-threatening events, which, as Appley and Trumbull (1967) noted, are universal stressors. The consensus that such events are highly stressful is, presumably, largely biologically determined. For most life events, such as losing a job or getting a divorce, however, there is no such biological reality underlying the perception of the event. Yet most people have ideas about how positive or negative events such as divorce or loss of a job are, and how much change they entail. These ideas must be learned. The question of how they are learned is central to resolution of the issue of idiographic versus nomothetic conceptualization of stressful life events.

In dealing with this question it is crucial to distinguish between the meaning of an event to an individual after he or she has experienced it as against its meaning to him or her beforehand. If we rely on the meaning of an event after it has been experienced to define stressful life events, we risk becoming ensnared in a tautology: events that are followed by dysfunctional behavior or illness are stressful; stressful events induce dysfunctional behavior or illness. In practice, some investigators advocating idiographic measures of stressful life events have done just this, since they have taken their measures of stressfulness after subjects have experienced particular events in association with, for example, an automobile accident (Vinokur and Selzer, 1975) or a heart attack (Theorell, 1974). These investigators have, moreover, further confused the issue by arguing for their idiographic definition of life events on the ground that it yields higher correlations with outcomes than a nomothetic definition, a result to be expected from the tautology involved (cf. Paykel and Uhlenhuth, 1972, p. SS93).

If we reject post hoc idiographic definitions of stressful life events, we come to the question of what is learned that would give idiographic meanings to stressful life events before they are experienced. Our reading of the literature indicates that this question has not been answered directly, since, for those who advocate idiographic definition, it is not the perception of the event as such that is conceived in idiographic terms but rather the relation between the individual's acquired coping skills, among other resources (e.g., Lazarus and Launier, 1978), and the demands of the event. Thus, for example, one group of investigators who advocated idiographic scoring as "more accurate" argued that "It may also reflect the subject's perception as well as his way of coping with life change events" (Ander, Lindström, and Tibblin, 1974, p. 123). In terms of the psychosocial stress model in Figure 1.1, this relational type of conception provides no basis for measuring stressful life events apart from the context of internal and external mediating factors in which they occur. Its limitations are, moreover, indicated in the rationale for it offered by Lazarus and Launier: "The continuous flow of such person-environment relationships in stress, emotion, and coping cannot comfortably be encompassed within the traditional S-O-R, linear causation models.... Such a flow, and the changing relationships involved in it, need to be examined in purely descriptive terms before one asks the more analytic questions about the respective causal roles of variables of person and environment" (1978). The time has come, we think, to ask these analytic questions.

We return, then, to the question of the learned basis for defining the stressfulness of life events. As a general principle we know that much learning that occurs in a social context depends on vicarious rather than direct experience. Moreover, this vicarious experience can be transmitted through many persons or generations as social norms (e.g., Bandura and Walters, 1963, p. 72). In this way individuals who have not personally experienced an event could come to have definite expectations concerning its stressfulness.

We are likely to recognize the existence of culturally determined expectancies about the meaning of certain events in the case of exotic phenomena such as voodoo and hex deaths (Seligman, 1975, pp. 176–177). We are, however, not as likely to be aware of less dramatic expectancies that also appear to be culturally determined. An example of such an expectancy is suggested by the finding of Miller and his colleagues (1974) that the amount of readjustment required by marriage was ranked much lower by residents of a rural area than by residents of urban areas in the United States. In interpreting their finding Miller and his coauthors noted: "In rural North Carolina when one marries the expectation is to move only a few miles and to stay where you move—or at least to stay in the locale. In an urban area marriage may mean the uprooting of one or the other of the couple, a change in living abode for more space, and a change in recreation because of a change in expenses'' (1974, p. 271).

As part of the answer to the question of how to conceptualize stressful life events, we hypothesize that the stressfulness of most life events is defined by group norms (cf. Hinkle, 1973, p. 46). We are therefore proposing a nomothetic conception of the stressfulness of life events, but one that implies that the stressfulness of a particular life event may vary from group to group and may change over time. Note, also, that we are not suggesting that the normative expectancy concerning its stressfulness will necessarily be the major determinant of the impact of a life event on an individual; internal and external mediating factors may be more important. However, other things equal, we hypothesize that the impact of a life event on an individual will be determined by a learned normative expectancy concerning the stressfulness of that event.

SOME PROCEDURAL IMPLICATIONS OF A NORMATIVE CONCEPTION OF THE STRESSFULNESS OF LIFE EVENTS

Given a normative conception, the basic question to be answered by procedures for measuring the stressfulness of a life event is whether there is consensus about it. A number of investigators have addressed this question using a variety of analytic techniques (especially Dohrenwend, Krasnoff, Askenasy, and Dohrenwend, 1978; Holmes and Rahe, 1967; Paykel, Prusoff, and Uhlenhuth, 1971).

Their data, though not identical in form, have all been numerical ratings of life events obtained from a substantial number of informants, usually more than 100. Note that informants were not asked to judge simply whether a life event is stressful or not, but how stressful it is. This procedure avoids the possible implication that only a limited number of highly visible events are stressful, an implication that experienced clinicians have rejected (e.g., Parkes, 1972, p. 4). Moreover, it yields more information than the simple dichotomous question, while not precluding later tests of the hypothesis that events at the low end of the rating scale are not stressors.

Turning to the analytic techniques employed to determine whether a set of numerical ratings reflect consensus about the stressfulness of life events, Holmes and his colleagues noted first that the dispersion of individual judgments of particular events followed Ekman's law, since they increased with the mean of the judgments of an event. This lawfulness, they implied, indicated that individual differences between informants could be ignored. In addition, Holmes and his colleagues tested for group differences in judgment by calculating the mean judgment for each event given by contrasting status groups, and correlating these means. They showed that the correlations between contrasting groups such as men and women, blacks and whites, and young and old, as well as between judges of different nationalities, were on the order of .90 (Holmes and Masuda, 1974). Despite the fact that correlations between groups do not necessarily indicate agreement in their absolute judgments (cf. Askenasy, Dohrenwend, and Dohrenwend, 1977), Holmes and his colleagues, while noting some cross-cultural differences concerning particular events, concluded that their data revealed "remarkable consensus" (Holmes and Masuda, 1974, p. 57).

Paykel, Prusoff, and Uhlenhuth examined the standard deviations of the ratings of each of their events in order to evalute the level of individual differences among their informants. They concluded, "When compared with the scale range these standard deviations appear moderate in magnitude" (1971, p. 342). In order to answer the question of whether there were group differences, they computed *t* tests on individual events for various dichotomized social statuses. They found significant differences on a substantial minority of events despite the fact that correlations between mean ratings by contrasting status groups, like those reported by Holmes and his colleagues, were in the range of .90. In evaluating these significant differences, however, they noted: "Most of the differences between means of individual events were between one and four points on a scale of 20-point range. In terms of magnitude such differences were of limited importance, and the very high correlations reflect these small magnitudes" (1971, p. 313). They concluded from their examination of individual and group differences that, in general, ". . . the findings indicate that there is a substantial common core in the way events are perceived that is shared by most persons, at least within one society" (1971, p. 347). With respect to use of these scores, however, they cautioned: "For use in a single individual scores would be unreliable, since two standard deviations on either side of the mean span a moderate range. For use in groups they appear more adequate" (1971, p. 342).

In a third variation in analytic procedure, Dohrenwend and her colleagues (1978) tested for group differences in much the same way as

Paykel and his colleagues had, using F tests where statuses such as ethnicity could not readily be dichotomized. They calculated the coefficient of variation rather than using the standard deviation as the measure of individual variability. This individual difference measure was calculated, however, only for events that did not show significant group differences. Furthermore, the decision as to whether the amount of individual variability permitted the conclusion that the judgments were consensual was left to the user, depending on his purpose.

The dilemma faced by all of these investigators is that there is no statistical criterion for identifying consensual judgments. The finding that there are statistically significant differences between groups can be used as a basis for concluding that community-wide consensus does not exist. It does not, however, prove total lack of consensus, since there may be group-specific norms concerning the stressfulness of some life events. Moreover, in practice this test has been implemented in a way that is inconclusive, since, with two exceptions (Dohrenwend et al., 1978; Miller et al., 1974), the rule has been to use informants recruited through personal connections, often in academic or medical institutions, rather than a sample representing the population whose consensus is being tested. Thus, for example, the friends and associates of two Japanese professors were the informants for a study designed to determine the extent of agreement between Japanese and United States norms. After the Japanese sample was obtained, the United States sample was selected to match it on social characteristics. As the authors noted: "Both samples were drawn from a university population of professional and technical status. It is obvious that any conclusions that can be drawn are tentative in view of the relative restriction in the samplings from the Japanese and American populations" (Masuda and Holmes, 1967, p. 230). In particular, the similarities in Japanese and American ratings may reflect the shared perspectives of the educationally elite segments of these populations rather than a general cross-cultural similarity.

Suppose, however, that a representative sample of the population is used to determine whether differences exist between status groups. We return to the question of how to decide whether there is consensus, either community-wide, where group differences have not been found, or within groups that differ significantly from each other. The decision in statistical terms as to how large a standard deviation or a coefficient of variation is tolerable, will be arbitrary. We suggest, therefore, that the decision should also be based on substantive tests of predictions about properties of the informants' judgments derived from the conception that they represent social norms.

For example, we suggest that such a prediction can be derived from the model shown in Figure 1.1 about judgments made by persons who have experienced a particular life event as against those who have not. Those who have not experienced the event should base their judgment of its stressfulness on information passed on to them by others who have experienced it, or who are, for some other reason, considered knowledgeable. This information should represent a distillate from which effects due to specific personal and situational contexts have been at least partially removed. In contrast, the experienced person's judgment will to a much greater degree reflect the particular values of these contextual factors as he experienced them. Therefore, we predict that the judgments of the inexperienced about a given event will be less variable than the judgments of those who have experienced this event.

Results reported to date that relate to this counterintuitive hypothesis are mixed, some showing more variability among experienced informants, some more variability among inexperienced informants, and some no difference between them (Grant, Gerst, and Yager, 1976; Horowitz, Schaefer, and Cooney, 1974). These analyses have not, however, been sufficiently well controlled to provide a rigorous test of the hypothesis that the ratings reflected consensual norms in a particular community or group.

It is possible to envision still other tests by recognizing that some categories of individuals have more than usual experience and influence as norm-senders with regard to certain events. The perceptions of a representative sample of a particular community or demographic group can be tested against such knowledgeable and influential norm-senders within the group. For example, physicians are in a strategic position as norm-senders about the amount of change in usual activities and pain that a particular injury would involve. Union officials are likely to be expert about change resulting from layoffs. And so on.

That consensual norms concerning the stressfulness of life events exist in some groups about some life events, is clearly suggested by correlational and other analyses of informants' ratings that have been presented in studies to date. The building of confidence in measures of this kind depends, however, on testing their construct validity by means of substantive tests of the sort that we have illustrated.

CONTENTS OF NORMS CONCERNING STRESSFUL LIFE EVENTS

Studies of ratings of stressfulness and of relations between life events and health have differed in their specification of the characteristics of these events that indicate their stressfulness. Most definitions of stressful life events are somewhat abstract as we showed above, but they all allude to one or more of three characteristics, each of which has been treated by at least one research group as the critical dimension of stressful life events. These three chracteristics are:

1. Change in the life pattern or activities of the individual, for better or for worse (Dohrenwend, 1974; Holmes and Rahe, 1967)
2. Undesirability (Gersten, Langner, Eisenberg, and Orzek, 1974; Vinokur and Selzer, 1975)
3. Upsettingness (Paykel, Prusoff, and Uhlenhuth, 1971)

Several questions about this set of life event characteristics are:

1. Do they represent an exhaustive list of possible indicators of stress-fulness?
2. How are they related to each other?
3. Are they all valid indicators of stressfulness?

The answer to the first question is probably "No." For example, interesting further distinctions have been made within the undesirability characteristic, involving exits of significant others (e.g., Paykel, 1974). And it is possible to envision further subdivision of the change charac-teristic in terms of types of activities involved.

The second question has been answered in part intuitively and in part empirically in studies of stressful life events. Apparently on an intuitive basis, the last two characteristics have been treated by some investigators as interchangeable ways of describing the dimension of emotional distress (Paykel and Uhlenhuth, 1972; Tennant and Andrews, 1976). In contrast, two studies have investigated the relation between the first characteristic, the amount of change, for better or for worse, entailed in an event, and a dimension conceived as embodying the other two characteristics. In these studies informants rated the same sets of events on the amount of change each entailed and on upsettingness or emotion distress. In one study

Paykel and Uhlenhuth (1972) showed that 8 of 19 events were rated significantly differently when the two dimensions were compared. In a study designed to compare and consolidate the work by Holmes and Rahe and by Paykel and his colleagues, Tennant and Andrews (1976) showed that the correlation between ratings of 66 events on change and on emotional distress was .44. Thus we must proceed on the assumption that these two dimensions, while not independent, cannot be substituted one for the other.

This assumption of some degree of independence has been implicit in a controversy in the literature about whether change or desirability is the actual basis for the stressfulness of life events. While attempts have been made to resolve this issue by determining which yields better predictions of health-related outcomes, the results of these studies are mixed (Dohrenwend, 1973; Gersten, Langner, Eisenberg, and Orzek, 1974; Vinokur and Selzer, 1975). Taking another tack, Paykel and Uhlenhuth suggested that desirability may be particularly relevant to precipitation of depression, and change to precipitation of somatic disorders (1972, p. SS99). However, Theorell's (1974) finding that scores on upsettingness were more closely associated with the occurrence of myocardial infarctions than scores on amount of change or adjustment, does not support this suggestion. It is apparent, then, that some useful work has been done on specification of the dimensions underlying the stressfulness of life events, but that more systematic investigation will be needed to answer the three questions posed about them earlier.

CONCLUSION

As we promised at the beginning, we have not dealt with all of the details of sampling, scaling, and other aspects of the procedures used in measuring stressful life events that have previously been subjected to methodological criticism. Instead of reviewing problems concerning how to carry out these measurements, we have focused on issues that are crucial for clarifying what we are measuring.

If stress researchers take seriously the idea that studies of human stress are concerned with the impact of the environment, a larger investment of time and effort will have to be made in conceptualizing and measuring the pervasive class of stressors referred to as stressful life events. This investment will, we have argued, do much to advance both our qualitative and our quantitative understanding of the effects of stress on human well-being.

References

Allport, G. W. *Personality: A Psychological Interpretation*. New York: Henry Holt & Co, 1937.

Ander, S., Lindström, B., and Tibblin, G. Life changes in random samples of middle-aged men. In Gunderson, E. K. G., and Rahe, R. H. (eds.), *Life Stress and Illness*. Springfield, Illinois: Charles C Thomas, 1974.

Antonovsky, A., and Kats, R. The life crisis history as a tool in epidemiological research. *J. Health Soc. Behav. 8:* 15–21, 1967.

Appley, M. H., and Trumbull, R. On the concept of psychological stress. In Appley, M. H., and Trumbull, R. (eds.), *Psychological Stress*. New York: Appleton, 1967.

Askenasy, A. R., Dohrenwend, B. P., and Dohrenwend, B. S. Some effects of social class and ethnic group membership on judgments of the magnitude of stressful life events: A research note. *J. Health Soc. Behav. 18:* 432–439, 1977.

Bandura, A., and Walters, R. H. *Social Learning and Personality Development*. New York: Holt, Rinehart & Winston, Inc., 1963.

Brown, G. W. Meaning, measurement, and stress of life events. In Dohrenwend, B. S., and Dohrenwend, B. P. (eds.), *Stressful Life Events*. New York: John Wiley & Sons, 1974.

Brown, G. W., and Birley, J. L. T. Crises and life changes and the onset of schizophrenia. *J. Health Soc. Behav. 9:* 203–214, 1968.

Clayton, P. The effect of living alone on bereavement symptoms. *Am. J. Psychiatry 132:* 133–137, 1975.

Clayton, P., Desmarais, L., and Winokur, G. A. A study of normal bereavement. *Am. J. Psychiatry 125:* 168–178, 1968.

Cobb, S., and Kasl, S. V. *Termination: The Consequences of Job Loss*. Cincinnati, Ohio: National Institute for Occupational Safety and Health, Division of Biomedical and Behavioral Science, 1977.

Dohrenwend, B. P. The social psychological nature of stress: A framework for causal inquiry. *J. Abnormal Soc. Psychol. 62:* 294–302, 1961.

Dohrenwend, B. P. Problems in defining and sampling the relevant population of stressful life events. In Dohrenwend, B. S., and Dohrenwend, B. P. (eds.), *Stressful Life Events*. New York: John Wiley & Sons, 1974.

Dohrenwend, B. P., and Dohrenwend, B. S. The conceptualization and measurement of stressful life events: An overview of the issues. In Strauss, J. S., Babigian, H. M., and Roff, M. (eds.), *The Origins and Course of Psychopathology: Methods of Longitudinal Research*. New York: Plenum Press, 1977.

Dohrenwend, B. S. Life events as stressors: A methodological inquiry. *J. Health Soc. Behav. 14:* 167–173, 1973.

Dohrenwend, B. S., and Dohrenwend, B. P. (eds.). *Stressful Life Events: Their Nature and Effects*. New York: John Wiley & Sons, 1974.

Dohrenwend, B. S., and Dohrenwend, B. P. Overview and prospects for research on stressful life events. In Dohrenwend, B. S., and Dohrenwend, B. P. (eds.), *Stressful Life Events*. New York: John Wiley & Sons, 1974.

Dohrenwend, B. S., and Dohrenwend, B. P. Some issues in research on stressful life events. *J. Nerv. Ment. Dis. 166:* 7–15, 1978.

Dohrenwend, B. S., Krasnoff, L., Askenasy, A. R., and Dohrenwend, B. P. *Exemplification of a method for scaling life events: The PERI life events scale. J. Health Soc. Behav. 19:* 205–229, 1978.

Engel, G. L. Sudden and rapid death during psychological stress, folklore or folk wisdom? *Annals Int. Med. 74:* 771–782, 1971.

Gersten, J. C., Langner, T. S., Eisenberg, J. G., and Orzek, L. Child behavior and life events: Undesirable change or change per se? In Dohrenwend, B. S., and Dohrenwend, B. P. (eds.), *Stressful Life Events*. New York: John Wiley & Sons, 1974.

Gersten, J. C., Langner, T. S., Eisenberg, J. G., and Simcha-Fagan, O. An evaluation of the etiologic role of stressful life-change events in psychological disorders. *J. Health Soc. Behav. 18:* 228–244, 1977.

Glass, D. C., and Singer, J. E. *Urban Stress: Experiments on Noise and Social Stressors*. New York: Academic Press, 1972.

Grant, I., Gerst, M., and Yager, T. Scaling of life events by psychiatric patients and normals. *J. Psychosom. Res. 20:* 141–149, 1976.

Gunderson, E. K. E., and Rahe, R. H. *Life Stress and Illness*. Springfield, Illinois: Charles C Thomas, 1974.

Hamburg, D. A., and Adams, J. E. A perspective on coping behavior. *Arch. Gen. Psychiat. 17:* 277–284, 1967.

Harris, P. W. The relationship of life change to academic performance among selected college freshmen at varying levels of college readiness. Doctor of Education thesis. East Texas State University, Commerce, Texas, 1972.

Hinkle, L. E., Jr. The concept of "stress" in the biological and social sciences. *Soc. Science and Med. 1:* 31–48, 1973.

Hinkle, L. E., Jr. The effect of exposure to cultural change, social change, and changes in interpersonal relationships on health. In Dohrenwend, B. S., and Dohrenwend, B. P. (eds.), *Stressful Life Events*. New York: John Wiley & Sons, 1974.

Holmes, T. H., and Masuda, M. Life change and illness susceptibility. In Dohrenwend, B. S., and Dohrenwend, B. P. (eds.), *Stressful Life Events*. New York: John Wiley & Sons, 1974.

Holmes, T. H., and Rahe, R. H. The Social Readjustment Rating Scale. *J. Psychosom. Res. 11:* 213–218, 1967.

Horowitz, M. J., Schaefer, C., and Cooney, P. Life event scaling for recency of experience. In Gunderson, E. K. E., and Rahe, R. H. (eds.). *Life Stress and Illness*. Springfield, Illinois: Charles C Thomas, 1974.

Hough, R. L., Fairbank, D. T., and Garcia, A. M. Problems in the ratio measurement of life stress. *J. Health Soc. Behav. 17:* 70–82, 1976.

Hudgens, R. W. Personal catastrophe and depression: A consideration of the subject with respect to medially ill adolescents, and a requiem for retrospective life-event studies. In Dohrenwend, B. S., and Dohrenwend, B. P. (eds.), *Stressful Life Events*. New York: John Wiley & Sons, 1974.

Kasl, S. V., Gore, S., and Cobb, S. The experience of losing a job: Reported changes in health, symptoms and illness behavior. *Psychosom. Med. 37:* 106–122, 1975.

Langner, T. S., and Michael, S. T. *Life Stress and Mental Health.* New York: Free Press of Glencoe, 1963.

Lapin, B. A., and Cherkovich, G. M. Environmental change causing the development of neuroses and cortiocovisceral pathology in monkeys. In Levi, L. (ed.), *The Psychosocial Environment and Psychosomatic Diseases, Vol. 1.* New York: Oxford University Press, 1971.

Lazarus, R. S., and Launier, R. Stress-related transactions between person and environment. In Pervin, L. A., and Lewis, M. (eds.), *Internal and External Determinants of Behavior.* New York: Plenum, 1978.

Masuda, M., and Holmes, T. H. The Social Readjustment Rating Scale: A cross cultural study of Japanese and Americans. *J. Psychosom. Res. 11:* 227–237, 1967.

McGrath, J. E. A conceptual formulation for research on stress. In McGrath, J. E. (ed.), *Social and Psychological Factors in Stress.* New York: Holt, Rinehart & Winston, Inc., 1970.

Miller, F. T., Bentz, W. K., Aponte, J. F., and Brogan, D. R. Perception of life crisis events: A comparative study of rural and urban samples. In Dohrenwend, B. S., and Dohrenwend, B. P. (eds.), *Stressful Life Events.* New York: John Wiley & Sons, 1974.

Myers, J. K., Lindenthal, J. J., and Pepper, M. P. Social class, life events, and psychiatric symptoms: A longitudinal study. In Dohrenwend, B. S., and Dohrenwend, B. P. (eds.), *Stressful Life Events.* New York: John Wiley & Sons, 1974.

Parkes, C. M. *Bereavement.* New York: International Universities Press, 1972.

Paykel, E. S. Life stress and psychiatric disorder. Applications of the clinical approach. In Dohrenwend, B. S., and Dohrenwend, B. P. (eds.), *Stressful Life Events.* New York: John Wiley & Sons, 1974.

Paykel, E. S., Prusoff, B. A., and Uhlenhuth, E. H. Scaling of life events. *Arch. Gen. Psychiat. 25:* 340–347, 1971.

Paykel, E. S., and Uhlenhuth, E. H. Rating the magnitude of life stress. *Can. Psychiatric Assoc. J. 17:* SS92–SS100, 1972.

Rahe, R. H. The pathway between subjects' recent life changes and their near-future illness reports: Representative results and methodological issues. In Dohrenwend, B. S., and Dohrenwend, B. P. (eds.), *Stressful Life Events.* New York: John Wiley & Sons, 1974.

Scott, R., and Howard, A. Models of stress. In Levine, S., and Scotch, N. A. (eds.), *Social Stress.* Chicago: Aldine Publishing Company, 1970.

Seligman, M. E. P. *Helplessness: On Depression, Development, and Death.* San Francisco: W. H. Freeman & Co, 1975.

Selye, H. *Stress Without Distress.* New York: J. B. Lippincott Co, 1974.

Selye, H. *The Stress of Life.* New York: McGraw-Hill, 1976.

Tennant, C., and Andrews, G. A. A single scale to measure the stress of life events. *Australian and New Zealand J. Psychiatry 10:* 27–32, 1956. (Rev. ed. 1976.)

Theorell, T. Life events before and after the onset of a premature myocardial infarction. In Dohrenwend, B. S., and Dohrenwend, B. P. (eds.), *Stressful Life Events.* New York: John Wiley & Sons, 1974.

Vinokur, A., and Selzer, M. L. Desirable versus undesirable life events; their relationship to stress and mental distress. *J. Personality Soc. Psychol. 32:* 329–337, 1975.

Weick, K. E. The "ess" in stress: some conceptual and methodological problems. In McGrath, J. E. (ed.), *Social and Psychological Factors in Stress.* New York: Holt, Rinehart & Winston, Inc, 1970.

Wolff, H. G., Wolf, S. G., Jr., and Hare, C. C. (eds.). *Life Stress and Bodily Disease.* Baltimore: The Williams & Wilkins Co., 1950.

2
Perspectives on Social Stress

Barbara B. Brown
formerly Chief, Experiential Physiology, V.A. Hospital, Sepulveda, California

During the past decade or so, a number of events have strategically converged at the interface between medicine and psychology to focus considerable interest on the role of higher-order mental processes in health and illness. A large part of the new interest has stemmed from both the recognition of the increasing pervasiveness of stress illnesses in society and the therapeutic impact of newly appreciated psychophysiological techniques such as biofeedback, progressive relaxation, autogenic training, meditation, and related procedures. These techniques are, in fact, responsible for an important improvement in identifying and characterizing many diverse psychological and physiological disturbances originating from psychosocial causes.

Modern medicine has had relatively little interest in cognitive functions, psychological techniques, or the effects of nuances of belief, faith, self-suggestion, or yogic exercises on internal functions in treatment regimes. On the other side of the therapeutic coin, psychology has fostered few formal applications for medicine. There are, however, emerging concepts of the cause and treatment of emotional, psychosomatic, and related problems, now popularly designated as stress-related problems, that are directed toward both psychophysiological relationships in health and illness and the influences of higher-order mental functions. And although relationships between psychosocial causes and psychophysiological effects are increasingly assumed and experimentally supported, little in the way of unifying concepts has been offered by theorists. The bioscientific isolationism between psychology and medicine has been so great as to make their respective research and approaches mutually exclusive in theory if not in practice. As a result there are a number of noticeable shortcomings in concepts about reactions to stress of psychosocial origin and about therapeutic approaches to their treatment.

The most obvious conceptual hiatus concerns the mechanisms operating between the external psychosocial factors and the activation of the internal psychophysiological mechanisms during reactions to psychosocial stress. Not only is it true that cognitive mediation is known, experientially and subjectively, to occur; but considerable research literature exists as well that implies a major influence of cognitive factors in psychosocial stress reactions. Despite the tacit understanding and pragmatic acceptance of cognitive mediation, the most popular notion of psychosocial stress is the vast oversimplification that psychological stressors excite the varieties of neural, endocrine, and immune systems that implement stress reactions, as defined by Selye.[1,2] The theoretical omissions are several. In general, current concepts lack adequate definitions; and systematic analyses of the nature of psychosocial stressors fail to suggest how such stressors are processed neurally or cognitively to result in activation of physiological processes that manifest the reactions, or how therapeutic interventions not directly affecting physiological mechanisms nonetheless reverse the effect of psychosocial stress.

CURRENT CONCEPTS OF PSYCHOSOCIAL STRESS

Although research and clinical thinking about stress problems of psychosocial origin is undergoing revision, most of the evidence and concepts derive from three peculiarly segregated disciplines: psychology, psychophysiology, and psychosomatic medicine. Each of these related but separate and unconsolidated specialties subscribes to the same two principles: first, that in general if human emotions are inappropriately or inadequately expressed, tension occurs, resulting in either emotional or psychosomatic disorders; and second, that the implementing mechanisms involve general or selective activation of aspects of neurophysiologic, neuroendocrine, or immune systems. The three disciplines, however, deal with quite different aspects of psychophysiological relationships on both conceptual and practical levels. Psychology concentrates on subjective factors of emotion; psychophysiology concentrates on physiological correlates of emotion; and psychosomatic medicine concentrates on psychosocial factors related to specific psychosomatic disorders. All three specialties rest on very insubstantial notions of emotions and emotional reactions.

There are, for example, many more than 20 current theories of emotion, the majority based on psychophysiological and neurophysiological indices. They generally begin with the assumption that environmental situations activate the physiological mechanisms manifesting the signs and symptoms of stress disorders, and do not deal with factors activating the emotions. In general, neurophysiological research extrapolates from experimentally induced, exaggerated emotional behavior; psychophysiological research is often poorly controlled, inappropriately reductionist, and subjectively evaluated; and psychodynamic research assumes unconscious mechanisms largely on the basis of clinical narrative, and deals neither with the nature of the unconscious mechanisms nor with the process by which unconscious activity might interface with the physiological mechanisms that express the disordered emotions. The obvious inability of the theories of emotion yet proposed to explain the mechanisms of emotion has been critically reviewed by Strongman.[3] Any serious analysis of theories and the data of emotions leaves many more questions than answers.

Inadequate understanding of the mechanisms of emotions means inadequate understanding of disorders of emotions. Clinical psychologists, psychodynamic theorists, and theorists of psychosomatic medicine tend to describe emotional problems and disorders as the result of unconscious conflicts or frustrations. Psychological theory, for example, suggests that behavioral, perceptual, and subjective distress are emotional reactions to the individual's desire for, but inability to achieve, a more satisfying way of life, to function in society, and to live with himself. It is generally agreed in psychology that episodes of normally occurring anxieties and unhappiness are dealt with by varieties of unconscious processes of mind, processes known as defense mechanisms, since they are believed to act principally to distort to deny the source of the anxiety. These defense mechanisms are usually classified as repression, regression, rationalization, and sublimation; when these defense mechanisms fail, it is said, behavior becomes neurotic.

For researchers and theorists of stress disorders, these well-accepted concepts leave many unanswered questions. When and how, for example, does the unconscious recognize a dissatisfaction that seems to require a defense? What are the processes involved in elaborating and selecting a defense? What are the internal factors that allow the unconscious to accept the success or nonsuccess of a defense strategy? What is the nature of communication between such sophisticated unconscious cognitive activity and conscious awareness? What is the mechanism by which the unconscious activity evokes physiological change?

The missing link in theories of emotion and emotional distress is the identification and characterization of the internal information processing of psychosocial data leading to development of effective or ineffective defense devices. For the most part, theoreticians and researchers interested in cognitive factors are hampered by the inaccessibility to study of unconscious activities. As well, the plethora of social, psychological, constitutional, and other factors that influence cognitive activity predisposes researchers and theorists to build concepts on one or another of the influences, and rarely to attempt unifying concepts.

In conceptualizing the psychophysiological mechanisms of emotions, for example, Arnold[4] emphasizes instinctive cognitive (cortical) appraisal of all encounters as the chief determinant of emotional expression; Duffy[5] has emphasized conscious awareness as a major factor modifying emotional expression; Schachter[6] has tended toward viewing cognitive activity as determining emotional states through mutual interaction between physiological arousal and cognitive appraisal; Leeper[7] suggests that emotions function both as motives and perceptions, i.e., as perceptions, emotions supply cognitive information about physiological reactions and as motives they provide goal-directed behavior; Lazarus[8] expands considerably on the role of appraisal and gives a much fuller description of interactions among cognitions, emotions, and biological-cultural considerations. Hechhausen and Weiner,[9] in a review of proposed cognitive determinants of emotion, perception, and self-perception, present an interesting scheme of interacting cognitive sequences during behavior, and assume that cognitive events determine the physiological expression of emotions.

Each of these major theories of emotion relates cognitive activity to physiological arousal as either initiating or modulating arousal. Evidence to support a primary role of arousal in emotional behavior is, however, weak. Physiological arousal does not account for all emotional behavior, nor is arousal a necessary condition for emotion. Moreover, arousal fails to explain idiosyncratic emotion.

In reviewing the data and diverse theories of emotionally related stress disorders, it seemed appropriate to begin to conceptualize psychosocial stress in a more systematic way that could relate psychosocial events more exactly to the disorders they are believed to cause. This essay, therefore, deals first with the rationale for greater precision in defining and describing that psychosocial distress deriving from individual interactions with the social environment; and second, with the rationale for identifying and systematizing the events intervening between psychosocial factors and those psychological and physiological reactions classified as stress-related disorders. It attempts to provide a logical base for the conclusion that disturbances due to psychosocial stress are caused by the supervention of cognitive functions in homeostatic regulating functions. It is also argued that when the cognitive functions are supplied with "relevant" information, cognitive activity supervenes in the feedback-regulating systems to reverse the disturbances through a prevention process of learned stress resistance.

CLASSIFICATIONS OF STRESS

In attempts to organize sources of human stress, the general class is usually designated as environmental stress with subclasses of psychological stress (e.g., loss of love, unconscious conflicts), social stress (e.g., cultural restrictions, technological change), economic stress (unemployment, poverty), and physiological stress (physical, chemical, bacteriological). This classification scheme catalogs the possible sources of stress and does not attempt to identify the nature of stress. Current evidence for common mechanisms of the multiple varieties of stress-related disturbances suggests that a more exact, prognostic classification would be more helpful in understanding the stress process.

Stress can also be classified according to whether it affects human behavior and function by direct or indirect means. This distinction identifies stressors as "physical" or "nonphysical," with nonphysical stress for the present purposes being subsumed under the heading of social stress.*

One reason for combining psychological, social, and economic stress into the single entity of social stress is that each subclass contains interact-

*Physical stressors can, of course, have nonphysical effects; but when they do, there is generally a conscious identification of the stressor by the person involved, and an awareness of the consequent psychophysiological change. For example, consider the person who moves to a sunny climate because he can no longer tolerate a depression associated with prolonged gloomy weather. These kinds of conscious reactions do not generally result in disordered psychological or physiological functions and are not initiated by social activities.

ing and overlapping elements, and so cannot be independently qualified. Another reason is that the term psychological stress often emphasizes primarily behavioral responses to specific environmental stimuli, and causes semantic confusion.

The notion of social stress, moreover, directly implies that nonphysical stress reactions are highly complex and dynamic interactions between individuals and the highly variable dimensions of the structure and operations of societies. The distinctive duality of the individual–society relationship requires separate attention to the nature of each as well as to the nature of the interaction. In the context of social stress, it is generally agreed that social situations and relationships are not inherently stressful. Nonetheless, social situations and relationships do result in stress disorders, suggesting intervening agencies that invest human social activities with qualities of stress. For social stress, the intervening agencies are aspects of the human organism, either as individuals or as groups, having the capability of supplying forms of associations among social variables and of imposing extraneous, extrinsic qualities on the objective nature, structure, and sequences of social events, resulting in subjective and physiological confusion, disorder, or distortion of the social events.

Despite a lack of consensus on definition, there is little doubt that the chief intervening agency is the interpretive, integrative, conceptualizing decision-making, action-directing functions of human beings. For reasons noted below, I have designated this agency as the "stressor processor," or in terms of process, the "stressor processing phase" of social stress reactions, preferring this to the phrase "cognitive mediator," which has become muddied by theoretical disputes. Once this distinction is made, the processes involved in the physiological expression of psychosocial reactions, such as the arousal response, can be discriminated and designated as the "physiological implementation phase" of the reactions.

DISTINCTIONS AMONG STRESS SYSTEMS

It is an enlightening and, I think, productive exercise to return to the abstract scientific meaning of stress, both as a basis for a more systematic analysis of social stress and in the interests of greater conformity to descriptions as defined by Selye.[10] Although the word "stress" was originally used as an expression of human difficulties caused by outside forces beyond one's control, it became formalized in science to mean any change within a system induced by an external force. To scientists it is

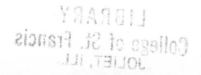

now a generic term for a class of cause–effect relationships, implying the existence of subclasses defined in terms of the elements involved in the relationship.

Table 2.1 lists the major categories of stress systems, the several elements implied by the general concept, and examples of stress in order of increasing complexity. Systems subject to stress may be physical, physiological, and nonphysical with both subjective and physiological expression. The elements implied are: (1) the system involved; (2) the nature of the external force; (3) the response; (4) the mechanisms involved in producing the response; and (5) the mechanisms involved in resisting the external force.

This analytic classification provides the basis for greater precision in defining the reactions involved in different stress systems, and also provides the foundation for two of the main issues with which this essay is concerned. These issues are: (1) that, contrary to general opinion, the characteristics and reactions of social stress are distinctively different from those of direct or imminent physical stress; and (2) that the mechanisms underlying both the reactions and the resistance to social stress are of a different order from that of reactions to direct or imminent physical stress.

The nature of stress for simple inorganic systems can be easily described, as in Table 2.1. Stress reactions of animal physiological systems are also well understood from the work of Cannon[11] and of Selye,[2] who have documented the physiological and biochemical responses to direct and imminent physical stress. Beyond this, difficulties arise when the concept of stress is applied to phylogenetically higher animals and to the complex systems of modern man.

Important differences in the stress phenomenon emerge as organic systems become more complex and variable. Animals that possess coordinating, interacting centralized neural networks and specialized organs react not only to direct physical assaults by a neurally coordinating mechanism regardless of the type of assault (largely according to the formula described by Selye) but also to physical elements that signify jeopardy to the *total* organism.

The differences between responses to local physical assaults and responses to assaults endangering the total organism are not generally the subject of theoretical analysis, since the two types of reaction share certain responding actions of the neural, hormonal, and immune systems. Significant differences do exist, however, in the modes of initiating,

Table 2.1 Operational Classification of Stress

SYSTEM	EXTERNAL FORCE (STRESSOR)	RESPONSE	INTERNAL MECHANISMS (PRODUCING DISTRESS)	RESISTING MECHANISMS (ADAPTATION)
simple inorganic	physical (pressure, heat, cold)	strain (change in shape, structure)	inorganic elements; molecules	opposite force
low organic (bacteria, plants)	physical	change in shape, structure, direction, or location	ion exchange; simple reflexes	secretions; regeneration; inclusion
higher animals, primitive man	physical; threats to physical well-being; threats to group	local and general physical arousal; fight-or-flight; aggregation	interacting neural networks; specialized organs; fostering systems	coordinated neural and hormonal systems; primitive control of external sources
socialized man	predominantly nonphysical; threats to social well-being and survival; intellectual pressure	primarily intellectual, emotional perceptual, change of consciousness; secondarily, physiological arousal	higher-order brain functions; abstract thought; ability to order and to project; language	awareness; understanding; social coping; exploring resources and alternatives; securing relevant information

mobilizing, and directing the responses and resistances. These differences suggest the existence of mechanisms capable of discriminating the direction and coordination of effectors required for a response. With increasing complexity and evolution, this discrimination capability appears to develop into a more highly organized and versatile ability that differentiates between physical stress and threat of general physical stress, implying an increased influence of intervening agencies between environment and the physical elements of organisms, and an increased capacity for complex kinds of adaptation.

It is the species man, and particularly modern man, developing into a complex social animal, that brings with it a further distinction with respect to stress. In modern society, direct and imminent physical stress has become a remarkably minor cause of stress reactions. Most hazardous physical stressors and their threats have come under control, both through control of elements of the physical environment and through chemical, immune, or physical assistance to the internal resisting mechanisms.

Suspiciously coincident with the growing effectiveness of techniques that lessen the potential for physical stress, stress reactions of psychosocial origin have increased substantially in incidence, variety, and severity, and have outdistanced the development of resisting mechanisms. The result is that social stress has become a dominant source of modern man's distress.

Table 2.1 illustrates the clear-cut differences among physical, physiological, and nonphysical instances of stress for socially complex human beings. The social stress system is modern man; the dominant stressors are derived from the social environment; and the responses are principally alterations in perceptual, intellectual, emotional, and consciousness activities, with physiological changes secondary. The internal mechanisms implementing social stress reactions are primarily those concerned with mental functions, including selective perception, direction of attention, reasoning, judgment, experiential organization, states of consciousness, and related activities; the internal mechanisms of resistance or adaptation are primarily mental activities, such as consciously or unconsciously altered perceptualizing, intellectual coping, understanding, and other varieties of selected cognitive processing, all of which can result in effective or ineffective control of both cognitive and physiological functions.

The crucial difference between physical and nonphysical stress first emerging in reactions to threats of physical stress, is that while physical stressors are extrinsic to the organism, nonphysical stressors require intrinsic factors of the organism to transform the external elements into significant stressors. Social stressors might be viewed as analogous to enzymes requiring the presence of coenzymes for reaction. The social environment supplies the extrinsic factors, while the intervening agency within the reacting system supplies the intrinsic factors, the result constituting the external force that activates the internal mechanisms producing both the psychological and physiological reactions to stress.

While social stress systems are decidedly complicated because of the labyrinthine feedback systems involved, it is ultimately the activity of higher-order mental processes that furnishes social activities with meaning. The force of social stress occurs only through an intervening system that invests social activities with qualities of stress, the action I have called "stressor processing." In other words, social stress is stressful only after cognitive processing.

SOCIAL STRESS

Social stress can be defined as an unfavorable perception of the social environment and its dynamics. Nearly all currently designated stress-related disturbances of psychosocial origin develop out of the way in which social situations are perceived. The term "stress-related" to describe these related entities has become increasingly popular in describing disorders and emotional problems benefited by biofeedback, cognitive therapies, and the relaxation, imagery, and meditation procedures. General scientific neglect or parochialism about psychosocial factors and the illnesses they cause has discouraged the use of descriptive terms and system analysis; thus the phrase "stress-related problems" has come in through the scientific back door. It is, nonetheless, an organizing term for variously designated emotional and psychosomatic disorders, and can be easily supported by the findings of commonalities of stress factors in their etiology and mechanisms. We are only now beginning to realize the relationship of many illnesses to social difficulties and the stress of living in complex and rapidly changing societies.

Table 2.2 lists disorders frequently believed either to have a social stress origin or to be significantly modified by social stress. They are classified according to dominant psychological or physiological signs and symptoms, process, or general severity of disturbance (e.g., neuroses vs. social adjustment problems).

Table 2.2 Some Psychological and Physiological Disturbances Believed to be Caused by, Related to, or Aggravated by Psychosocial Stress

Emotional: anxiety, insomnia, tension headaches, aging, sexual impotency, neuroses, phobias, alcoholism, drug abuse, learning problems, general malaise

Psychosomatic: essential hypertension, auricular arrhythmias, ulcers, colitis, asthma, chronic pain, acne, peripheral vascular disease

Organic, triggered by stress: epilepsy, migraine, herpes, angina, coronary thrombosis, rheumatoid arthritis

Psychological adjustment problems: e.g., anxiety of classroom learning (moderate interference in satisfying/fulfilling human potential)

Sociological problems: e.g., chronic unemployment; delinquency (socially undesirable; socioeconomic impoverishment and instability)

Aggravated or prolonged distress in illness of any origin

The existence of many and diverse reactions to social stress has made it difficult to apply a specific term or descriptive definition to designate the major determinants, and most neologisms are confusing. Therefore I have resorted to a nonscientific term that is widely understood and succinctly approximates the crucial process: (''worry'' or ''worry syndrome''). This term encompasses all of the subjective emotional activities concerned in social stress reactions and, further, implies the dominant role of cognitive activity. Worry covers both conscious and unconscious worry, and is made up of the well-known elements of apprehension, anxiety, feelings of insecurity, uncertainty, inadequacy, conflict, frustration, and related emotions. All of these expressions of subjective emotion are rooted in an intellectual concern about social activity, such as adequate social performance, meeting social criteria, or ensuring a sense of social well-being and social survival. All the subjective sensations are, in effect, expressions of a disturbed intellect, i.e., a disturbance about the way in which social relationships are appreciated and interpreted. Intellectual mechanisms, moreover, can relieve or intensify the worry.

The study and systematic analysis of the role of intellectual functions in reactions to social environments is surprisingly meager and unconsolidated. For the most part, reactions to social influences are characterized by overt behavioral reactions linked to excessive emotional reactions or to reported subjective anguish, with supporting research generally following reductionist approaches and clinical documentation focusing on quite severely disordered functions. In psychophysiological research, for example, experimental stressors are often limited to unnatural or single-variable stimuli, such as electric shock to induce expectancy, specific orienting instructions, or commonly learned and immediately appreciated values such as achievement, induced failure, or observing stress experienced by others. The experimentalist's correlations of emotions of anxiety, expectancy, frustration, and conscious conflict with changes in physiological activity are several orders of reactions removed from the kinds of psychophysiological reactions to psychosocial elements that result in stress-related disorders and problems. Learning theorists tend to attribute social stress reactions to learned responses, but fail to supply evidence for facilitating intermediaries between stimulus and response, although it is experientially and descriptively reasonable to assume that certain components of stress reactions can be deeply imprinted, learned reactions, particularly where alternative possibilities are restricted.

In contrast to laboratory or clinical research designs that use well-defined influencing variables and measures of reactions, the stress signals in life's activities are characterized in general by degrees of remoteness and obscurity, prolonged temporal accumulation and selection processes in their perception, and often little quantifiable change in the social environment.

And in contrast to psychophysiology, the psychodynamic perspective relies on deducing influences of unconscious conflicts and variously designated mental-emotional defenses against anxiety such as denial, repression, or isolation. Such reactions imply higher-order mental activities, vexingly inaccessible to observation. The psychodynamic perspective thus also assumes for social stress little quantifiable change in the social environment. It would seem only logical that if psychodynamic theorists deduce complex reactions occurring in the unconscious, then the mental processes required to develop them are complex intellectual activities. In most stress disorders, given a particular though erroneous assumption about a social problem, quite logical processes do indeed accomplish purposes decided upon by the individual as a result of intelligent action, albeit unconsciously, such as psychological defense mechanisms. The fact that the result of the intelligent action is not usually an intelligent decision when distress results, does not deny the probability that the same intellectual activities are used as for making a useful, satisfying decision. The judgment as to whether the decision is intelligent or not is a function of the individual's society, not of the process.

MENTAL EVENTS MEDIATING REACTIONS TO SOCIAL STRESS

Since complex intellectual functions can be assumed to be involved in reactions to social stress, it would seem important to describe them in operational terms rather than as consequences, such as defense reactions, unconscious conflict, frustration, guilt, neuroses, and so on. These latter qualifiers describe responses rather than process. An operational classification of cognitive processes leading to these responses could aid importantly in identifying and characterizing the order and progression of the critical cognitive activities involved, and could materially assist in selecting appropriate treatment procedures.

The classification scheme in Table 2.3 is designed to identify the general types of intellectual activities that form a sequence in the processing of social data leading to emotional and physiological distress. Each step of the process contains multiple prior determinants relating to individual experiential and constitutional background. Further, as the sequence progresses, each phase increasingly interacts with and influences preceeding phases, a feedback action that tends to concentrate the cognitive activities within an increasingly closed system. Application of the cognitive sequence for the understanding of the development and for the treatment of specific disorders would, of course, require in-depth definition of the specific contributions to each component process, a determination of the principal, presenting stage of the mediating process, and the recognition that both psychological and physiological changes occur concomitantly.*

a. Expectations. If reaction to social stress is a "fault" of a disturbed intellect, i.e., distress from processing social data, then the process is contingent upon the way social environments are perceived and appreciated. How the social environment is perceived, however, depends in large part upon what the perceiver expects to perceive.

If events of the social environment are consonant with expectations or preconceived concepts, or if effective psychological defenses are de-

---

*An important physiological effect usually overlooked is the feedback system between neural and mental data processing. Paraphrasing Sperry,[12] neural events determine mental events, and mental events determine neural events. Thus for every cognitive reaction to social stress, central neural activity is concurrently affected and vice versa, accounting in part for the physiological changes accompanying cognitive reactions to social stress. The physiological changes often dominate the clinical picture because they are more visible and readily measurable in contrast to the less obvious, often covert and only marginally measurable subjective changes of social distress.

Table 2.3 Steps in the Intellectual Processing of Social Data Leading to Psychosocial Distress

1. Expectations
2. Perceptions
3. Interpretation of disparity between expectations and perceptions
4. Rumination
   a. generates social threats; physiological arousal.
   b. constructs mental images; physiological tensions.
   c. elaborates unconscious defenses.
5. Perceptual distortion
   a. reinforces arousal.
   b. limits problem-solving potential.
6. "Cortical inhibition"
   a. interferes with appreciation of internal physiological signals.
   b. reinforces rumination.
   c. narrows attentional focus.
   d. limits cognitive activities.

veloped when they are not, and provide reasonable satisfaction with respect to expectations for achievement or continued or improved well-being, then few problems arise. However, expectations are multidimensional, subjective activities, depending upon individual history; and they are determined, modified by, and linked to aspirations, motives, and situational clues with either immediate or long-range implications, all of which can contribute toward satisfying or not satisfying the expectations. It is the complex origin of expectations and the expectational set that can initiate the stream of mental processes leading to emotional and physiological distress if relative satisfaction is not attained, or if offsetting or neutralizing strategies are not developed for the social situation perceived.

b. Perceptions. Any perception of the social environment is literally a global activity, since not only the total environment but also subtle distinctions within the social dynamics and social relationships are perceived. Obviously, perception of social scenes requires extensive interpretation because of the variability and diversity of social behavior and the dependence of interpretation on the way in which social behavior is expressed. One of the socially undesirable effects of modern communications is that they have become more distal and less personal. Complex concepts affecting human behavior are often symbolized in abstruse language and behavior, requiring mental effort to relate to individual social activities. Communications within the social environment are thus broad, layered, symbolic, elite, caste-developed, and rife with opportunities for misinterpretation. Moreover, social activities are increasingly competitive and charged with innumerable rewards and penalties. A perceiver must constantly interpret varying human behavior, motives, social customs, personality influences, emotional expressions, body language, and language itself.

Thus, in order for one to "perceive" a social situation, a number of interacting social events must be observed, associated, analyzed, and judged. Since the social environment and dynamics are complex, multidimensional, and variable, any perception of a social situation requires multidimensional construction and reconstruction of events, their significance, and their implications. The reconstruction of any set or of related sets of social dynamics and relationships requires both the perceptual data and some kind of customary or logical or desirable mental appreciation of relationships among events. The appreciation of social situations is thus an interpretation and a mental construction of social events and their significance, and as well it is invariably a mental projection of the situation into past and future.

c. Interpretation of a Disparity. When a significant disparity between expectations and perceptions occurs, it sets in motion intense cognitive activity with direct effects upon both subjective sensations and physiological activities. In the language of psychodynamics, the disparity represents a conflict between the emotions and appraisals of expectancy and the emotions and appraisals of denial or lack of satisfaction. In the development of most social stress reactions, conscious appreciation of either component is vague and only marginally in conscious awareness, since the social situations and relationships leading to stress disorders are fluid and generally develop over appreciable periods of time. Moreover, failures to be rewarded or fulfilled are often unconsciously repressed as a habitual defense developed during prior experience. The mental activities, therefore, that underlie the understanding of social realities operate under two considerable difficulties: first, the incomplete and often tenuous nature of the perceived information stemming from inadequate social communications; and second, the uncertainty created by the perceived conflict itself.

d. Rumination. When the disparity between expectations and perceived social activity is recognized, mental action is taken both consciously and unconsciously to attempt to resolve or understand the reasons for the disparity. Depending upon the background of the social situations and the personality traits of the individual, the mental action may be persistent and either conscious or unconscious. The mental effort involved is commonly called "worry," but a more psychologically descriptive term is rumination. The mental activities employed to understand the disparity are problem-solving activities to develop coping devices or resistance to the perceived stress. When, however, the perceived information is, or is believed to be, inadequate to arrive at a satisfactory solution, the developing unconscious conflicts begin to bias the problem-solving process, which becomes unsatisfactory; and rumination becomes more persistent, intense, and circular. Because of informational poverty, unconscious bias, uncertainty, and developing anxiety, rumination is not a simple, straightforward process of logic; it expands into pondering, speculating, projecting, imagining, and reacting to each possible alternative solution to the perceived problem.

There are two effects of rumination on physical functions. First, the uncertainty about answers constitutes a threat to social well-being and generates anxiety or apprehension, the neural product of which directly activates the physiological defense mechanisms that result in muscle, visceral, and subjective tension, i.e., the physiological responses that are the partly innate, partly learned responses to threats to the well-being of living organisms.

At the same time, rumination involves the almost constant creation and re-creation of the social situation and problem as mental images. Each re-creation also involves projection of various alternative solutions to the problem into both past and future imagined situations. These images, involving social postures if not social activity, directly evoke physiological activation, as Edmund Jacobson[13] showed so extensively. If I project eating a sour lemon in my imagination, the salivary juices flow, and the gut may recoil. Conscious or unconscious images (memories) of anxiety-producing situations can excite physiological postures that mimic the original reactions. All organs of the body respond to mental images involving those organs, and, with certain predisposing factors, the images may evoke any or all of the physiological arousal responses accompanying anxiety. Thus, learned or even accidentally associated stimulus-response relationships may account for the specific physiological changes.

   e. Perceptual Distortion. Another mental activity during reactions to social stress is the distortion of perception.* The rumination process,

---

*How unconscious motives skew perception is described in detail by Murphy.[14]

working with inadequate and often unrealistic information about the social situation, tends to generate "worst case" answers to the problem, which intensify apprehension and uncertainty. With this cognitive-emotional mind-brain processing load, perceptual attention becomes directed toward those elements in the social environment that are related to the mental construction of the problem, and perceptions become skewed. The individual sees and hears predominantly those elements of the social dynamics that fit preconceived pictures and images of the situation and problem. The selected perceptions intensify the dimensions of the problem and strengthen inappropriate solutions, resulting in an increase of distress.

f. "Cortical Inhibition." Finally, as cognitive activity becomes more narrowly focused, normal homeostatic mechanisms regulating neural conduction to muscles and viscera become impaired. Increasing physiological tensions appear no longer to be effective in evoking normalizing mechanisms as they do under normal circumstances of functional activity. Since the physiological systems are inactivated as part of the social stress reaction, and degrees of activation are often maintained at high levels, it has been inferred that cortical or higher-order processes are responsible for the failure to relay proprioceptive information to the primary muscle regulatory systems. Hefferline[15] called this "cortical inhibition," indicating that the cortex inhibits the normalizing actions of lower brain regulatory systems, an effect which sustains activation. Regardless of its mechanism, the sustained activation has a threefold effect: a decrement in the subjective appreciation of cause–effect relationships of the tensions, but with a paradoxical increase in the sensation of tension of unknown origin, and physiological adaptation.

The cortical inhibitory effect is often extrapolated to indicate that cortical cognitive activity is also inhibited, or, in psychopathological terms, that a distortion in the perceptions of social realities takes place. Certainly, when the bulk of cognitive activity is concerned with problem-solving, conflicts, and frustrations, the focus of cognitive attention is so intense that conscious recognition of the peripheral source or possible causes of body tensions is likely to be restricted. Moreover, with physiological adaptation to increased muscle or visceral tension, proprioceptive impulses would be decreased, or at least not significantly increased.

Summary of Sequence. The sequence of mental activities from expectation through perceptual distortion constitutes a phase of cognitive activity that processes social data in such a way that elements ot th social environment are interpreted as posing alarming threats to social well-being; hence, I have called it the "stressor processing phase" of the social stress reaction. Rumination in particular generates both threats to well-being and accompanying emotional sensations, along with mental images exciting defense postures. These appear to be the primary processes activating the mechanisms implementing the physiological and psychological manifestations of stress responses. Figure 2.1 illustrates this process.

GENERAL COGNITIVE MEASURES MODIFYING THE COGNITIVE DEFECTS IN SOCIAL STRESS REACTIONS

If the cognitive processing scheme outlined has validity, it should enable us to identify areas of defective function and to suggest appropriate and effective treatment procedures. Both the processing and implementing phases of social stress reactions can be analyzed for specific defects that lead to problems and illnesses. The first defect is the lack of information for the cognitive intellectual processes adequately to perceive the reality of social situations, relationships, and dynamics, and hence the lack of adequate information to understand or solve or cope with the perceived social problems. The second defect is the lack of physiological pro-

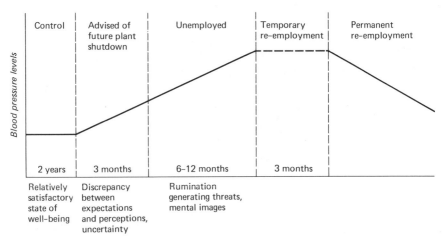

Figure 2.1. Relationship between cognitive actions and physiological stress reactions. (Schematized from a report by Kasl and Cobb, 1970,[18] on blood pressure changes in factory workers as they might relate to cognitive events in reactions to social stress. Times are approximate.)

prioceptive information to the homeostatic regulating systems as a result of the failure of the mind-brain to recognize the body's physiological reactions, i.e., the failure to appreciate the information about body changes related to the perceived problem. If what the reacting systems need to resist stress is information, then treatment should supply the information needed.

Information about the social reality, about the inappropriateness of certain emotional reactions, and about social coping mechanisms can be supplied through a variety of sources such as psychotherapy, cognitive therapies, counseling, meditation, and related techniques. To remedy the defect in recognizing body tensions and physiological reactions, information about how and when the body is reacting to stress, about the inappropriateness of excessive body reactions, and about how to discriminate productive from unproductive physiological activity can be supplied through techniques such as biofeedback, yoga, progressive relaxation, autogenic training, imagery practice, and other body awareness techniques. Since the physiological and psychological reactions are actually concurrent, both psychosocial and physiological information in the treatment procedures might be expected to provide greater benefits than either alone.

STRESS REDUCTION WITH BIOFEEDBACK

Currently biofeedback is emerging from its initial stage of overexploitation and misunderstanding to take its place as a valuable tool in both medicine and psychology. As a fundamental phenomenon of man's ability to learn and exert voluntary control over virtually any physiological activity of the body, biofeedback has far-reaching applications. One of its principal uses is in the treatment of psychosocial stress reactions. The following brief discussion of biofeedback is confined to the muscle-tension component of social stress reactions, since more definitive information exists for muscle tension-relaxation processes than for visceral tension-relaxation mechanisms, and also because muscle biofeedback is more widely used in treating social stress reactions than are other biofeedback modalities.

Biofeedback is the technique by which individuals can exert control over selected physiological functions. The bottom line appears to be that human beings can learn how to regulate the flow of impulses in any nerve of their choosing. The evidence for this rather extraordinary phenomenon is that (a) biofeedback learning successfully decreases the rapid impulse flow responsible for tension states (muscle tension, autonomic hyperactivity), and (b) biofeedback learning equally increases the flow of nerve impulses (increasing motor unit activity, heart rate).

In clinical use, biofeedback procedures vary from therapist to therapist and with the type of disorder being treated, but all procedures generally have the following elements in common: reasonably accurate, sensitive, and continuous displays of an index of the selected physiological activity via an appropriate instrument; instructions to the patient to find some way to change the physiological activity by some subjective manipulation; a variety of learning aids in the form of relaxation exercises, self-suggestion, imagery, or meditation; and a variety of measures designed to support, reinforce, and consolidate the learning.

The nature of biofeedback learning has posed some problems for learning theorists, particularly since considerable biofeedback research is an outgrowth of the application of operant conditioning techniques. The available evidence for biofeedback learning, however, clearly implies the crucial role of cognitive information-processing. In muscle (EMG) biofeedback learning, for example, muscle tension levels detected by the instrument represent unfelt muscle tension, i.e., tension not consciously appreciated by the patient. It is this information that appears to substitute for proprioceptive information, and along with suggestions and auxiliary techniques for becoming aware of smaller degrees of tension, learning apparently proceeds by higher-order cognitive activity that appreciates the significance of the information and makes it available to the homeostatic regulating systems. The system is self-regulating and self-reinforcing, the "new" element of the system being the supravention of cognitive and subjective factors in the automatic feedback systems. A simplified scheme of this process is diagrammed in Figure 2.2.

As with most learning involving intellectual activities, the cerebral processes involved are complex, diverse, and rarely appreciated in conscious awareness. Thus the sequence of events that effect tension reduction can only be postulated on the basis of fragmented and indirect evidence.

The first assumption needs to deal with the fate of the visually—or auditorially—perceived feedback information of unfelt muscle tension. Apparently the disposition of the information is facilitated both by the usual instructions to use mental strategies to reduce tensions and by the augmenting relaxation procedures, all of which are designed to foster

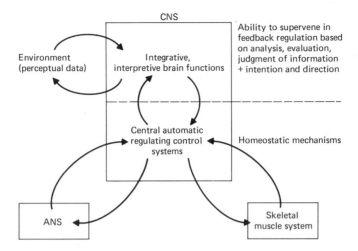

Figure 2.2. Feedback interactions among higher-order mental functions, central regulatory systems, and receptor-effector systems.

awareness of feeling states accompanying low tension levels. Presumably the attention directed toward the unfelt but perceived tension, plus attention toward detecting internal feeling states associated with tension and relaxation, enables one to process the substitute proprioceptive information and within the higher-order systems such that the information becomes incorporated into the channels normally concerned with the regulation of tension. The result is a corrective response of the control system and a decrease in tension.

It is somewhat more difficult to speculate why or how the subjective tension (anxiety and related sensations) is reduced by learned reduction of physiological tension. The most likely explanation seems to be that the learned reduction and the consequent reduction of proprioceptive tension information largely eliminate the cause of the sensations. This must be qualified, however, since neither the symptoms nor the relief from subjective tension may localize the physiological tension. It also seems quite likely that the attention paid to the information about muscle tension levels, and the task of both subjectively appreciating and trying to change the tension level without conscious effort, replaces the preoccupation with the social stress cause of the tension. Both effects contribute to the increased ability to discriminate levels of tension and relaxation, and hence to be aware of tension as it is developing and take appropriate action. This is a significant difference in the operation of biofeedback from that of previous stress-reduction treatments, since it is primarily a learning how to prevent the effects of future social stress rather than how to actively reverse or block the effects.

STRESS REDUCTION WITH PROGRESSIVE RELAXATION AND RELATED TECHNIQUES

It has been the research of Edmund Jacobson[16] that has shed the most light on the relationship between anxiety and relaxation. As a medical physiologist Jacobson detected residual muscle tension in patients with symptoms of anxiety, and developed the thesis that anxiety and true relaxation were mutually exclusive states. He demonstrated what he called "tension-image patterns" in individuals with anxiety, and further demonstrated that mental images universally evoke activation of physiological systems, particularly the muscle groups involved in the images. Jacobson called the difference between felt and unfelt muscle tension "residual tension" and hypothesized that individuals could become aware of the unfelt tension. The relaxation technique he developed was based largely on muscle manipulations that would lead to the patient's increased ability to detect and become aware of smaller and smaller levels of tension by a process of comparison while vigorously tensing muscle groups and then relaxing them. Because his experimental work showed the quantifiable increased muscle tension with mental images, Jacobson incorporated the use of images in his relaxation treatment programs. The images were used to enable the subject to recall the tension reactions during actual tension-producing situations and then to learn to discriminate levels of tension during therapy. The ultimate objective was to accomplish deep levels of relaxation without the images. A brief summary of Jacobson's concepts[13] of events during social stress reactions and their treatment is given in Table 2.4.

Both clinical and experimental evidence tend to confirm Jacobson's thesis that anxiety and relaxation are mutually exclusive states. The thrust of Jacobson's work that has not been adequately recognized as crucial until recently is the importance of the cognitive processes. The two critical elements, awareness of previously unfelt tension and the physiological effects of mental images, apply directly to the sequence of mental events outlined for the stressor processing phase of social stress reactions. Awareness of tension, whether via biofeedback or by comparing tense–relax sensations, results in diminution of the alerting effect (response to

Table 2.4 Jacobson's Anxiety-Relaxation Thesis

Major assumptions
  1. Anxiety and relaxation states are mutually exclusive.
  2. Comparing tension to relaxation (tense–relax exercises) develops awareness of feelings of relaxation.
  3. Anxiety is not caused by a problem "out there," but results from unproductive energy expenditure in trying to solve the problem.
  4. The imagery during problem solving evokes physiological activity and expends energy.

Anxiety(tension)-reducing procedure
  1. Identify the tension-producing situations.
  2. Identify the reactions, the tension-image patterns.
  3. Use the images during relaxation learning.
  4. Eliminate the images while maintaining relaxation.

threat) and a return toward normal homeostatic control. Further, the use of mental images both confirms the source of the tension and aids in identifying relationships between social situations and tension states. Although experimental proof is largely subjective, clinical documentation suggests that awareness of and attention to internal functions evoke mechanisms resistant to the assaults of social stress. Also relying largely on subjective reports, it appears that the awareness and understanding of the reaction process and how to resist it contribute toward subjective relaxation with consequent improvement in perception, broadening of focus, and more productive thought.

Schultz and Luthe's Autogenic Training technique[17] is a stress-reduction procedure that relies mainly on directing attention toward internal functions and changing states of awareness and consciousness. The principal elements of autogenic training are, first, varieties of self-suggestion relating to sensations of relaxation, followed by meditation exercises; and second, emphasis on the concept of "passive concentration." The voluminous literature on autogenic training sees its effects as decreasing muscle proprioceptive information activating cortical alerting activity, thus diminishing the alerting action on lower muscle control relays. To support this contention, the release of tension as an anxiety reaction is cited; that is, it is said that frequently in Autogenic Training therapy marked shaking and muscle twitching occur, believed to be due to a "sudden" release of the cortical activation effect, resulting in a burst of "stored" activating impulses from the lower muscle control relays.

Many other procedures having components utilizing cognitive mediation are presently being found effective in relieving social stress problems. The common denominators of the procedures appear to be principally the development of awarenesses of the stress potential of social activities and the development of awareness of internal tensions relating to these occasions, with the mechanism underlying the effect primarily a learning how to prevent the impact of potential social stress both psychologically and physiologically.

SUMMARY

In an attempt to understand the means by which psychosocial influences can activate the psychological and physiological processes that evidence reactions to social stress, I undertook two analyses. The first was a systematic analysis of stress both to define terms and to indicate that the predominant stress for modern man is social stress, with cognitive concerns about social activity being the primary cause of all the disorders of psychological and physiological function now called stress-related problems. The second was an analysis of a sequence of interacting mental events leading to social stress reactions which can be identified and characterized to provide a basis for selecting appropriate treatment of stress-related problems.

References

1. Selye, H. A syndrome produced by diverse nocuous agents. *Nature (Lond.) 138:* 32, 1936.
2. Selye, H. *Stress in Health and Disease.* Reading, Massachusetts: Butterworths, 1976.
3. Strongman, K. T. *The Psychology of Emotion.* New York: Wiley & Sons, 1973.
4. Arnold, M. B. In *Feelings and Emotions: The Loyola Symposium.* New York: Academic Press, 1970.
5. Duffy, E. *Activation and Behavior.* New York: John Wiley & Sons, 1962.
6. Schachter, S. In *Feelings and Emotions: The Loyola Symposium.* New York: Academic Press, 1970.
7. Leeper, R. W. In *Feelings and Emotions: The Loyola Symposium.* New York: Academic Press, 1970.
8. Lazarus, R. S., Averill, J. R., and Opton, E. M., Jr. In *Feelings and Emotions: The Loyola Symposium.* New York: Academic Press, 1970.
9. Hechhausen, H., and Weiner, B. The emergence of a cognitive theory of emotion. In Dodwell, P. D., (ed.), *New Horizons in Psychology* 2. New York: Penguin Books, 1972.
10. Selye, H. *The Stress of Life,* 2nd ed. New York: McGraw-Hill, 1976.
11. Cannon, W. B. *The Wisdom of the Body.* New York: W. W. Norton & Co., 1939.

12. Sperry, R. W. Mental phenomena as causal determinants in brain function. In Globus, G., Maxwell, G., and Savodnik, I. (eds.), *Consciousness and the Brain.* New York: Plenum Press, 1976.
13. Jacobson, E. *Progressive Relaxation.* Chicago: University of Chicago Press, 1938.
14. Murphy, G. *Outgrowing Self-Deception.* New York: Basic Books, 1975.
15. Hefferline, R. F. The role of proprioception in the control of behavior. *Trans. N.Y. Acad. Sci. 20:* 1338, 1958.
16. Jacobson, E. *Tension in Medicine.* Springfield, Illinois: Charles C Thomas, 1967.
17. Schultz, J., and Luthe, W. *Autogenic Training: A Psychophysiologic Approach in Psychotherapy.* New York: Grune & Stratton, 1959.
18. Kasl, S. V., and Cobb, S. Blood pressure changes in men undergoing job loss: A preliminary report. *Psychosom. Med. 32:* 19–38, 1970.

3

Psychoneuroendocrine Approaches to the Study of Stressful Person-Environment Transactions

Marianne Frankenhaeuser

Experimental Psychology Unit, Department of Psychology, University of Stockholm

This chapter reviews some experimental approaches to the psycho-neuroendocrinology of human stress and coping, centered on research concerning the sympathetic-adrenal medullary system carried out in our laboratory at the University of Stockholm.

CONCEPTUAL FRAME AND RESEARCH STRATEGY

The susceptibility of the sympathetic-adrenal medullary system to psychological factors was first demonstrated by Walter B. Cannon and his associates at Harvard during the early part of this century. Results from a series of experiments on cats led Cannon (1914, 1932) to formulate the "emergency function" theory of adrenal-medullary activity, stating that many of the physiological effects of adrenaline serve the goal of preparing the organism to meet threatening situations involving fear or rage or pain. Some decades later, von Euler (1946, 1956) showed that noradrenaline, the nonmethylated homologue of adrenaline, is the adrenergic neuro-transmitter as well as an adrenal-medullary hormone. These findings, together with Selye's (1950) pioneering work on the pituitary-adrenal cortical system and the general adaptation syndrome, form the basis of today's psychoendocrine stress research.

Our approach to human stress and coping problems combines two research strategies. One involves extracting specific sub-problems from natural settings and bringing them into the laboratory for examination under controlled conditions. The other takes our laboratory-based experimental techniques into the field, and applies them to the study of people engaged in their daily activities. Both approaches involve examining individual response patterns in carefully designed situations, securing *concurrent* measures of responses at the psychological and physiological levels, and relating them to more permanent characteristics of the person.

Stress, in this context, is regarded as a process of transactions between the individual and his environment (cf. Lazarus, 1966, 1977), and hormonal measurements are seen as tools by which new insights can be gained into the dynamics of these transactions. The key notion guiding our research (reviewed by Frankenhaeuser, 1971, 1975a,b, 1976) is that the effectiveness of psychosocial factors in arousing the adrenal-medullary system is determined by the individual's cognitive appraisal of their meaning and the context in which the stimuli are embedded, rather than by the physical properties of the stimuli. These ideas, which will be discussed in relation to our experimental data, are in accord with those of Mason and his associates (e.g., 1976), and the reader is referred to their analysis of the relative influence of psychological and physical factors on adrenal-medullary and adrenal-cortical secretion, as well as to other reviews by Mason (e.g., 1968, 1975).

Methodological Considerations

Research on the psychological significance of the adrenal-medullary hormones has been greatly facilitated by the development of fluorimetric techniques (Euler and Lishajko, 1961; Andersson, Hovmöller, Karlsson, and Svensson, 1974) for estimating free catecholamines in urine, with the result that relevant data can be obtained by sampling urine while persons are engaged in their ordinary daily activities. Thus, as first demonstrated by von Euler and Lundberg (1954), these methods are well suited to the study of psychosocial influences in everyday life. Only a small fraction of the liberated amines is excreted in urine as free adrenaline and noradrenaline, but this fraction shows a high degree of intraindividual constancy over time (e.g., Pátkai, 1970; Johansson, 1973). For a comprehensive review of adrenal-medullary secretion and its neural control, the reader is referred to von Euler (1967). A detailed review of sources of error in urinary catecholamine measurement, e.g., dietary and chemical factors, is given by Levi (1972).

Catecholamine excretion rates of healthy subjects are generally low during recumbency and rest. In males, adrenaline secretion doubles during daily routine activities, and rises three to five times above the resting level under conditions of "mild" to "moderate" stress, regardless of whether these conditions are perceived as pleasant or unpleasant (Levi, 1965; Pátkai, 1971a). The rise is generally lower in females. Severe emotional stress elicits a further pronounced increase of adrenaline secretion, and noradrenaline may rise markedly too. In other words, noradrenaline also reflects behavioral arousal, but the threshold for its release in response to psychological stimuli is higher than that of adrenaline. It is also noteworthy that, of the two amines, adrenaline shows the more pronounced diurnal variation, secretion being lowest between midnight and the early morning hours, and highest in the afternoon (Levi, 1972; Fröberg, Karlsson, Levi, and Lidberg, 1975). For studies concerning interindividual differences in the diurnal pattern, the reader is referred to Pátkai (1971b,c).

Provided the conditions under which urine is sampled are carefully standardized, catecholamine excretion rates constitute sensitive indices of the psychological impact of the environment.

EXPERIMENTAL MODELS

Exposure to Underload and Overload

The concepts of underload and overload refer to the inability of the organism's homeostatic mechanisms to maintain an optimal arousal level at high and low levels of stimulus input. Hence, conditions of underload and overload, although opposites in terms of physical characteristics, may be psychologically similar in that both are perceived as disturbing deviations from the level of stimulation to which the person is cognitively set and emotionally tuned. Insofar as this psychological resemblance dominates situational perception, we expect the adrenal-medullary response to be the same in both conditions.

Support for this assumption has been obtained in several experiments.

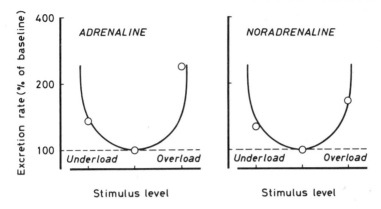

Figure 3.1. Mean adrenaline and noradrenaline excretion (log scale) at different levels of stimulation in laboratory situations. Values obtained under conditions of stimulus underload and overload are expressed as percentages of those obtained under conditions of "medium" stimulation. (Based on Frankenhaeuser, Nordheden, Myrsten, and Post, 1971.)

Results from a laboratory study (Frankenhaeuser, Nordheden, Myrsten, and Post, 1971) are presented in Figure 3.1, showing that underload (represented here by a repetitive, monotonous vigilance task) and overload (represented by a complex audiovisual choice-reaction task, requiring selective attention and rapid response) both induced an increased catecholamine secretion compared with a situation designed to match the "medium" input level of an "ordinary" environment. Psychologically, the two situations were similar in that both induced stress and both required effort. We shall return to this question when discussing underload and overload in natural settings.

Repeated Exposure

The psychoendocrine changes accompanying repeated exposure to one and the same stressful event, provide an excellent model for assessing the relative influence of situational versus emotional factors. For this purpose, the human centrifuge is a suitable tool, since exposure to gravitational stress, when a novel experience, is perceived as theatening and potentially dangerous, requiring the mobilization of physiological defenses, whereas once a person has gone through the experience and found that it can be coped with adequately, the person's emotional and physiological responses are rapidly toned down. This adaptational process is illustrated in Figure 3.2, showing data obtained in six objectively

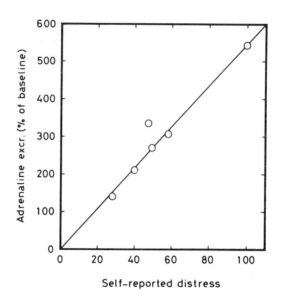

Figure 3.2. Mean values for adrenaline excretion (expressed as percentages of baselines) plotted against mean self-reports of distress in six sessions (one week apart) in a human centrifuge. (Based on Frankenhaeuser, Sterky, and Järpe, 1962.)

identical sessions, separated by one-week intervals (Frankenhaeuser, Sterky, and Järpe, 1962). The results show that adrenaline excretion was almost directly proportional to the degree of subjective distress as measured by a ratio-estimation technique.

It is worth noting that noradrenaline was markedly elevated in all sessions but that, unlike adrenaline, it showed no tendency to decrease with repeated exposure. The dissociation between the two adrenal-medullary hormones in this particular situation is consistent with their different adaptive functions, noradrenaline being involved in maintaining cardiovascular homeostasis under gravitational stress.

The point we want to underscore is that repeated exposure to a particular situation is accompanied by adrenal-medullary deactivation only insofar as the repetition is associated with a decrease in psychological involvement. To this end, it is interesting to compare the centrifuge data with results from a study of parachute jumping (Bloom, Euler, and Frankenhaeuser, 1963). Parachute jumping is an activity which probably never becomes routine in the sense that it demands less acute attention and concentration. Unlike the centrifuge situation, where the person remains passive, the parachute jump requires active effort. In accordance with the psychological demands inherent in parachute jumping, our results showed that the increase in catecholamine excretion during jump periods, as compared with periods of ground activity, was as high in experienced officers as in trainees making their first jump. In other words, under conditions where a high degree of involvement was maintained, the level of adrenaline secretion remained high.

Manipulating Controllability

The possibility of exercising situational control is recognized as a major determinant of the stressfulness of person–environment transactions. It is generally agreed that, over the long run, controllability facilitates adjustment and enhances coping effectiveness, although the effort involved in exerting control may be associated with a temporary increase in arousal (cf. review by Averill, 1973). We have been particularly interested in the issue of personal control, on the assumption that a person who is in a position to regulate stimulus input may be able to maintain both physiological arousal and psychological involvement at an optimal level over a wide range of stimulus conditions.

Conditions characterized by uncertainty, unpredictability, and lack of control usually produce a rise in adrenaline output. The influence of situational control on the adrenal-medullary response can be studied in laboratory experiments, designed to permit systematic variation of the uncertainty experienced by the subject. In one study (Frankenhaeuser and Rissler, 1970) the subjects were given different degrees of situational control in successive sessions. In the first session, high uncertainty was induced by telling the subject that each change in his heart rate, which was recorded continuously, would automatically release an electric shock to his left hand. In actual fact, shocks were given according to a predetermined schedule, the same routine being followed for all subjects. Under these conditions of high uncertainty, adrenaline excretion rose threefold from baseline level. Reducing the subjects' uncertainty by giving them more control counteracted the rise in adrenaline output. In two subsequent sessions the subjects performed a choice-reaction task, where quick performance reduced the shock punishment; the last session was designed so that the subject exercised almost complete control. As shown in Figure 3.3, adrenaline output decreased successively as uncertainty was reduced from a state of helplessness to an ability to master the disturbing influences. Noradrenaline excretion, however, was not much affected.

Although the ability to exert control counteracted the adrenal-

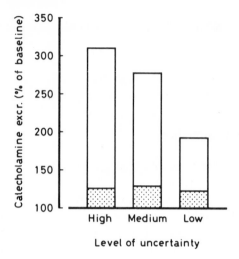

Figure 3.3. Mean excretion of adrenaline (dotted + open bars) and noradrenaline (dotted bars), expressed as percentages of baseline values, in laboratory situations where subjects experienced different degrees of uncertainty. (Based on Frankenhaeuser and Rissler, 1970.)

medullary response to uncertainty, the level remained elevated, as one would expect during attention-demanding activity. It is also to be expected that these conditions would produce a dissociation between catecholamine and cortisol secretion. The pituitary-adrenal cortical system is particularly interesting in relation to the helplessness-mastery dimension, since it is highly susceptible to all aspects of control (cf. Mason, 1975; Henry, 1976). Typically, lack of control is accompanied by a pronounced increase of cortisol secretion, whereas secretion may be suppressed in conditions characterized by control and predictability (e.g., Weiss, 1972; Coover, Ursin, and Levine, 1973; Vernikos-Danellis, Goldenrath, and Dolkas, 1975).

Recent data from our laboratory (Frankenhaeuser, Lundberg, and Forsman, 1978b) illustrate the dissociation between the adrenal-medullary and the adrenal-cortical response to an achievement situation characterized by feelings of complete mastery, safety, and control (Figure 3.4). This was attained by giving each participant a carefully designed preparatory period in which he was encouraged to try out different stimulus rates on a choice-reaction task in order to arrive at his own "preferred work pace." The task proper did not begin until the subject felt confident about the pace at which to begin a period of sustained work. Every five minutes he was then given the opportunity to modify the

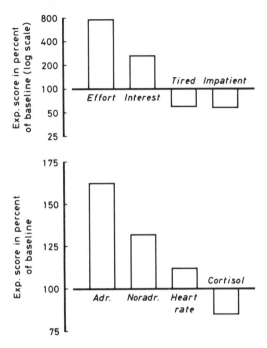

Figure 3.4. Mean changes (log scale) from baseline level in mood variables (upper diagram) and physiological variables (lower diagram) in an achievement situation characterized by high controllability and "confident task involvement." (Frankenhaeuser, Lundberg, and Forsman, 1978b.)

stimulus rate so as to maintain an optimal work pace. Hence, the situation was both predictable and controllable to a very high degree. Self-reports indicated that these experimental arrangements were successful in creating an atmosphere which was both pleasant and stimulating, providing excellent possibilities for sustained work. Under these conditions of "confident task involvement," cortisol showed a tendency to decrease to a level below the baseline. In contrast, adrenaline showed the increase typical of this hormone in situations requiring effort and concentration.

In another recent study (Lundberg and Frankenhaeuser, 1978), interest focused on psychological and physiological effects of control over noise intensity in a situation where the subject performed mental arithmetic under noise exposure. Every other subject was offered a choice between noise intensities, while the next subject, serving as his yoked partner, had to submit to the same noise. An interesting feature of the results was that the participants tended to respond to the control versus no-control situation in accordance with their general expectations about control as assessed by the internal-external locus of control scale (Rotter, 1966). Thus, for "internals" the increase from baseline was smaller (indicating a lower stress level) when they had control over noise intensity than when they did not, whereas for "externals" the pattern was reversed. It thus appears that stress responses to noncontrollable situations may be related to the extent to which persons generally tend to perceive life-events as lying beyond or within their sphere of influence.

We shall return to the modifying influence of control when discussing highly mechanized work processes. For other examples of research on perceived control in natural settings, the reader is referred to our studies of urban commuting (Lundberg, 1976; Singer, Lundberg, and Frankenhaeuser, 1974).

THE COST OF ACHIEVEMENT

"Raising the Body's Thermostat of Defense"

When a person performing a task is confronted with an increase in task demand, he may adopt one of two principally different strategies, either maintaining performance at a constant level by increasing his effort, or keeping his effort constant and letting performance deteriorate. The former strategy exacts a higher "subjective cost," as reflected in self-reports of various aspects of psychological involvement, positive (e.g., effort, interest) as well as negative (e.g., distress, discomfort). The "physiological cost" will be higher, too, as reflected in neuroendocrine, autonomic, muscular, and cortical indices of arousal.

In general, the participants in our experiments, under laboratory as well as natural conditions, chose to meet situational demands by investing the effort needed to maintain a high performance level, often showing a remarkable ability to "pull themselves together." An example is provided by experiments (Frankenhaeuser and Johansson, 1976) in which a color-word conflict task (a modified form of the Stroop test) was performed at two levels of difficulty; one denoted "single conflict," the other "double conflict" (Figure 3.5). In the latter case, where interfering auditory color words were added to those presented visually, the mental load was markedly higher, as reflected in self-reports of involvement as well as in increased adrenaline excretion. In other words, the subjects met

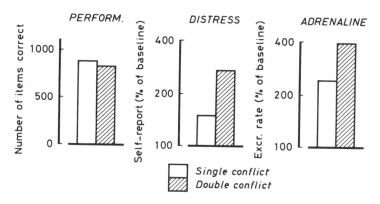

Figure 3.5. Mean performance in a color-word task under conditions of "single" and "double" conflict, and mean changes (log scale) in subjective distress and adrenaline excretion, expressed as percentages of baseline values. (Based on Frankenhaeuser and Johansson, 1976.)

the increase in task demand by "raising the body's thermostat of defense" (Selye, 1974), and, under these circumstances, performance remained intact.

The picture was similar in experiments with noise stress (Lundberg and Frankenhaeuser, 1978), where subjects performed mental arithmetic while exposed to one of two intensities of white noise. As predicted, more effort was invested in doing arithmetic at the higher noise load, physiological arousal increased, and performance remained intact. The trend was the same for all arousal indices, i.e., adrenaline, noradrenaline, and cortisol excretion, as well as heart rate.

It is instructive to compare these results with those from another noise experiment (Frankenhaeuser and Lundberg, 1977), where the subjects' cognitive set was manipulated so as to induce a less ambitious response style. In essence, this was done by introducing the subjects, right at the start of an experimental series, to a lower noise load than that used in the main part of the experiment. In keeping with the notion that conditions in the initial phase of stress exposure tend to have a lasting effect on a person's mode of adjustment, the subjects responded to the increased noise intensity by letting their performance drop instead of striving to meet the rise in demand. Under these circumstances increases in noise intensity were *not* accompanied by increased catecholamine output. (For a discussion of relations between performance, noise, and catecholamines, see Lundberg, 1978.)

Catecholamine Output and Behavioral Efficiency

Considerable interindividual differences are found in catecholamine secretion, and by relating them to behavioral parameters we can analyze the
action of peripheral catecholamines on psychological functions. Our
findings show that, among normal healthy persons, those who secrete
relatively more catecholamines tend to perform better in terms of speed,
accuracy, and endurance than those who secrete less. This relationship is
particularly marked for adrenaline secretion under low to moderate stimulation, but seems to hold for noradrenaline too (see review by Frankenhaeuser, 1971; O'Hanlon and Beatty, 1976). The example given in
Figure 3.6 (Frankenhaeuser and Andersson, 1974) shows that performance in a learning task was consistently superior in high-adrenaline
compared to low-adrenaline subjects (i.e., subjects above and below the
median adrenaline-excretion value).

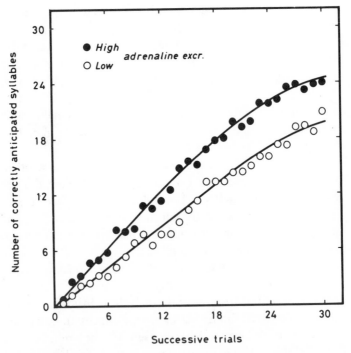

Figure 3.6. Mean performance on successive trials in a verbal-rote learning task in subjects with
high (above median) and low (below median) adrenaline excretion. (Based on Frankenhaeuser and
Andersson, 1974.)

When the conditions of stimulus load were varied (Frankenhaeuser, Nordheden, Myrsten, and Post, 1971), subjects with relatively high adrenaline levels were found to perform better under monotonous conditions, whereas those with relatively low levels performed better under conditions of audiovisual overload requiring selective attention. The impaired ability of high-adrenaline subjects to select relevant signals is consistent with an interpretation of the Yerkes-Dodson law in terms of a narrowing of the range of cues utilized at high levels of arousal (Easterbrook, 1959).

The positive relationship between adrenaline secretion and psychological efficiency at low to moderate stimulus levels is not confined to acute situations but applies to cognitive functions in general. For example, studies of children show that school achievement and measures of intelligence correlate positively with catecholamine secretion (Johansson, Frankenhaeuser, and Magnusson, 1973). Moreover, according to teachers' ratings and self-ratings, high-adrenaline children are happier, livelier, and better adjusted to the school environment than their low-adrenaline peers.

Thus, interindividual differences in the capacity to regulate catecholamine release to suit environmental demands may account, in part, for differences in the ability to tolerate conditions characterized by low and high stimulus loads. The "paradoxical" reaction, i.e., a decrease of adrenaline secretion evoked by a stressor, is an example of adaptive failure. This phenomenon, observed from time to time in apparently healthy subjects, probably reflects a denial of environmental demands (cf. Frankenhaeuser, 1975b).

We do not yet understand the precise mechanisms by which circulating catecholamines modify mental capacity. However, the available evidence does indicate that the catecholamines cross the blood-grain barrier in some regions only, but presumably penetrate sufficiently to exert a central effect. In addition, the perception of the peripheral changes that accompany catecholamine release may have an alerting effect.

The experimental finding that those healthy individuals who secrete relatively more adrenaline tend to cope better with both cognitive and emotional stresses, raises the question of possible long-term effects of adrenaline-mediated adjustment to the psychosocial environment. Although there is no direct evidence of a causal relationship between catecholamines and disease, data from several sources suggest that increased catecholamine secretion is in fact potentially dangerous, since, if

it lasts too long or is repeated too often, it may cause functional disturbances in various organs and organ systems, which, in turn, may lead to
disease (cf. Kagan and Levi, 1974; Theorell, Lind, Fröberg, Karlsson,
and Levi, 1972; Henry, 1976).

SLOW "UNWINDING"—A CRITICAL ASPECT OF COPING

Recovery from Short-Term Stress

In the studies reviewed above we have seen how a person who deals with
acute environmental demands by "raising the thermostat" may have to
"pay a price" in terms of increased psychological involvement and
physiological arousal. It may then be asked whether adjustment to short-
term demands is likely to have lasting aftereffects, reducing the person's
ability to cope with subsequent requirements and, probably, threatening
his health and well-being.

It seems reasonable to regard the *duration* of the response evoked by
temporary disturbances in daily life as a key determinant of their potential
harmfulness. In other words, the speed with which a person "unwinds"
after stressful transactions with his environment, will influence the total
wear and tear of the organism. In this context it is noteworthy that individuals tend to differ with regard to the temporal pattern of their
catecholamine release during stress. Comparisons between persons
classified as rapid and slow "adrenaline decreasers" support the assumption that a quick return to physiological baselines, after energy mobilization induced by short-term exposure to a heavy mental load, implies an
"economic" mode of response. Conversely, a slow return to baseline
indicates poor adjustment in the sense that the person "overresponds" by
spending resources which are no longer called for. In agreement with this
reasoning, results from a laboratory study (Johansson and Frankenhaeuser, 1973) showed that "rapid decreasers" tended to be psychologically better balanced and more efficient in achievement situations.

In this context it is also interesting that the coronary-prone behavior
pattern A (cf. Jenkins, Rosenman, and Zyzanski, 1974) appears to be
characterized by low flexibility in physiological arousal relative to situational demands (Frankenhaeuser, Lundberg, and Forsman, 1978a;
Lundberg, 1979). Thus, in a situation with alternating periods of mental
work and inactivity, Type A persons tended to maintain the same arousal
level (as measured by catecholamine excretion and heart rate) under both
conditions; Type B persons, on the other hand, adapted to inactivity by
lowering their arousal, raising it again when required to be active.

An equally important finding is that the time for "unwinding" varies predictably with the individual's state of general well-being. Thus, in a group of industrial workers, the proportion of "rapid decreasers" was significantly higher after a vacation period that had improved the workers' physical and psychological condition (Johansson, 1976), than before.

Cumulative Aftereffects of "Overtime" at Work

The findings described above led us to focus on possible aftereffects of overload at work. A recent study of female employees in an insurance company (Rissler and Elgerot, 1978) concentrated on stress and coping patterns during an extended period of "overtime." The extra time (an average of 73 hours per employee) was spread over two months, but most of it occurred during a four-week period. No new duties were involved, only an increase in the quantity of regular work. The employees were free to choose the schedule for their extra hours, and most of them opted for work on Saturdays and Sundays, rather than doing more than eight hours on weekdays. Since these women ordinarily devoted several weekend hours to household duties, they faced a conflict between responsibilities at home and those at work.

It was argued that the additional overtime load would call for intense adaptive efforts, the effects of which would not be restricted to the extra work-hours, but would also manifest themselves during and after the ordinary work-days. The results supported this hypothesis, in that adrenaline excretion was significantly increased throughout the overtime period both during the day and in the evening. Figure 3.7 shows daytime and evening measures of adrenaline excretion on nine Tuesdays, one before, six during, and two after the overtime period. The daytime values were determined in samples obtained at the place of work, the evening values in samples taken at home. Each value during and after the overtime period was expressed as a percentage of the corresponding daytime or evening value before the overtime period. As shown in the diagram, the adrenaline level was consistently elevated during the overtime period, after which it declined and approached the levels typical of ordinary work conditions. The most remarkable finding was the pronounced elevation of adrenaline output in the evenings, which were spent relaxing at home. This was accompanied by markedly elevated heart rate as well as feelings of irritability and fatigue. It is also worth noting the time lag between the work-load peak, which occurred in the middle of the overtime period, and the peak adrenaline excretion, which came at the very end of the period.

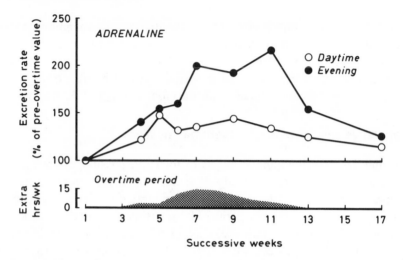

Figure 3.7. Mean adrenaline excretion in office workers during the day and evening (two-hour urine samples) on nine occasions before, during, and after a period of "overtime" at work. Values obtained during and after the overtime period are expressed as percentages of those obtained before this period. Most of the extra hours were worked at weekends, and urine samples were obtained on Tuesdays. (Based on Rissler and Elgerot, 1978.)

Hence, the results show that the effects of overload may spread to leisure hours, and that they may accumulate gradually, delaying their full impact.

STRESS ON THE ASSEMBLY LINE

There is a conceptual link between our laboratory models for the study of psychoendocrine aspects of underload, overload, and lack of control (cf. p. 000ff), and the social-psychological approach to job stress (e.g., Gardell, 1976). One of our research projects, concerned with stress in working life, is based on the assumption that new knowledge can be gained by combining methods and data from social psychology and experimental psychoendocrinology (Frankenhaeuser and Gardell, 1976; Frankenhaeuser, 1977). This approach will be illustrated by data from a study of the stress involved in highly mechanized work.

Catecholamine Excretion in High-Risk Workers

Work on the assembly line, organized in terms of the "moving belt," is characterized by the machine-system's rigorous control. The job is understimulating in the sense that there are no options for variety in either pace or content, and the opportunities for social interaction are minimal. At the same time the work contains elements of overload, such as rapid pacing, coercion, and demands for sustained attention.

In a pilot study (Johansson, Aronsson, and Lindström, 1978) interest was focused on a group classified as high-risk workers on the basis of the extremely constricted, machine-paced nature of their assembly-line job. This group was compared with a control group of workers from the same mill, whose job was not as constricted physically and mentally.

Figure 3.8 shows successive measurements of catecholamine excretion, taken during an eight-hour work shift and expressed as percentages of baseline values obtained under work-free conditions at home. The average adrenaline excretion was significantly higher in the high-risk group than in the controls. Furthermore, the time course was strikingly different for both amines, catecholamine release decreasing toward the end of the work day in the control group, but increasing in the high-risk group. The difference between the groups in the last measurement of the day was significant for both amines. Such a buildup of catecholamine arousal during a long work day should be regarded as a warning signal, indicating that the organism is forced to mobilize "reserve capacity," which in the long run is likely to add to its wear and tear. In other words,

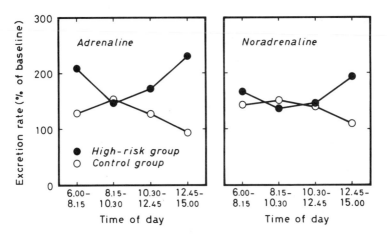

Figure 3.8. Successive mean values for adrenaline and noradrenaline excretion during an eight-hour work shift in two groups of sawmill workers. Values are expressed as percentages of baselines obtained under non-work conditions. (Reprinted with permission of the publisher: Frankenhaeuser and Gardell, *Journal of Human Stress, 2:* 35–46, 1976.)

the cost of adaptation may be exceedingly high. These assumptions were supported by interview data indicating that an inability to relax after work was a common complaint in the high-risk workers. Moreover, the frequency of psychosomatic symptoms as well as absenteeism was exceptionally high in this group.

Critical Aspects of the Work Process

The next step was to try to identify those aspects of the work process that induced the psychological and neuroendocrine stress responses. It was hypothesized that the common origin of the high catecholamine level and the high frequency of psychosomatic symptoms in our high-risk group was the monotonous, coercive, machine-paced nature of the job. In agreement with this, correlational analyses showed consistent, statistically significant relationships between psychoendocrine response patterns and job characteristics referring to different aspects of monotony and machine control. These relationships were examined further by comparing subgroups of workers differing with regard to specific job characteristics, e.g., degree of repetitiveness and physical constraint, as determined by expert ratings. Most subgroups were rather small and the differences between them not statistically significant, but the trends were consistent and formed a meaningful pattern as illustrated in Figure 3.9. Stress, as reflected in adrenaline and noradrenaline excretion as well as in self-reports of irritation, was most severe when the job was highly repetitious, when the worker had to maintain the same posture throughout working hours, and when the work pace was controlled by the machine. (For a full account, see Johansson et al., 1978.)

These examples from conditions in a sawmill—examples which are representative of a wide range of mass-production industries—point to potential uses of psychoendocrine techniques in assessing the stressfulness of different aspects of technologically advanced work systems. Presumably, these techniques have wide-ranging applications in the area of working life.

DO WOMEN COPE MORE "ECONOMICALLY" THAN MEN?

Comparisons between male and female stress-response patterns under various psychosocial conditions have revealed consistent sex differences in adrenal-medullary activity (reviewed by Frankenhaeuser, 1978). (Note

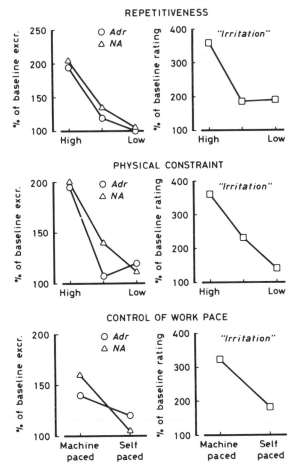

Figure 3.9. Mean values for adrenaline and noradrenaline excretion and self-ratings of irritation in a group of sawmill workers under conditions differing with regard to repetitiveness, physical constraint, and control of work pace. Values obtained during work have been expressed as percentages of baselines obtained under non-work conditions. (Based on Johansson, Aronsson, and Lindström, 1978.)

that the data presented so far in this chapter were obtained in studies with male participants only, except for the "overtime" study, p. 000.)

Under conditions of rest and relaxation, sex differences are generally slight, provided one allows for body weight. It is only in stressful and challenging situations that consistent sex differences appear, indicating a lesser reactivity of the adrenal-medullary system in females than in males. Thus, in a series of experiments involving moderately stressful conditions (e.g., Johansson and Post, 1974; Frankenhaeuser, Dunne, and Lundberg, 1976), we found little, if any, increase of adrenaline excretion in women, whereas males in the same situation showed a significant rise.

Our next step was to compare the sexes under more severe, real-life stress conditions, and to include measures of adrenal-cortical activity (Frankenhaeuser, Rauste von Wright, Collins, von Wright, Sedvall, and Swahn, 1978). Figure 3.10 shows the catecholamine and cortisol excretion of male and female high-school students during a six-hour matriculation examination. In this very challenging achievement situation, adrenaline output was significantly elevated in both sexes compared to the level during an ordinary school day. But the rise for adrenaline was significantly greater in the males than the females, and the rise for cortisol was significant only in the male group. In other words, under conditions of severe stress, the females did respond in a manner similar to the males, but to a lesser degree.

These results prompt the question of whether the neuroendocrine sex differences are mediated by differences on the psychological level. With regard to performance, our experiments have not revealed any significant sex differences. But as the slight differences found in various studies do consistently favor the females, there is no support for an interpretation of their lower adrenaline level in terms of lower motivation. It is worth noting, however, that self-reports of various aspects of psychological

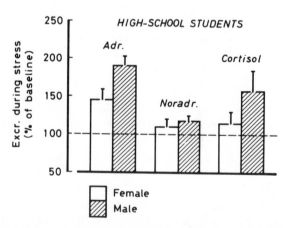

Figure 3.10. Means and standard errors for adrenaline, noradrenaline, and cortisol excretion during examination stress in female and male high-school students. Values obtained during examination are expressed as percentages of those obtained during a day of ordinary school work. (Based on Frankenhaeuser, Rauste von Wright, Collins, von Wright, Sedvall, and Swahn, 1978.)

involvement in achievement situations show consistent *qualitative* differences between the sexes. Thus, in males, feelings of confidence, effort, and satisfaction with one's own performance tend to dominate, whereas females express more negative feelings, such as distress, worry, and dissatisfaction with own performance. It is also interesting that high discomfort tends to correlate with poor performance in males and with good performance in females. Moreover, in a sample of school children where boys had a higher adrenaline output during stress than girls (Johansson, Frankenhaeuser, and Magnusson, 1973), "overachievement" correlated positively with adrenaline level in the boys only (Bergman and Magnusson, 1979).

As yet, as we do not have the knowledge necessary to evaluate the relative influence of psychological versus biological factors in the regulation of neuroendocrine stress responses in the two sexes. One way of tackling this problem might be to study neuroendocrine stress responses in patients with hormonal disturbances, e.g., women with high androgen or low estrogen levels (Frankenhaeuser, Eneroth, Lundberg and Collins, in progress). Another approach involves the study of women who have adopted typical "male work roles," the assumption being that their stress responses might be more "male-like" than those of more "traditional females." With this question in mind, we compared male and female engineering students, all chosen from the most male-dominated study courses, where fewer than 5% are female (Collins and Frankenhaeuser, 1978). Results from an achievement situation (Figure 3.11) show that the increase in adrenaline excretion was significant for both sexes, and nearly as large in the female as in the male engineers. The trend was the same for cortisol, but here the increase from baseline was significant only for the males.

These results, while suggestive, do not tell us anything about the causal relations. In other words, we do not know to what extent a constitutional tendency to respond to stress and challenge in a "male-like" fashion had influenced the vocational choice of the female engineers, and to what extent they had acquired a masculine way of responding as a result of exposure to the same challenges as their male colleagues. A better understanding of sex-role identity as a determinant of stress and coping responses may be gained in ongoing studies (Frankenhaeuser et al.), focusing on psychological differentiation—in terms of agency, communion, and androgyny (cf. Bem, 1974)—as related to neuroendocrine response patterns in males and females. Research along these lines may aid an

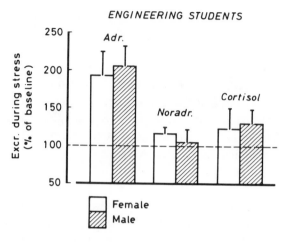

Figure 3.11. Means and standard errors for adrenaline, noradrenaline, and cortisol excretion in female and male engineering students in an achievement situation, expressed as percentages of baseline values. (Collins and Frankenhaeuser, 1978.)

evaluation of possible health consequences, for both sexes, of new sex-role patterns.

ACKNOWLEDGMENTS

The research reported in this chapter has been supported by grants from the Swedish Medical Research Council (Project No. 997), the Swedish Work Environment Fund, and the Swedish Council for Research in the Humanities and Social Sciences. Special thanks are due to Dr. Ulf Lundberg and Dr. Gunn Johansson for invaluable contributions and collaboration over several years.

References

Andersson, B., Hovmöller, S., Karlsson, C.-G., and Svensson, S. Analysis of urinary catecholamines: An improved auto-analyzer fluorescence method. *Clinica Chimica Acta 51:* 13–28, 1974.

Averill, J. R. Personal control over aversive stimuli and its relationship to stress. *Psychological Bulletin 80:* 286–303, 1973.

Bem, S. L. The measurement of psychological androgyny. *Journal of Consulting and Clinical Psychology 42:* 155–162, 1974.

Bergman, L. R., and Magnusson, D. Overachievement and catecholamine output in an achievement situation. *Psychomatic Medicine 41,* 1979, in press.

Bloom, G., Euler, U. S. v., and Frankenhaeuser, M. Catecholamine excretion and personality traits in paratroop trainees. *Acta Physiologica Scandinavica 58:* 77–89, 1963.

Cannon, W. B. The emergency function of the adrenal medulla in pain and the major emotions. *American Journal of Physiology 33:* 356–372, 1914.

Cannon, W. B. *The Wisdom of the Body.* New York: Norton, 1932.

Collins, A., and Frankenhaeuser, M. Stress responses in male and female engineering students. *Journal of Human Stress, 4:* 43–48, 1978.

Coover, G., Ursin, H., and Levine, S. Corticosterone and avoidance in rats with basolateral amygdala lesions. *Journal of Comparative and Physiological Psychology 85:* 111–122, 1973.

Easterbrook, J. A. The effect of emotion on cue utilization and the organization of behavior. *Psychological Review 66:* 183–201, 1959.

Euler, U. S. v. A specific sympathomimetic ergone in adrenergic nerve fibers (sympathin) and its relation to adrenaline and noradrenaline. *Acta Physiologica Scandinavica 12:* 73–97, 1946.

Euler, U. S. v. *Noradrenaline.* Springfield, Illinois: Charles C Thomas, 1956.

Euler, U. S. v. Adrenal medullary secretion and its neural control. In Martini, L., and Ganong, W. F. (eds.), *Neuroendocrinology,* Vol. 2. New York: Academic Press, 1967, pp. 283–333.

Euler, U. S. v., and Lishajko, F. Improved technique for the fluorimetric estimation of catecholamines. *Acta Physiologica Scandinavica 51:* 348–355, 1961.

Euler, U. S. v., and Lundberg, U. Effect of flying on the epinephrine excretion in air force personnel. *Journal of Applied Psychology 6:* 551–555, 1954.

Frankenhaeuser, M. Behavior and circulating catecholamines. *Brain Research 31:* 241–262, 1971.

Frankenhaeuser, M. Sympathetic-adrenomedullary activity, behaviour and the psychosocial environment. In Venables, P. H., and Christie, M. J. (eds.), *Research in Psychophysiology.* New York, London & Sydney: John Wiley & Sons, 1975a, Chapter 4, pp. 71–94.

Frankenhaeuser, M. Experimental approaches to the study of catecholamines and emotion. In Levi, L. (Ed.), *Emotions—Their Parameters and Measurement.* New York: Raven Press, 1975b, pp. 209–234.

Frankenhaeuser, M. The role of peripheral catecholamines in adaptation to understimulation and overstimulation. In Serban, G. (ed.), *Psychopathology of Human Adaptation.* New York and London: Plenum Press, 1976, pp. 173–191.

Frankenhaeuser, M. Job demands, health and wellbeing. *Journal of Psychosomatic Research 21:* 313–321, 1977.

Frankenhaeuser, M. Psychoneuroendocrine sex differences in adaptation to the psychosocial environment. In Zichella, L. (ed.), *Clinical Psychoneuroendocrinology in Reproduction* (Serono Symposia Series). New York and London: Academic Press, 1978. pp. 215–223.

Frankenhaeuser, M., and Andersson, K. Note on interaction between cognitive and endocrine functions. *Perceptual and Motor Skills 38:* 557–558, 1974.

Frankenhaeuser, M., Dunne, E., and Lundberg, U. Sex differences in sympathetic-adrenal medullary reactions induced by different stressors. *Psychopharmacology 47:* 1–5, 1976.

Frankenhaeuser, M., and Gardell, B. Underload and overload in working life: Outline of a multidisciplinary approach. *Journal of Human Stress 2:* 35–46, 1976.

Frankenhaeuser, M., and Johansson, G. Task demand as reflected in catecholamine excretion and heart rate. *Journal of Human Stress 2:* 15–23, 1976.

Frankenhaeuser, M., and Lundberg, U. The influence of cognitive set on performance and arousal under different noise loads. *Motivation and Emotion 1:* 139–149, 1977.

Frankenhaeuser, M., Lundberg, U., and Forsman, L. Note on arousing Type-A persons by depriving them of work. Reports from the Department of Psychology, University of Stockholm, No. 539, 1978a.

Frankenhaeuser, M., Lundberg, U., and Forsman, L. Dissociation between adrenal-medullary and adrenal-cortical responses to an achievement situation characterized by high controllability: Comparison between Type A and Type B males and females. Reports from the Department of Psychology, University of Stockholm, No. 540, 1978 b.

Frankenhaeuser, M., Nordheden, B., Myrsten, A.-L., and Post, B. Psychophysiological reactions to understimulation and overstimulation. *Acta Psychologica 35:* 298–308, 1971.

Frankenhaeuser, M., Rauste von Wright, M., Collins, A., von Wright, J., Sedvall, G., and Swahn, C.-G. Sex differences in psychoneuroendocrine reactions to examination stress. *Psychosomatic Medicine 40:* 334–343, 1978.

Frankenhaeuser, M., and Rissler, A. Effects of punishment on catecholamine release and efficiency of performance. *Psychopharmacologia 17:* 378–390, 1970.

Frankenhaeuser, M., Sterky, K., and Järpe, G. Psychophysiological relations in habituation to gravitational stress. *Perceptual and Motor Skills 15:* 63–72, 1962.

Fröberg, J. E., Karlsson, C.-G., Levi, L., and Lidberg, L. Circadian rhythms of catecholamine excretion, shooting range performance and self-ratings of fatigue during sleep deprivation. *Biological Psychology 2:* 175–188, 1975.

Gardell, B. Technology, alienation and mental health. Summary of a social psychological research programme on technology and the worker. *Acta Sociologica 19:* 83–94, 1976.

Henry, J. P. Understanding the early pathophysiology of essential hypertension. *Geriatrics 31:* 59–72, 1976.

Jenkins, C. H., Rosenman, R. H., and Zyzanski, S. J. Prediction of clinical coronary heart disease by a test for the coronary-prone behavior pattern. *New England Journal of Medicine 290:* 342–347, 1974.

Johansson, G. Activation, adjustment and sympathetic-adrenal medullary activity. Field and laboratory studies of adults and children. (Dissertation summary.) Reports from the Psychological Laboratories, University of Stockholm, Suppl. 21, 1973.

Johansson, G. Subjective wellbeing and temporal patterns of sympathetic–adrenal medullary activity. *Biological Psychology 4:* 157–172, 1976.

Johansson, G., Aronsson, G., and Lindström, B. O. Social psychological and neuroendocrine stress reactions in highly mechanized work. *Ergonomics,* 1978. (In press.)

Johansson, G., and Frankenhaeuser, M. Temporal factors in sympathoadrenomedullary activity following acute behavioral activation. *Biological Psychology 1:* 63–73, 1973.

Johansson, G., Frankenhaeuser, M., and Magnusson, D. Catecholamine output in school children as related to performance and adjustment. *Scandinavian Journal of Psychology 14:* 20–28, 1973.

Johansson, G., and Post, B. Catecholamine output of males and females over a one-year period. *Acta Physiologica Scandinavica 92:* 557–565, 1974.

Kagan, A., and Levi, L. Health and environment—psychosocial stimuli: A review. *Social Science and Medicine 8:* 225–241, 1974.

Lazarus, R. S. *Psychological Stress and the Coping Process.* New York: McGraw-Hill, 1966.

Lazarus, R. S. Psychological stress and coping in adaptation and illness. In Lipowski, Z. J., Lipsitt, D. R., and Whybrow, P. C. (eds.), *Psychosomatic Medicine: Current Trends and Clinical Applications.* New York: Oxford University Press, 1977, pp. 14–26.

Levi, L. The urinary output of adrenaline and noradrenaline during pleasant and unpleasant emotional states. *Psychosomatic Medicine 27:* 80–85, 1965.

Levi, L. Stress and distress in response to psychosocial stimuli. Laboratory and real life studies on sympathoadrenomedullary and related reactions. *Acta Medica Scandinavica,* Suppl. 528, 1972.

Lundberg, U. Urban commuting: Crowdedness and catecholamine excretion. *Journal of Human Stress 2:* 26–32, 1976.

Lundberg, U. Psychophysiological aspects of performance and adjustment to stress. Reports from the Department of Psychology, University of Stockholm, Suppl. 45, 1978. (Also in Krohne, H. W., and Laux, L. (eds.), *Achievement, Stress and Anxiety.* Washington, D.C.: Hemisphere Publishing Corporation, 1979.)

Lundberg, U., and Frankenhaeuser, M. Psychophysiological reactions to noise as modified by personal control over noise intensity. *Biological Psychology 6:* 51–59, 1978.

Mason, J. W. A review of psychoendocrine research on the sympathetic-adrenal medullary system. *Psychosomatic Medicine 30:* 631–653, 1968.

Mason, J. W. Emotion as reflected in patterns of endocrine integration. In Levi, L. (ed.), *Emotions—Their Parameters and Measurement.* New York: Raven Press, 1975, pp. 143–181.

Mason, J. W., Maher, J. T., Hartley, L. H., Mougey, E., Perlow, M. J., and Jones, L. G. Selectivity of cortiocosteroid and catecholamine response to various natural stimuli. In Serban, G. (ed.), *Psychopathology of Human Adaptation.* New York: Plenum Press, 1976, pp. 147–171.

O'Hanlon, J. F., and Beatty, J. Catecholamine correlates of radar monitoring performance. *Biological Psychology 4:* 293–304, 1976.

Pátkai, P. Relations between catecholamine release and psychological functions. (Dissertation summary.) Reports from the Psychological Laboratories, University of Stockholm, Suppl. 2, 1970.

Pátkai, P. Catecholamine excretion in pleasant and unpleasant situations. *Acta Psychologica 35:* 352–363, 1971a.

Pátkai, P. The diurnal rhythm of adrenaline secretion in subjects with different working habits. *Acta Physiologica Scandinavica 81:* 30–34, 1971b.

Pátkai, P. Interindividual differences in diurnal variations in alertness, performance, and adrenaline excretion. *Acta Physiologica Scandinavica 81:* 35–46, 1971c.

Rissler, A., and Elgerot, A. Stressreaktioner vid övertidsarbete. (Stress reactions related to overtime at work.) Department of Psychology, University of Stockholm, Rapporter No. 23, 1978.

Rotter, J. B. Generalized expectancies for internal versus external control of reinforcement. *Psychological Monographs, 80,* No. 1 (Whole No. 609), 1966.

Selye, H. *The Physiology and Pathology of Exposure to Stress.* Montreal: ACTA, Inc., 1950.

Selye, H. *Stress without Distress.* Philadelphia and New York: Lippincott, 1974.

Singer, J. E., Lundberg, U., and Frankenhaeuser, M. Stress on the train: A study of urban commuting. In Baum, A., Singer, J. E., and Valins, S., (eds.), *Advances in Environmental Psychology,* Vol. I. Hillsdale, N.J.: Erlbaum, 1978, pp. 41–56.

Theorell, T., Lind, E., Fröberg, J., Karlsson, C.-G., and Levi, L. A longitudinal study of 21 subjects with coronary heart disease: Life changes, catecholamine excretion and related biochemical reactions. *Psychosomatic Medicine 34:* 505–516, 1972.

Vernikos-Danellis, J., Goldenrath, W. L., and Dolkas, C. B. The physiological cost of flight stress and flight fatigue. *U.S. Navy Medicine, 66:* 12–16, 1975.

Weiss, J. M. Psychological factors in stress and disease. *Scientific American 226:* 104–113, 1972.

4
Stress in Israel

Shlomo Breznitz
*University of Haifa, Israel**

Israel's special conditions as a country under a high level of stress are described, and the question is posed of whether prolonged exposure to such conditions will lead to psychological exhaustion or to immunization. Research is reported on the effects of successive wars, threat to life, and continuous tension on a variety of behaviors. Prominent among them are: combat reactions, stress reactions of women and children, widows and orphans, and physical disability. Morale under stress is discussed in the context of a community with a high level of personal and social involvement. It is argued that Israel offers a unique opportunity to serve as a "natural laboratory" for stress research.

In view of its recency, the degree to which the stress concept has succeeded in transcending the boundaries of its original discipline is significant. The integrative properties of Selye's modern formulation of the General Adaptation Syndrome (1956, 1974) invited a broad multidisciplinary approach, which was quickly forthcoming. Besides experimental medicine, other branches of science joined in the common venture, the quest for understanding the complex intricacies of stress and adjustment. The psychological aspect of the problem, while always present, got its current impetus with such major contributions as those of Grinker and Spiegel (1945), Janis (1958), and Lazarus (1964, 1966). The intensity

*I am indebted to Mrs. Ben Zur and Mrs. Maos for their invaluable help in the preparation of this chapter.

and diversity of research effort in the area of psychological stress today is, of course, very evident.

This chapter will deal almost exclusively with the psychological aspects of stress, for two reasons, one technical and one substantive. The technical reason is that, being a psychologist myself, I have of course a strong bias in that direction; but more important, the substantive reason has something to do with the particular nature of the stress of life in Israel.

What makes Israel an especially interesting case in the context of stress research are the particular living conditions and events taking place in this country, all of which point researchers toward the psychological dimension. There is nothing outstanding about the physical and biological conditions in Israel. It happens to be a place with a mild climate, and free of unique diseases. The psychological conditions, however, are exceptional indeed, and they are the clue to understanding the research effort in the area of stress in this country. Let us sketch them briefly.

SOURCES OF PSYCHOLOGICAL STRESS IN ISRAEL

Life everywhere is often visited with difficulties, misfortune, and tragedy. We ought to bear in mind that by virtue of having additional problems of their own Israelis are not exempted from "the thousand natural shocks that flesh is heir to." What follows is therefore a short description of the *extras* that in Israel are superimposed upon the usual quota of stress.

First and foremost among them is the continuous state of war between Israel and its Arab neighbors. Since its establishment thirty years ago, Israel has fought four major wars, but they could easily be described as one long "thirty years war." Between the major outbreaks were two long episodes of war of attrition, and a ceaseless chain of hostilities. Terrorist activity inside the country adds to the sense of insecurity. The continuous need to take precautions and be on guard makes the subjective perception of threat omnipresent in the day-to-day routine of life. Even in the case of gradual habituation, the occasional explosion and loss of life remind one of the realities in which he lives.

Israel is an immigration country par excellence. The overwhelming majority of the citizens were born elsewhere, and are newcomers to the land. Immigration is a major stressor even when one's conditions are improved by it. The uprooting of an individual from some of his relatives, most of his friends, the familiar surroundings, customs, and language, is not a small matter. Often he was allowed to leave only after a long period of uncertainty, and without his family and his possessions. To complicate matters, the immigrants are not of a single origin. On the contrary, their diversity turns the country into a true melting pot of languages and cultures.

Economic hardships constitute another facet of stress. With an inflation rate of about 35% per year there is little trust in the economy, and few ways exist to provide safely for present and future.

In addition to active military service for three years for young men and two years for young single women, every Israeli serves on reserve duty. This consists of approximately a month a year in "normal times," provided there are no special emergencies. One serves until the age of 50, then switching to civil defense. These reserve duties often totally disrupt one's activity for long periods of time.

Last but not least, it ought to be remembered that Israel is a very small place with a small population. This implies that whatever is happening always becomes to a great extent a *personal affair*. Thus, for instance, when somebody is injured or killed, chances are good that he was personally known by any randomly chosen individual, or by one of his friends. This smallness means that everybody is attuned to names and details, and effectively amplifies the impact of casualties.

It is, therefore, not surprising that Israelis live by the news. They start their day with the news, go to sleep with the news, and listen to it many times in between. Their state of mind can rightly be described as one of continuous vigilance.

The personal history of many Israelis includes the tragedy of the Holocaust in Europe. Sole survivors of entire families surely feel a hypersensitivity to personal loss nourished by psychological wounds of Gargantuan dimensions, unprecedented in modern times. The specter of another national holocaust exponentially magnifies the subjective experiences of the various objective stressors of the community.

These then are some of the specific causes of stress in the lives of many Israelis. Add to them the ever-important dimension of time, the prolonged exposure to all of this, and the central question concerning adaptation comes into focus:

On the basis of available knowledge of psychological stress, what would be the expected impact of such prolonged bombardment with multiple traumas? Would the individuals living in such conditions necessarily break down eventually under the strain, or would they rather develop a certain immunity against stress?

This is an open question on both the empirical and the theoretical level, and we shall return to it after surveying some of the stress research in this country.

PSYCHOLOGICAL STRESS RESEARCH IN ISRAEL

Until the traumatic surprise of the Yom Kippur war, there was a conspicuous absence of research on psychological stress in this country. With the exception of some basic research on the effects of threat upon fear (Breznitz, 1967, 1968, 1971, 1972, 1973; Kugelmass, 1966) and studies of morale and social integration during the six-day war (Kamen, 1971), very little was done in this area. What followed during and in the wake of the Yom Kippur war can best be described as a flood of interest in researching the various facets of that trauma. This dramatic contrast tempts one to look for psychological reasons for both the earlier absence of interest and its subsequent eruption. If I may be allowed a brief speculation on this matter, I submit that there was a prolonged attempt of *denial of stress* on the part of both the population at large and the behavioral scientists in particular. With the sudden outbreak of the most frightening of all our wars, denial was not tenable any more as a coping device. In a matter of days it turned into massive preoccupation with psychological stress, preferably in the emotionally neutral disguise of objective research. Thus, for many Israeli scholars, researching the tragedies in the midst of which they found themselves became, I believe, a convenient strategy of coping.

I would have been more cautious in this respect were it not that a rather similar thing happened in relation to studies of the Holocaust. For years Israeli scholars were curiously absent in much of the research done on the survivors of the Holocaust, in spite of obvious advantages in doing the work here. The entire topic was taboo, until the beginning of the Eichmann trial in 1961. Then too, all at once, denial turned into an active preoccupation of both the general public and scholars from the various relevant disciplines. Being themselves part of a scene dominated by anxieties, it is perhaps only natural that scientists orient themselves to such anxiety-provoking topics at least in part according to their personal psychological needs.

The International Conference on Psychological Stress and Adjustment in Time of War and Peace, which took place in Tel-Aviv during January 1975, attracted thousands of professional and semiprofessional participants. It became the focus for many who attempted during the Yom Kippur war and in the period following it to be involved with the various helping programs, most of which were initiated by volunteers. There was an obvious need to report and discuss these experiences with active research in the domain of psychological stress. Under such circumstances it is quite obvious that by taking advantage of a serious natural stress much of this research lacked planning and methodological rigor. At the same time it reflects the enormous potential of Israel as a natural laboratory for stress research.

Combat Reactions and Their Treatment

During the six-day war there were very few psychiatric casualties among the Israeli soldiers. Leo (1968) mentions the high standards in the selection of manpower and extremely high motivation and identification with the cause as the main explanatory factors for this low incidence of breakdown in battle. Were it not for the Yom Kippur war, these "explanations" might still have been taken seriously. During the Yom Kippur war, however, with the same highly select manpower, and with the same if not higher motivation and identification with the cause, combat reactions became a much more frequent phenomenon and reached serious proportions. This indicates that at least some of the variance is under the control of *the exact nature of the stressor itself*. Thus, while the six-day war erupted following a relatively long period of tension and preparation, the Yom Kippur war came as a total and shocking surprise. The course of the battle itself was also different, and, instead of advancing, troops were often subjected to periods of passivity and local defeat or retreat. The death or wounding of comrades played, of course, a key role in the formation of battle reactions. Last but not least, the Yom Kippur war consisted of a much longer period of intensive fighting than six days, and stress accumulates in time. Combat reactions can be seen as indicating the stage of exhaustion in the course of the G.A.S.

Merbaum and Hefez (1976) compared the MMPI profiles of physically wounded patients with those labeled as psychiatric casualties. They also utilized American controls of both groups. They claim that: "... the psychiatric casualty groups can be unequivocally distinguished from hospitalized medical controls in both the Israeli and American samples" (p. 5). Interviewing the patients, they found that: "Insofar as combat stress is concerned, virtually all of the Israeli medical and psychiatric casualties were directly exposed to extreme stress in combat. The results from the psychiatric group are intensely disturbing and include sustained shelling, watching the death and injuries of comrades, persistent fears for personal survival, and utter bewilderment over the mysterious onset of uncontrollable sensory-motor tremors and shaking that powerfully reinforced feelings of anxiety and helplessness" (p. 5).

After posing the critical question of why the medical group did not experience emotional collapse as well, the authors indicate the fairly high incidence of premorbid problem behavior in the psychiatric group. And yet, over 60% of the psychiatric casualty group appeared to be clear of premorbid problems. This, again, suggests the need for more detailed investigation of the parameters of stressful events themselves. In any event, since the frequency of high-risk soldiers who did not break down is unknown, it is practically impossible actually to predict psychiatric breakdowns.

A case study described by Perla (1975) reveals the complex etiology of psychological stress reactions. The adjustment difficulties of the young man in question actually started only after the fighting when he attempted to return to his studies at the University. In the course of therapy he related that during the six-day war as an eleventh grader he worked as a volunteer in a hospital and described in great detail his feelings at helping a badly burned soldier. He later revealed that his mother had been killed in 1948 in a bomb explosion when he was several months old, and it became clear that he went about with a horrible premonition that such a terrible fate was also awaiting him. "In retrospect," claims Perla, "the early trauma of losing his mother and the fears associated with the nature of her death, or the confrontation with a severely injured soldier when he was an adolescent, were reactivated by the events of the Yom Kippur war" (p. 48).

This clearly illustrates the cumulative nature of stress reactions, as well as the fundamental issue of the long-range effects of the stress of life in Israel.

Schlosberg (1975) studied the sleep patterns of three combat-fatigued patients who suffered from severe insomnia and nightmares. They had no nap during the day and spent the night in the sleep laboratory. He reports increased sleep latency, very long REM latency, fewer REM periods, with stage 4 sleep nearly absent. Nightmares usually appeared in stage 2 sleep.

Sohlberg (1976), while pointing out the basic similarity between the combat reactions found in Israeli soldiers and those reported elsewhere, indicates the need to weigh variables like ego-involvement and commitment to one's country beyond more general variables, which are related to the unavoidable stress and strain of combat conditions and war. In view of our earlier comment about this, it might be argued that while motivation does not necessarily significantly reduce the risk of combat reactions, it might play a central role in therapy and readjustment. Since there appears to be a consensus among many therapists that early return to one's outfit is an important ingredient in the therapeutic process, high motivation can certainly facilitate such a process.

Teichman and Frischoff (1978), studying 53 combat exhaustion patients, found that "family relationships, apparently prove to be a prerequisite for better readjustment following a traumatic experience" (p. 5). Their data lend support to the importance of interpersonal relationships as a central dimension in the recovery process.

Kipper (1975) reports attempts to utilize desensitization therapy to treat combat reactions. Group psychotherapy was used and studied by Litman and Yaffe (1975). They report some differences between post-six-day groups and the Yom Kippur group. While the symptoms were similar, a more active and emotional attitude was observed in the Yom Kippur groups. Bodenheimer (1975) claims that psychotherapy of stress conditions and war neuroses indicates the need of respect for the individual's freedom and dignity as a possible access to an otherwise inaccessible personality. Inbar, Weingarten, and Bar-Or (1975) report that physical activity programs were found to be helpful in rehabilitating battle-shocked patients.

Winokur (1975) suggested a taxonomy of combat reactions, while Amit and Greenfield (1975) proposed a comprehensive battery for evaluation of combat-affected soldiers.

The above discussion gives a glimpse into the intensive preoccupation with the various aspects of the problems of combat fatigue. Basic research, quest for antecedents, taxonomy, clinical case-histories, therapy, and evaluation are all represented. The Israeli army itself became aware of the need for "field psychologists" whose main task is to prevent major emotional difficulties by means of professional advice and on-the-spot intervention, and their status and actual deployment were upgraded accordingly (Greenbaum, Rogovsky, and Shalit, 1975).

Stress Reactions of Women and Children

The frequent and long absence of the father and the husband in times of danger is of course a primary source of stress for the rest of the nuclear family. The particular kind of family involved and its relationship with its immediate social surroundings became crucial parameters in the attempt to adjust. Sometimes, the society successfully assumes a certain portion of the parent role. Krasilovsly, Ginoth, London, and Bodenheimer (1972) summarize clinical observations between 1968 and 1970 from six Israeli Kibbutzim (collective settlements) and two cooperative farming communities, all on the Jordanian border. These villagers were subjected to frequent shelling and other kinds of terrorist activity during this period. They report that the highly organized Kibbutz society, by being able to take more responsibility upon itself for its members than the independent family, has proved its advantage in hostile circumstances.

Children living in this area were also the subjects of studies by Kristal (1975) and Ziv, Kruglanski, and Shulman (1974). Ziv et al. compared the psychological reactions of 51 children in Israeli settlements subjected to frequent artillery shellings with those of 287 children never subjected to shelling. The shelled children exhibited more local patriotism, more covert aggression, and greater appreciation of courage than their non-shelled controls. No differences were found in attitudes towards the war, desire for peace, and overt aggressiveness towards the enemy. Specific modes of coping seemed to be partly affected by the prevailing social norms.

Milgram and Milgram (1975) took advantage of existing data from pre–Yom Kippur (April 1973) testing of fourth- and fifth-grade Israeli children using the Sarason General Anxiety–Test Anxiety Scale. They retested the children in December 1973, five weeks after the ceasefire of the Yom Kippur war. The general anxiety level of the children nearly doubled, with the children who reported the lowest prewar anxiety levels reporting the highest postwar levels. *Contrary to expectation, the rise in anxiety level was not related to war-related stress.* The authors offer the explanation that Israel is a small and highly integrated society, implying that even those who did not lose a close relative lost many personal friends and acquaintances. This argument lends support to one of the basic considerations stated at the beginning of this chapter.

The rise in test anxiety scores paralleled that of general anxiety, indicating that the heightened general anxiety level was reflected in increased anxiety about school matters as well. The negative correlation between initial anxiety levels and rise in anxiety was explained in terms of higher postwar legitimacy for expression of anxiety. In addition, those who were highly anxious before, could now find a focus for their anxiety, and that actually helped them or even reduced their diffuse anxiety.

Kedem, Gelman, and Blum (1975) studied the effect of the Yom Kippur war on the attitudes of young adolescents. Their results indicated a strong effect on the political-social attitudes of all their subjects, but the *extent of active participation of family members in the war did not effect the attitudes.* This "no effect of higher personal involvement" was also reported by Cohen and Dotan (1957). Interviewing mothers during the war and again eight months later, they found that while considerably more stress could be ascertained during the war than after it was over, *whether or not the male head of the family was drafted did not have any detectable effect.*

Goldberg, Yinon, Saffir, and Merbaum (1977) developed the Israeli Fear Survey Schedule, and found that in periods of national stress, responses in all categories (not just those dealing with war) were higher. The IFSS had proved sensitive to intensity of national stress. When subjects were divided into groups who had or had not a relative killed or wounded, *no significant differences were found in their fear scores.*

While one is tempted to account for those "no difference" effects in terms of the "small country" argument, it should be mentioned that there are other, quite plausible explanations. Thus, where anxiety—as contrasted with objective fear—is concerned, the objective intensity of the stressor might become less relevant. Another possibility is that the overall high level of anxiety does not lend itself to fine discriminations. These alternative formulations are not, however, mutually exclusive, and might all play a certain role in contributing to these interesting empirical findings.

A key factor in children's reactions to stress is, of course, the way their parents react to it. Baider and Rosenfeld (1974) claim that parental fear reactions are especially traumatic for the small child when the parents try to protect him by denying the facts of war. They cite illustrations of small children reacting to unexplained and hidden causes of stress in their environment with great distress. Children notice and can be helped to comprehend events that affect their lives. When an adult is able to act as a mediator and interpreter of stressful events, the child's anxiety lessens, and both adult and child find a new source of comfort and strength in each other.

Interviewing a random sample of 184 women, Anson, Bernstein, and Antonovsky (1975) found that the most poorly-adapted women were found to be those of Asian-African origin, the more religious, and the less educated. Control analysis indicated that each of the three factors is contributory, though the effect of ethnicity disappears at the higher education level. Education would seem to be the most important and religiosity the least important variable in this respect.

Widows and Orphans

"The sudden, violent death of a soldier is a crisis-inducing event because no matter how psychologically geared a woman is to the possibility, it still is unexpected and irreversible and is an occurrence with which most survivors, particularly young ones, have had little prior experience. Such a death sets off a series of ever-widening reverberations in and among the soldier's wife, children, parents and siblings, all of whom function within interacting networks" (Golan, 1975, p. 369). In her major article entitled: "Wife to Widow to Woman," Golan then proceeds to analyze the various stages of widowhood in terms of emotional adjustment. Most of her material comes from the Israeli scene where since the War of Independence in 1948, some 2,130 women have lost their soldier-husbands. Among other issues she mentions the exceptional difficulties of families of those missing in action: "Families were almost unanimous in saying that this lack of certainty, of not knowing and experiencing what had happened, was the hardest aspect of the situation to bear. The tragic situation of the 'missing' delayed for many wives even the start of the bereavement process" (p. 371).

While religiously observant widows in Israel found their psychosocial tasks considerably eased in the first phase by the observance of the week of prescribed ritual mourning, women from a restrained Western background and those who were not religious found it harder to cope with the initial threat to past security. "In some Kibbutzim, although the death of a member is keenly felt and mourned by all members, the absence of meaningful rituals and the tendency to shield the widow from outside contacts or worries usually leaves her roleless and bottled up, unable to find a socially sanctioned way to grieve. She may be relieved of her work and child-caring responsibilities and often spends her time in loneliness or in putting up a facade'' (p. 372).

Golan claims that in groups of widows the inclusion as co-leader of a widow who had already passed successfully through the mourning process, is most effective. An identical conclusion is reached by Safir (1975). A nonprofessional woman who had been widowed in the six-day war and had successfully started a new life was chosen as a co-leader of a widow's group, an idea adopted from a ''Widow to Widow'' program developed by Silverman in Harvard. Katz (1975) also reports that with the outbreak of the Yom Kippur War, many widows, most of whom had participated in groups in the past, volunteered to visit the new widows.

Ashkenazi (1975) describes the application of operant conditioning principles to war widows and their children.

In a study aimed at assessing the relationship between family structure, social perception of self, parental figures and social milieu, and their behavioral integration in the classroom, Lifshitz (1976) included in her sample of boys and girls about 14 years old, children who had lost their fathers in war three to six years earlier. She found that fatherless subjects, especially those orphaned before the age of seven, tended to show significant contraction in awareness and differentiation of their broader social milieu, and tightening of diverse psychological indices. Another study by Lifshitz, Berman, Galili, and Gilad (1977) investigated the short-range effects of loss of father in Israeli children from the city, Kibbutzim, and Moshavim. Boys were found to be more affected than girls; generally, Kibbutz children were least affected. ''The relative stability of life in the Kibbutz and its organization, which provide the family with ample help and father substitutes, lead to a situation where change in the life-style of the bereaved family is relatively small compared to city families'' (p. 281). This is in direct contrast to the effect of Kibbutz life on the widowed woman, as described above. It is odd that a particular social framework helps the child while at the same time makes the mother's readjustment more difficult. Since the emotional state of the mother is crucial to the child, one wonders whether those findings are conclusive or whether they happen to focus on different samples of behavior.

This finding is supported by Wieder (1975), describing the parallel reactions of widows and their children following the war. Mothers' stress reactions were among the most severe stressors for the children. Thus, for instance, the children of the missing in action showed disturbances "... in response to the loss of their *mothers* who went into various stages of psychological suspension, depression, regression and rage" (p. 68).

Since children in Israel have to face the subject of death more than children in most other countries, Smilansky (1975) advocates helping children to conceptualize the notion of death. There is now a growing idea in this country to introduce death into the educational system. Two of its active proponents are Schwarcz (1975), who recommends utilizing drawing and art in general, and Koubovi (1975), who recommends using the medium of literature to promote "therapeutic teaching."

Adjusting to Physical Disability

A few studies have attempted to qualify the special problems caused by physical disability due to injury in war, as compared to physical disability caused by other factors. Thus, for instance, Avni (1975) reviews the particular psychiatric problems of burn patients of both kinds. Rosenbaum and Najenson (1975) surveyed wives of soldiers suffering various kinds of disability. The subjects were asked to assess the changes that had occurred since their hubands' injury in the following major areas: interpersonal relations with the husband, social activities, relations with the extended family, relations with the children, and household activities. The differences between role expectations and actual role performance were taken as another index of strain. These measures of stress were found to be a function of the type of injury suffered by the husband.

Shurka, Florian, and Katz (1975) point out that disability as a stress situation is possibly modified to a certain extent by public or social perception. War-disabled are in a better situation from this perspective than those disabled by accident or from birth.

Morale under Stress

Continuous exposure to threats of various kinds makes the issue of personal and collective morale central to any analysis of coping and adjustment. The importance of morale is demonstrated by the effort to ascertain the level of its components as often as possible. The Continuing Survey of the adult Israeli population by the Institute of Applied Social Research has been and remains a major tool in the attempts to measure morale since 1967. It offers a unique opportunity for social scientists to investigate the effects of a whole spectrum of events upon the mood of the population.

Analyzing data from the Continuing Survey, Guttman and Levy (1975) reached the conclusion that it is essential to distinguish between mood and morale, when the latter is defined in terms of ability to cope with the situation. The two are not highly correlated on a individual basis at each point of time, and there is no relationship between their population levels and changes over time. Under conditions that lead both to high and to low average mood, the feeling of being able to cope remains uniformly high. It also appears that ability to cope with expected difficulties is more central than present difficulties.

This relative independence of morale of the short-term fluctuations in one's mood is, of course, a major requirement for adjustment to prolonged periods of stress. If it were true that the ups and downs of one's personal fortunes and reactions to daily events drastically influence the subjective beliefs in the ability to cope, the sustained stress would quickly wear down one's resistance, leading to exhaustion.

In their attempt to boost the morale of the population immediately after the shock of the Yom Kippur invasion, the mass media almost made the big mistake of misrepresenting the facts. Peled and Katz (1975) point out that the resulting drop in the credibility of government spokesmen and of the media expressed itself only after the onset of the ceasefire, but was discerned during the fighting, in the high level of word-of-mouth communication and in listening to foreign stations. The afore-mentioned basic research done by the present author on the effects of credibility loss, indicates the long-term dangers of inaccurate information to morale and adjustment.

One important indicator of the high morale which characterizes the Israeli scene during acute outbreaks of hostilities is *civilian volunteering*. While volunteering is a "natural phenomenon" in times of community crisis (e.g., Halpern, 1974), in Israel it tends to reach almost epidemic proportions. This may in certain areas actually reduce efficiency owing to lack of the necessary infrastructure for the proper channeling of the volunteer's good will.

When in a situation of war and uncertainty an individual volunteers to work in the helping professions with people already hit by disaster, he might often find himself in need of help. Levy (1975) describes volunteer social workers who worked with bereaved families after the onset of the

Yom Kippur war. Since members of their own families were also serving in the front, the volunteers were confronted daily with the immediacy of death and were forced to deal with their own emotional reactions. This element of identification with the bereaved families constantly pervaded and affected their mutual relationships. Such phenomena considerably reduced the "professional distance" between client and worker. Levy reports that workers kept dropping out because the stress became unbearable. Teichman, Spiegel, and Teichman (1975), on the basis of a survey of volunteers in the helping professions, also found that many of the volunteers in crisis intervention themselves require help to carry on with their voluntary effort.

The above suggests that volunteering is perhaps of more than substantive instrumental value, and serves one's personal need to "do something," thus effectively reflecting social integration, solidarity, and morale.

Psychiatric patients are no exception to the general creation of a tightly-knit social framework under acute threat. Merbaum and Hefez (1975) studied the emotional adjustment of psychiatric patients following their unexpected discharge due to war. On the first day of the Yom Kippur war, all civilian psychiatric inpatients at a hospital in Israel were discharged to make room for war casualties. Thirty of these patients were followed up at one month and again ten months after discharge. Surprisingly, ten months after discharge only four had been rehospitalized, and only four were receiving drugs. Behavior ratings at both follow-up periods suggested mild-to-moderate emotional distress. Assuming that persons requiring psychiatric hospitalization are poor tolerators of stress, the findings are surprising indeed. The authors suggest that: "throughout the war and sometime thereafter, personal coping behavior was for some reason effectively mobilized. In addition, it appeared that the former patients' social environment tended to reinforce their presence in the home, thus causing or enhancing emotional improvement" (p. 713). In trying to explain this change in the social climate, Merbaum and Hefez point out that during the war: "Interpersonally there appeared to be an outburst of comradeship and closeness. People went out of their way to be considerate, helpful and concerned. Great sacrifice was not unusual. It is reasonable to speculate that the former patients released in the midst of this unique environment reaped certain positive emotional benefits" (p. 713). Falk and Mann (1975) similarly describe a patient who was mobilized and performed well until the end of the war, and only then broke down again.

Conceivably, while the national emergency lasts, social rewards can compensate for certain personal problems. It is when things gradually return to normalcy that the difficulties often surface once more.

Disturbed individuals were, however, not the only ones to find the return to normal routine difficult. Gluskinos and Gordon (1975) tell of organizations whose employees served in the war, many of which were experiencing readjustment difficulties upon their return. Post-traumatic coping is often as much a problem as coping while the events are actually taking place.

THE CUMULATIVE EFFECTS OF STRESS

Let us now return to the focal question concerning the long-range effects of living in a highly stressed environment. Are the persons exposed to such conditions gradually exhausting their reservoirs of "adaptation energy" with the ultimate result of reaching their individual breaking points, or are they developing a certain immunity to stress? The above description of the work on psychological stress in Israel does not, of course, lead to an obvious preference between these opposing conceptions. At the same time it does, however, point out certain features of the issue which are highly relevant.

Thus, much of the stress in this country belongs to the same category, that of inescapable threat to basic physical security. Prolonged exposure to the same kind of stressors was shown to be likely to produce high risk to health and well-being (Selye, 1956, 1974). The other kinds of stress mentioned at the beginning of this chapter, as well as personal sources of stress, are all superimposed upon it with the individual having very little control over the situation. Consequently, there is good reason to question the "endless" ability to cope with repeated wars and tensions, particularly in view of limited opportunities for proper relaxation. In Israel one cannot easily shut himself off from day-to-day national concerns for the purpose of recuperation and the replenishment of certain vitally needed resources.

The argument is not, however, that simple. Many of the studies indicate the surprising ability of certain people to mobilize their coping abilities very effectively indeed. In times of war, morale is exceptionally high, and the social rewards of a small nation closing ranks ought not to be dismissed lightly. Recent research in psychological stress demonstrates the importance of cognitive factors that mediate the actual impact of objective stressors. Thus, it is not the external reality as such, but rather the way the person construes and interprets that reality, that mostly accounts for the stress effects. *The same event which is a threat to one is a challenge to the other.* A challenge, while still producing stress, need not produce distress (Selye, 1974), and as Lararus (1966) demonstrated, a particular cognitive appraisal can short-circuit the stress properties of an a priori difficult situation.

Shifting the focus from the stimulus to the filtering devices of those perceiving and interpreting that stimulus complicates the methodology of the relevant research beyond recognition. Paradigms of study are called for that allow for detailed explanation of the intricate interactions between people and their so-called objective environments. Similarly, higher sophistication is needed at the dependent-variable side of the spectrum. The cost of adjusting to stressful living conditions may turn out to be multifaceted and often latent, hidden from the superficial observer or counter of simple phenomena. Very little such work has been done anywhere so far, and Israel offers a unique opportunity to serve as a natural laboratory for research on psychological stress.

References

Amit, M., and Greenfield, H. A comprehensive battery for evaluation of combat affected soldiers. Paper presented at the *International Conference on Psychological Stress and Adjustment in Time of War and Peace,* Tel Aviv, 1975.

Anson, O., Bernstein, J., and Antonovsky, A. Resistance resources and maladaptive responses to a natural stress situation; Israeli women, October, 1973. Paper presented at the *International Conference on Psychological Stress and Adjustment in Time of War and Peace.* Tel Aviv, 1975.

Ashkenazi, Z. The application of principles of operant conditioning to war widows and their children. Paper presented at the *International Conference on Psychological Stress and Adjustment in Time of War and Peace,* Tel Aviv, 1975.

Avni, J. Psychiatric care of burn patients during wartime. *Psychotherapy and Psychosomatics 26:* 203–210, 1975.

Baider, L., and Rosenfeld, E. Effect of parental fears on children in wartime. *Social Casework 55:* 497–503, 1974.

Bodenheimer, A. R. Psychotherapy: This side of freedom and dignity. *Psychotherapie and Medizinische Psychologie 25:* 109–123, 1975.

Breznitz, S. Incubation of threat: Duration of anticipation and false alarm as determinants of fear reaction to an unavoidable frightening event. *Journal of Experimental Research in Personality 2:* 173–180, 1967.

Breznitz, S. " 'Incubation of threat' in a Situation of Conflicting Expectations." *Psychological Reports 22:* 755–756, 1968.

Breznitz, S. A study of worrying. *British Journal of Social and Clinical Psychology 52* (4), November, 1971.

Breznitz, S., The effect of frequency and pacing of warnings upon the fear reaction to a threatening event. Research report. Jerusalem: Ford Foundation, 1972.

Breznitz, S., The effect of early vs. late cancellation of a threat upon the fear reaction to a second similar threat. Research report. Arlington, Virginia: U. S. Army Research Institute for the Behavioral and Social Sciences, 1973.

Cohen, A. A., and Dotan, J. Interpersonal behavior and mass communication consumption in the family as means of coping with stress in war and peace: The effects of socioeconomic status and the absence of the adult male. Paper presented at the *International Conference on Psychological Stress and Adjustment in Time of War and Peace,* Tel Aviv, 1975.

Falk, A., and Mann, R. War as therapy. Paper presented at the *International Conference on Psychological Stress and Adjustment in Time of War and Peace,* Tel Aviv, 1975.

Gluskins, V., and Gordon, Y. A management training module to facilitate the readjustment of military reserves to industrial work life. Paper presented at the *International Conference on Psychological Stress and Adjustment in Time of War and Peace,* Tel Aviv, 1975.

Golan, N. Wife to widow to woman. *Social Work 20:* 369–375, 1975.

Goldberg, J., Yinon, Y., Saffir, M., and Merbaum, M. Fear in periods of stress and calm among Israeli students. *Behavior Therapy and Experimental Psychiatry 8:* 5–9, 1977.

Greenbaum, C., Rogovsky, I., and Shalit, B. The role of the field psychologist during wartime. Paper presented at the *International Conference on Psychological Stress and Adjustment in Time of War and Peace,* Tel Aviv, 1975.

Grinker, R. R., and Spiegel, J. P. *Men under Stress.* New York: McGraw-Hill Book Company, 1945.

Guttman, L., and Levy, S. Mood, morale and stress. Paper presented at the *International Conference on Psychological Stress and Adjustment in Time of War and Peace,* Tel Aviv, 1975.

Halpern, E. Volunteering in times of community crisis: An integration within Caplan's theory of support systems. *The Canadian Psychologist 15:* 242–250, 1974.

Inbar, O., Weingarten, G., and Bar-Or, O. The role of physical activity in the rehabilitation program for acutely upset combat soldiers. Paper presented at the *International Conference on Psychological Stress and Adjustment in Time of War and Peace,* Tel Aviv, 1975.

Janis, I. L. *Psychological Stress.* New York: John Wiley & Sons, Inc., 1958.

Kamen, C. S. Crisis, Stress, and social integration. The case of Israel and the Six-Day War. Doctoral dissertation, The University of Chicago, 1971.

Katz, M. Background and development of the project. Paper presented at the *International Conference on Psychological Stress and Adjustment in Time of War and Peace,* Tel Aviv, 1975.

Kedem, P., Gelman, R., and Blum, L. The effect of the Yom Kippur War on the attitudes, values and locus of control of young adolescents. Paper presented at the *International Conference on Psychological Stress and Adjustment in Time of War and Peace,* Tel Aviv, 1975.

Kipper, D. A. The treatment of war induced fears through desensitization therapy. Paper presented at the *International Conference on Psychological Stress and Adjustment in Time of War and Peace,* Tel Aviv, 1975.

Koubovi, D. "Therapeutic teaching" in time of national crisis. Paper presented at the *International Conference on Psychological Stress and Adjustment in Time of War and Peace,* Tel Aviv, 1975.

Krasilovsky, D., Ginath, Y., London, R., and Bodenheimer, M. The significance of parent-male substitution by society in various social structures. *American Journal of Orthopsychiatry 42:* 710–718, 1972.

Kristal, L. The effects of a wartime environment upon the psychological development of children in border settlements. Paper presented at the *International Conference on Psychological Stress and Adjustment in Time of War and Peace,* Tel Aviv, 1975.

Kugelmas, S. Reactions to stress. Research report to the U.S. Air Force. Jerusalem: The Hebrew University, 1966.

Lazarus, R. S. A laboratory approach to the dynamics of psychological stress. *American Psychologist 19:* 400–411, 1964.

Lazarus, R. S. *Psychological Stress and the Coping Process.* New York: McGraw-Hill Book Company, 1966.

Leo, A. Military psychiatry, occupation and refugee problems in Israel. *Military Medicine 133:* 265–274, 1968.

Levy, S. Social work intervention in bereaved Israeli families. Paper presented at the *International Conference on Psychological Stress and Adjustment in Time of War and Peace,* Tel Aviv, 1975.

Lifshitz, M. Long-range effects of father's loss: The cognitive complexity of bereaved children and their school adjustment. *British Journal of Medical Psychology 49:* 189–197, 1976.

Lifshitz, M., Berman, D., Galili, A., and Gilad, D. Bereaved children. The effects of mother's perception and social system organization on their short-range adjustment. *Journal of Child Psychiatry 16:* 272–284, 1977.

Litman, S., and Yaffe, O. Group psychotherapy with veterans suffering from post traumatic reaction: Some comparative observations on veterans of the 1967 and 1973 wars. Paper presented at the *International Conference on Psychological Stress and Adjustment in Time of War and Peace,* Tel Aviv, 1975.

Merbaum, M., and Hefez, A. Emotional adjustment of psychiatric patients following their unexpected discharge due to war: Short- and long-term effects. *Journal of Abnormal Psychology 84:* 709–714, 1975.

Merbaum, M., and Hefez, A. Some personality characteristics of soldiers exposed to extreme war stress. *Journal of Consulting and Clinical Psychology 44:* 1–6, 1976.

Milgram, R. M., and Milgram, N. A. The effects of the Yom Kippur War on anxiety level in Israeli children. Paper presented at the *International Conference on Psychological Stress and Adjustment in Time of War and Peace,* Tel Aviv, 1975.

Peled, T., and Katz, E. Media functions in wartime. Paper presented at the *International*

Conference on Psychological Stress and Adjustment in Time of War and Peace, Tel Aviv, 1975.

Perla, B. A delayed combat stress reaction: A case study. Paper presented at the *International Conference on Psychological Stress and Adjustment in Time of War and Peace,* Tel Aviv, 1975.

Rosenbaum, M., and Najenson, T. Sources of stress in the life of wives of severely disabled soldiers a year after injury. Paper presented at the *International Conference on Psychological Stress and Adjustment in Time of War and Peace,* Tel Aviv, 1975.

Safir, M. A widowed students' group with a former widow as co-leader. A clinical report. Paper presented at the *International Conference on Psychological Stress and Adjustment in Time of War and Peace,* Tel Aviv, 1975.

Schlosberg, A. Disturbed sleep patterns in combat fatigue. Paper presented at the *International Conference on Psychological Stress and Adjustment in Time of War and Peace,* Tel Aviv, 1975.

Schwarcz, J. H. An instance of creative educational guidance in time of war. Paper presented at the *International Conference on Psychological Stress and Adjustment in Time of War and Peace,* Tel Aviv, 1975.

Selye, H. *The Stress of Life.* New York: McGraw-Hill Book Company, 1956. Revised ed., 1976.

Selye, H. *Stress without Distress.* Philadelphia: J. B. Lippincott Company, 1974.

Shurka, E., Florian, V., and Katz, S. Physical disability, stress and social perception. Paper presented at the *International Conference on Psychological Stress and Adjustment in Time of War and Peace,* Tel Aviv, 1975.

Smilansky, S. Development of the conceptualization of death in children—ages 4–10. Paper presented at the *International Conference on Psychological Stress and Adjustment in Time of War and Peace,* Tel Aviv, 1975.

Sohlberg, S. C. Stress experiences and combat fatigue during the Yom Kippur War (1973). *Psychological Reports 38:* 523–529, 1976.

Teichman, M., and Frischoff, B. Combat exhaustion: An interpersonal approach. Spielberger, C. D., and Sarason, I. (eds.), *Stress and Anxiety,* Clinical psychology series, V.5, New York: John Wiley & Sons, 1978.

Teichman, Y., Spiegel, Y., and Teichman, M. Volunteers' report about their work with families of servicemen missing in action. Paper presented at the *International Conference on Psychological Stress and Adjustment in Time of War and Peace,* Tel Aviv, 1975.

Wieder, S. Parallel reactions of widows and young children following the Yom Kippur War. Paper presented at the *International Conference on Psychological Stress and Adjustment in Time of War and Peace,* Tel Aviv, 1975.

Winokur, M. The aetiology and treatment of combat reaction. Paper presented at the *International Conference on Psychological Stress and Adjustment in Time of War and Peace,* Tel Aviv, 1975.

Ziv, A., Kruglanski, A., and Shulman, S. Children's psychological reactions to wartime stress. *Journal of Personality and Social Psychology 30:* 29–30, 1974.

5
Psychological Stress and Adaptation: Some Unresolved Issues

R. S. Lazarus, J. B. Cohen, S. Folkman, A. Kanner, and C. Schaefer
University of California, Berkeley

By about 1955, after enthusiastic beginnings in the 1920s, psychosomatic medicine had lost much ground as a scientific discipline. As Lipowski (1977, p. 235) puts it, "The field suffered a sharp drop in popularity and credibility and seemed to be heading for the annals of medical history." Yet in recent years there has been an extraordinary revival of interest and activity in stress phenomena and their links to disease at three separate but interconnected levels of analysis: the social, the psychological, and the physiological. We now seem again at the threshold of making important advances in our understanding of the complex relationships between stress processes on the one hand and adaptational outcomes, such as somatic illness, social functioning, and morale, on the other (see also Engel, 1974, 1977; Schwartz and Weiss, 1977).

This paper is designed to articulate some important issues underlying the relationships between stress and these adaptational outcomes from the perspective of psychological stress theory. We consider social functioning and morale to be relevant outcomes which must be considered along with somatic ones because an optimal outcome in the one area frequently

Writing of this paper was supported in part by research grants from the National Institute of Aging (AG-00002) and the National Cancer Institute (CA19362-01S1).

occurs at the expense of an optimal outcome in the other, as when denial or avoidance through heavy drinking helps to maintain morale, but at the expense of physical health and social functioning.

One broad issue possessing three aspects stands out in our minds as particularly interesting, important, and as yet under-examined, namely, how adaptational outcomes, especially somatic illness, are affected by mediating cognitions, emotions, and coping processes.

MEDIATING COGNITIONS

The key feature of psychological stress that distinguishes it from stress at the social and physiological levels is the presumption that cognitive activities—evaluative perceptions, thoughts, and inferences—are used by the person to interpret and guide every adaptational interchange with the environment. The person is said to *appraise* each ongoing and changing transaction (or bit of commerce) with the environment with respect to its significance for that person's well-being. This appraisal includes judgments (whether conscious or unconscious) about environmental demands and constraints as well as about the person's resources and options for managing them. At the human level, cognitive appraisal processes are complex and symbolic, permitting individuals to recognize and distinguish among harm-loss, threat, and challenge, and to make numerous other subtle cognitive distinctions that give human life its highly rich and complex emotional qualities.

There is elaborate empirical support for the mediating role of cognitive processes in psychological stress (cf. Lazarus, 1966, 1968; Lazarus, Averill, and Opton, 1970; and Lazarus and Launier, 1978). The general principle seems not to be greatly challenged or in doubt according to most recent writers (e.g., Mandler, 1975; Kemper, 1978; Bolles, 1974; Dember, 1974; Meichenbaum, 1977; Goldfried and Goldfried, 1975; Ellis, 1962). However, the nature of the link between cognitive processes, adaptational behavior, and physiological outcomes remains obscure. It is here that some of the most interesting and significant research issues concerning the role of stress in somatic illness, social functioning, and morale, appear to lie. We shall concentrate on whether different dimensions of appraisal have different adaptational consequences.

First it is necessary to consider carefully the distinction between the actual nature of a potentially stressful circumstance and, in contrast, the appraisal of that event. Many of the research reports now available do not make this distinction. Thus, Holmes, Rahe, and co-workers (Holmes and Masuda, 1974) see illness as the result of the general mobilization required for adaptation to the change, and do not address separately the psychological appreciation of the change. The assumption is that individual appraisal of the nature of these events is not relevant or does not vary enough to contribute to differences in adaptive consequences.

Selye (1974) has made a distinction between "good" stressors, such as commitment to accomplishment, and "bad" ones, such as frustration and resentment. In our terms, these are not stressors, but rather are reactions whose nature depends on the appraisal of transactions with the environment. Further, the same event or set of circumstances (e.g., an examination) could clearly be seen as a "good" stressor by one person and a "bad" stressor by another. Some persons appear to appraise environmental demands as largely *threatening,* while others, seeing mainly the positive potential in engaging them, appraise such demands as *challenging.* Although the environmental conditions themselves may provide a basis for this difference in cognitive appraisal, personality factors seem also to be important; that is, some persons feel constantly challenged, while others feel constantly threatened.

The possibility that threat and challenge have different adaptational outcomes makes the distinction in this example important. The common-sense expectation would be that those who are disposed to see demands in positive rather than threatening terms have two major advantages. First, they are apt to have higher morale than those who feel threatened, since they can see things in a positive light even when others would be dysphoric; second, they are likely to perform better under pressure because they are more confident, less emotionally overwhelmed, and more capable of drawing upon their resources than those who are inhibited or blocked.

There are, however, some arguments opposing the idea presented here as an example of differences in cognitive appraisal. Contrary to the common-sense viewpoint, clinical observers often assume that the person who seems to think positively is actually involved in self-deception, using denial or reaction formation as a defense. Such defenses could conceal conflicting inner states and actually increase the individual's psychological vulnerability. Moreover, self-deception may require considerable adaptational energy, as expressed in Otto Fenichel's (1945) lovely phrase, "silent internal tasks." These tasks supposedly leave the individual with reduced energy resources, a clinical syndrome once referred to as neurasthenia.

Though these negative outcomes of defensively positive thinking may indeed occur in some persons, the empirical case is not a strong one. Even less empirical support, however, can be generated for the alternative proposition, that challenge appraisals result in more benign or protective somatic processes than threat appraisals. Thus, at present, it is still an open question whether health, morale, and social functioning are harmed by or benefit from an accent on the positive in the face of demanding or unfavorable life conditions.

EMOTIONS

Emotions are intricately intertwined with the processes of cognitive appraisal and coping. For example, the way a person construes his or her plight (appraisal) influences the quality and intensity of the emotional reaction. The effectiveness with which a person resolves troubled social relationships and associated affective distress and somatic disturbance (coping) also influences that reaction. Moreover, the relationship between cognitive activity and emotion also operates in the other direction, as when strong emotions interfere with adaptive thought and skilled performance, alter the appraised significance of what is happening, or serve as rewards and punishments that have contemporary emotional as well as developmental significance.

There have been two major approaches to the study of the link between emotion and somatic illness, the generality model and the specificity model (see also Lazarus, 1977). The *generality model* assumes that the nature of the stress itself, and the particular forms of coping used, are less important than the general mobilization accompanying any emotion, which precipitates tissue damage or increased vulnerability to illness through the direct and indirect effects of associated neuroendocrine activity.

Psychosomatic medicine, however, actually began with a version of the *specificity model*. It held that each illness—hypertension, gastric ulcers, colitis, or whatever—has its own distinctive type of stress dynamics (cf. Lipowski, 1977; Alexander and Selesnick, 1966). Faulty management or discharge of anger, for example, was said to be implicated in hypertension, while concealment of dependency urges was said to dispose the person to duodenal ulcers. The logic of this position is not unreasonable if one assumes, for example, that psychodynamic variations can lead to different chronic or repeated emotional patterns and, further, that different emotions have distinguishable physiological response patterns.

The argument over generality and specificity has continued through the last several decades. One major psychophysiological version of the generality position has been arousal or activation theory, which flowered especially in the writings of Duffy (1962), Lindsley (1951), and Malmo (1959). It was Lindsley, for example, who linked physiological arousal (via EEG, reticular, and autonomic measures) to a behavioral dimension of drowsiness, alertness, and excitement, and tied these in turn to the theoretical concept of drive. Another major version was Selye's (1976) concept of the General Adaptation Syndrome, an orchestrated form of bodily mobilization against all forms of noxious agents. In the 1950s and 1960s, the generality position was still being seriously entertained though it was losing ground because research was beginning to suggest that there were different emotional correlates of adrenaline and noradrenaline, and divergent patterns of autonomic nervous system end-organ response (cf. Funkenstein, King, and Drolette, 1956; J. Schachter, 1957; Ax, 1953; and Elmadjian, Hope, and Lamson, 1958).

The dominant outlook today seems to favor a strong generality position. Some reasons for this are the seminal influence of Selye; the weakness of the early research on specificity, e.g., data linking fear to adrenaline secretion and anger to noradrenaline (see also Frankenhaeuser, 1976); and the demonstration of highly overlapping autonomic nervous system patterns in these emotions. One might also mention the impact on psychological thought of S. Schachter's (1966) treatment of emotions as a generalized form of arousal distinguished qualitatively only by the cognitive label a person puts on the situation; in effect, if one is aroused in a socially anger-centered situation, one thinks and feels anger, while the same arousal in a euphoric situation is labeled and felt as euphoria (cf. Schachter and Singer, 1962). Such a stance, however, equates emotion with the external social context and fails to deal with the internal mediating psychological processes shaping emotion (Lazarus and Averill, 1972). Besides, this research did not test whether these emotion-context patterns had similar physiological response profiles.

Additional evidence that general arousal theory is wrong, or at least overstated, comes from a number of important directions. First, studies of more than one autonomic nervous system end-organ reaction have reported negligible or very low correlations among them. For example, when skin conductance goes up, heart rate or blood pressure may or may not be dropping. Lacey's (1967) impressive work on the specificity of autonomic end-organ reactions to different types of stressful situations should have brought about the demise of general activation theory. Lacey found, for example, that while skin conductance always rose under stimulating or stressful conditions, heart rate rose simultaneously when a person was seeking to avoid stimulus input or trying to engage in mental work despite interference from the outside, and fell sharply just before the occurrence of an anticipated, time-locked stimulus. In effect, somatic responses may reflect the psychological impact of the person-environment relationship. And although Lazarus, Speisman, and Mordkoff (1963) showed that the relationship among autonomic indicators was higher if one studied the correlation within individuals rather than across individuals, at best the relationships among them were quite modest. Such findings fail to support activation theory.

Further support for specificity from research using autonomic nervous system measures is provided by: Graham's (1962) efforts to link given attitudes to physiological response patterns and somatic symptoms; the research of Engel (1960) and Engel and Bickford (1961) demonstrating stimulus specificity; and research by Shapiro, Tursky, and Schwartz (1970) on the specificity of autonomic end-organ responses in biofeedback studies.

One reason the case for specificity has been less impressive to researchers and theoreticians on the psychophysiology of emotion is methodological. Because of technological complications and high costs, individual laboratories have tended to study *either* autonomic end-organ reactions using electrophysiological instruments, *or* catecholamines by means of blood or urine measures, *or* corticosteroids, also assessed in the blood and urine. Rarely, if ever, does a single laboratory simultaneously examine somatic patterning across multiple hormonal or organ systems, that is, catecholamines *and* corticosteroids *and* autonomic nervous system reactions.

Thus, although it is not a distortion to state, as Schachter (1966) and others have, that the present evidence for somatic response specificity in qualitatively different emotions such as fear, anger, depression, guilt, anxiety, joy, love, or exhilaration is weak, it would indeed be cavalier to assert that the whole body responds in essentially the same way regardless of the emotion involved. To make such a claim requires that research include multiple somatic response systems and multiple research settings. Such a claim also requires better methods for assessing the quality of an emotional response, and the changing patterns of emotion and of coping activity occurring in the ordinary course of adaptation (Lazarus, 1978).

Nothing approaching this had been done until recently, when Mason and his colleagues (Mason, 1975; Mason et al., 1976) provided a useful model for how the relations between emotion, coping processes, and somatic response patterns might be profitably investigated. They obtained measures of many different endocrines and assessed their profile of response to a variety of physical stressors in both monkeys and humans. Physical stressors such as heat, cold, exercise, and fasting were compared, and a particular effort was made to control for any psychological threats that might have been confounded with these physical stressors. For example, any sudden change of temperature was avoided in the heat and cold situation; and in fasting, the psychological distress a monkey would experience on seeing a trainer pass him up while feeding other animals was prevented by using placebos for the experimental monkeys. In the human exercise situation, threats connected with doing poorly or with perceived physiological reactions were eliminated or at least reduced by keeping the exercise demand modest. Two findings are of interest: first, corticosteroid output in the absence of psychologically-based threat did not necessarily rise with physical stressors; second, a different profile of hormonal response was found for each type of physical stressor. In short, there was a high degree of stimulus specificity, but little evidence of an overall, general response as predicted by the General Adaptation Syndrome theory of Selye.

Mason has not yet tested systematically the relationships of hormonal patterns with specific emotional response qualities, though he is convinced that his data suggest that such relationships will indeed be found (Mason, personal communication). He has studied the hormonal response of monkeys in situations that should have quite distinct psychological implications, for example, those characterized by unpredictability and which generate coping efforts. The inferred psychological factors seem to produce different hormonal secretion patterns. Summarizing this work, he writes cautiously (1975, p. 170):

Research on psychological stimuli has so far, then, yielded only preliminary and limited indications that different, relatively specific emotional states may be correlated with different, specific patterns of multiple hormonal responses, although several promising leads along these lines appear worthy of further study.

Mason also (1975, p. 149) suggests, more forcefully, that:

It appears . . . the hormonal trend is a resultant of a balance of opposing and cooperating forces and can be predicted with increasing accuracy as the multiple factors involved, including affective state, defensive organization, social setting, prior experiential or developmental factors, and current activities, can all be evaluated in a psychodynamic perspective for each individual subject.

And further (1975, p. 169):

There appears to be little doubt that a broad range of hormones and endocrine systems respond concurrently to psychological influences, including the pituitary-thyroidal, pituitary-gonadal, growth hormone, and insulin systems, as well as the pituitary-adrenal cortical and sympathetic-adrenal medullary systems.

Clearly, what is needed is research designs in a variety of environmental contexts using enough diverse types of somatic response measures to construct patterns or profiles while simultaneously varying the key mediating psychological processes in stress, emotion, and illness, including appraisal, coping, and the emotion quality (see also Lazarus, 1966, 1977). We think future research will show that quite divergent, though perhaps overlapping, somatic response patterns are associated with different emotional states. Such findings would bring to the fore again the earlier notion that psychodynamic factors do have causal significance in individual differences in psychosomatic disease etiology.

There is another fascinating facet to the generality-specificity issue that has received little serious attention, and yet is potentially of great importance. It is a variant of the distinction made earlier in this paper between positively-toned and negatively-toned emotions. There has been some interest in positive emotions, mainly from the standpoints of psychological well-being (Bradburn and Caplowitz, 1965), marital happiness (Orden and Bradburn, 1968), and life tedium (Kanner, Kafry, and Pines, 1977). However, the unresolved practical issue implied in the discussion above is whether or not it matters for adaptation that positive emotions enter or predominate in a person's life. It is widely assumed (though not conclusively demonstrated) that negatively-toned emotions may result not only in lower morale and social disability, but also in diseases of adaptation through the hormones they produce. The provocative question we would raise is whether positive emotions might have an opposite, positive or constructive effect, at the physiological level as well as the social and psychological, possibly helping to prevent, lessen, or cure stress-linked disorders.

Norman Cousins, Editor of the *Saturday Review,* has raised this question in *The New England Journal of Medicine* (1976), where he describes his bout with a collagen disease, the normal course of which is severe and rapid deterioration. He suggests that his self-generated program of producing laughter and positive emotions in himself significantly helped him to overcome his illness. Though recognizing that such a single case could have little scientific validity, he writes engagingly of it as follows:

The inevitable question arose in my mind: What about the positive emotions? If negative emotions produce negative chemical changes in the body, wouldn't the positive emotions produce positive chemical changes? Is it possible that love, hope, faith, laughter, confidence and the will to live have therapeutic value? Do chemical changes occur only on the downside?

The idea suggested by Cousins is, of course, not new. It forms part of the belief system of the field that some refer to as "holistic medicine," the thrust of which is to focus attention upon the whole person who is experiencing a health crisis rather than upon the diseased tissues only; it is found in most or all of the current crop of inspirational guides to living, e.g., relaxation, meditation, search for oneness with the world, and other spiritualistic movements. Unfortunately, its potential value is greatly limited by the failure to test and discover the rules by which ongoing psychological processes such as emotional states affect health and illness. It is time, however, for serious researchers to take up the challenge implied in layman Cousins' well-stated question. We think that there are substantial theoretical and empirical grounds for believing that such research could yield important insights into psychosomatic theory and practice.

In the above discussion of the links between emotions and physiological responses, we have been talking about short-range outcomes—momentary or acute changes in physiological functioning due to psychological stress or emotional states. However, mammals are constructed to be capable of "emergency reactions," and such reactions, in themselves, are not disease. One important issue is whether they are, as Levi and Kagan (1971) have intimated, "precursors" of disease. For example, blood pressure can rise sharply under stress, but hypertension represents a long-term change in tissue activity. Similarly duodenal ulcer and colitis are diseased tissue states, and many diseases involve irreversible changes. The crucial question is how we go from acute, short-range emergency reactions or patterns of physiological mobilization to long-range disease processes. The answer to this question is really not known, since research has not been designed to attack concurrently the psychosocial and physiological processes contributing to illness and the emergence, exacerbation, or cessation of illnesses.

Epidemiological studies using such longer-range outcomes have shown the importance of psychosocial factors in rates of disease and overall mortality. For example, Marmot and Syme (1976) demonstrated the importance of acculturation among Japanese-Americans in explaining differential rates of myocardial infarction and angina pectoris. Low socioeconomic status has been repeatedly found to be a risk factor for many diseases, as has the status of being unmarried (Syme and Berkman, 1976). Bereavement, too, has been cited as an antecedent of many diseases (Weiner, 1977). In fact, the evidence supporting these psychosocial variables as risk factors in widely varying disease outcomes has led at least one investigator (Syme, 1977b) to propose that such an observation supports a generality model. It is Syme's contention that these psychosocial factors, as well as others, create a generally raised susceptibility to all disease.

The problem with this idea, in our view, is that it leaves unexamined the mechanisms which underlie such population phenomena as increased or decreased probability of illness as a result of low socioeconomic status, acculturation, or being unmarried. After all, all three of these phenomena imply a large number of associated psychological and social factors that might be at work in producing the relationship to illness. What is needed is research that would establish the link between the correlations observed among momentary or acute phenomena and longer-range, population relationships. This "missing link" has been remarked upon by a number of researchers, including Luborsky, Docherty, and Penick (1973), Stahl et al. (1975), Herd (1977), and Lazarus (1978). The case is most easily made for the example of hypertensive cardiovascular disease, where, to quote Herd (1977):

We have some knowledge concerning the mechanisms whereby psychological processes may influence cardiovascular function during short periods of time. However, we do not know the mechanisms whereby a susceptibility to transient elevations in blood pressure may convert to sustained arterial hypertension. Finally, we do not know what psychological and physiological characteristics might predispose an individual to develop hypertensive cardiovascular disease when exposed to certain environmental situations over long periods of time.

What is left out here is the possibility that recurrent or stable psychological characteristics, regardless of the environmental situation, entail certain physiological consequences which might eventually result in disease. If, for example, one observed repeated patterns of appraisal, emotion, or coping among the same individuals over time and across diverse environmental situations, one might also find that, depending on the content of the repetitious behavior, this group of individuals also had distinctive adaptational outcomes. This is one way to conceptualize the possible connection between momentary or acute phenomena and longer-range or chronic, disease-related ones. Discovery of such mechanisms requires certain measurement and design innovations which we will discuss later under methodological issues.

COPING PROCESSES

It is coming to be recognized widely that coping processes, set in motion when a person is having a stressful transaction, greatly affect adaptational outcomes at the social and physiological levels, including the prospect of somatic illness. Some coping processes can *increase* the risk of maladaptation or illness, while others can *decrease* it, though the psychophysiological mechanisms underlying these effects are far from clear.

Coping and Increased Risk of Illness

There are at least three ways in which coping can add to the risk of social, psychological, or physical malfunctioning. The first is by direct damage to tissues. Obvious examples of this include smoking, drinking, overeating, and undereating. Such behavior, often generated as ways of dealing with stressful conditions of life, can result in damage to morale or social relationships, or in physiological damage, say, to the liver, the lungs, or the cardiovascular system. This, in turn, may increase general vulnerability to disease or directly result in disease itself, as in esophageal or lung cancer, or cirrhosis of the liver.

A second way is more indirect, and involves the bodily effects on the internal milieu of the mobilization often required for coping. Epidemiological research implicates such mobilization in disorders such as hypertension (Syme, 1977a; Ostfeld, 1967). The well-known findings concerning the relationship between Type A Behavior and coronary heart disease belong in this category (Rosenman et al., 1976). Type A Behavior is a coping response arising from the socialization process in a society emphasizing the Protestant Ethic. Note that Type A Behavior is an extremely stable, self-induced response in individuals exemplifying it. We can speculate that it is the repeated physiological mobilization associated with the behavior pattern which leads to the bodily changes that eventually lead to increased risk of coronary disease and infarction. Just beginning now is research on the situations that do or do not elicit Type A Behavior, the physiological mechanisms linking Type A Behavior to the long-term atherosclerotic process, and the immediate, short-term events surrounding a heart attack (cf. Glass, 1977).

In any case, the hormonal secretions that accompany mobilization can cause *direct damage,* as in one element of Selye's General Adaptation Syndrome triad of the alarm stage, namely, ulceration of the gastrointestinal tract (Selye, 1976); or they can cause *indirect damage,* as illustrated by another G.A.S. element, the shrinkage of the thymus gland and reduction in the number of lymphocytes in the blood. This mechanism, which weakens the immune system's capability of resisting infection, thereby increasing the likelihood of illness, is favored by some (e.g., Cassel, 1976) in explaining the role of unfavorable social relationships in morbidity and mortality.

Less obvious is a third mode of effect in which coping processes interfere with adaptive behaviors that could help to preserve life or normal adaptive functioning. Katz et al. (1970) have observed many women who, on finding a suspicious breast lump, denied its serious health implications and delayed seeking medical attention. Similar observations have been made by Von Kugelgen (1975) in the case of men experiencing the symptoms of a heart attack. And Hackett and Cassem (1975) have described some illustrative cases of men who, during a heart attack, did vigorous pushups or ran up a flight of stairs, reasoning that they could not be experiencing a heart attack, since exertion did not cause them to drop dead. These palliative methods of coping, that is, methods whose intention is to make the person feel less threatened and distressed, increase the person's vulnerability to a truly life-threatening illness by interfering with or delaying actions that might save or prolong his life. Similar examples could be cited of palliative coping which interferes with psychological health or social relationships.

Coping and Decreased Risk of Illness

Coping has been gaining center stage in the study of stress and illness mainly because of growing evidence that some forms of coping decrease morbidity and mortality by reducing vulnerability or by being highly conducive to the person's well-being. It will be instructive to examine briefly some of the major examples of research that demonstrate this.

Nuckolls, Cassel, and Kaplan (1972) obtained information on life stress and psychosocial coping assets from women early in their first pregnancies. The prognosis for pregnancy complications was made most accurately for women who had high life stress levels along with low psychosocial assets for coping with them. On the other hand, women with equally high life stress levels, but who were characterized by high assets, had only one third the complication rate of their peers with low psychosocial assets.

Other studies, while also not addressing the mechanism by which somatic illness might have been influenced, nevertheless demonstrate quite clearly the potent role of coping. One of the most interesting is a study of coping and mortality in an aged population who were moved from one institution to another (Aldrich and Mendkoff, 1963). In this type of dislocation it is customary to find very great increases in mortality rates (Parkes et al., 1969), and, indeed, this was observed by the study. However, when the ways these elderly people coped with the dislocation were taken into account, large differences in mortality rates were noted. Those who did most poorly were the manifestly psychotic, and those responding with depression were not far behind. The lowest mortality rates were found for persons taking the dislocation philosophically, and nearly as favorable rates were observed for persons who responded angrily; so it is not just a matter of controlled arousal. It is quite possible that the major mechanism underlying these relationships involved life-maintenance behavior, such as eating and caring for oneself in other ways, rather than centering on hormonal secretions associated with mobilization for coping with stress. While the mechanisms remain obscure, we see again the profound consequences that coping has for somatic health or illness, in this case operating on the most severe criterion of adaptation, namely, survival itself.

In another study of coping, Cohen and Lazarus (1973) assessed how patients were coping with the threat of surgery the night before their operation. The interviewer determined how much the patient knew about his or her illness, the nature of the surgery itself, and the extent to which information about this was sought or avoided. Patients were found to vary greatly from one extreme of avoidance to the other extreme of vigilant search for information. The score on this "dimension" of coping was then related to a variety of measures of outcome, including the number of days spent in the hospital, extent of negative psychological reactions, pain medication, and minor medical complications. The vigilant group showed a poorer picture of postoperative recovery than the avoiders, especially in regard to the outcome criteria of number of days in the hospital and the extent of minor complications.

If we ask why the avoiders should have the best postsurgical outcome, one possible speculation is that continual vigilant attention to signals of trouble and search for active ways of coping are likely to lead nowhere in the hospital setting, where passivity and conformity are highly valued, and in which literally nothing constructive can be done through efforts at active mastery. In a postsurgical hospital stay, as perhaps distinguished from other stressful contexts, avoidant modes of cognitive coping seem to be a more adaptive solution than vigilant ones. Here, too, the psychophysiological mechanisms involved are unknown. It is possible that the difference in recovery indexes for the two groups reflect more on features of the environmental or institutional setting, and on social behavior, than on hormonal or other tissue processes. For example, physicians may release patients who are anxious to leave and who seem comfortable faster than vigilant worriers. And since in the hospital where the research took place, pain medication was given more or less on demand, we would expect that avoiders would demand less medication than vigilant patients. In sum, assuming the replicability of this finding, a variety of biological, social, and psychological mechanisms could easily be operating.

Another illustration of the role of coping comes from recent research by Weisman and Worden (1975) with patients suffering from advanced cancer. These researchers were interested in differences in coping between two groups of patients, those who survived longer than expected on the basis of the severity of the disease, and those whose outcomes were unexpectedly poor. Using a survival quotient (SQ) based on observed survival in months minus expected survival, divided by the standard error of estimated survival for the particular cancer site, Weisman and Worden found that longevity depended heavily on coping. Survival was better among patients "who could maintain active and mutually responsive relationships, provided that the intensity of demands was not so extreme as to alienate people responsible for the patient's care" (1975, p. 74). On the other hand, survival was poorer for patients who showed long-standing alienation, deprivation, and depression, and maintained destructive relationships with others extending into the terminal stages of the illness. The latter group displayed these social and interpersonal difficulties in despondency, desire to die, contemplation of suicide, and inordinate complaints, all of which increased their isolation and feelings of self-defeat.

Here too, as in the Aldrich and Mendkoff (1963) study, the psychophysiological mechanisms underlying earlier or delayed death were not assessed. Moreover, behavioral and social processes may offer good prospects for understanding health outcome. That is, they may have to do with coping behavior that is damaging to health, such as failing to do what is necessary for survival as opposed to increasing or ameliorating the destructive effect of the hormonal secretions associated with stress emotions. Present evidence does not permit us to determine the mechanisms operating in these relationships between coping and adaptational outcomes, or even to be sure of the cause-and-effect link between them. Nevertheless, a considerable body of observation suggests strongly that coping processes are central factors in adaptational outcome.

Several studies seem to indicate that successful coping can affect levels of stress hormone production, which, if they were elevated chronically or repeatedly over a long time, might produce "diseases of adaptation." One example is a study by Wolff et al. (1964) of coping in parents facing the tragedy and stress of having a child die of leukemia. Through psychological assessment, the parents were rated on the extent to which they were well defended (usually through various forms of denial), and a high correlation was found between this rating and corticosteroid production. The most well-defended parents showed the lowest levels of adrenal cortical hormone production during the period prior to the death of the child. Although unfortunately this study confounded the measure of coping with evidence of distress, it does give support to the idea that successful coping can be inversely related to the somatic stress response. Later studies (Hofer et al., 1972) of this same group of parents have suggested that those who showed low corticosteroid levels before the child died were more disturbed six months later, raising the question about the costs of coping, and highlighting the problem of time relations in evaluating coping outcomes.

Weiner, Singer, and Reiser (1962) exposed hypertensives and normotensives to an emotional interview and found, paradoxically, that the hypertensives had lower blood pressure than the normotensives during the interview. Clinical assessment suggested that this was the result of a process the authors refer to as ''insulation.'' The hypertensives defended themselves against threatening interactions with the interviewer to which they were especially vulnerable by remaining ''consistently impersonal, distant, and wary.'' (See Sapira et al., 1971; Singer, 1974.)

We have defined three broad areas that we believe are both interesting and important for an understanding of the relationship between stress and adaptation: mediating cognitions, emotion, and coping. We have also made a number of distinctions and raised issues within each of these areas, namely, the importance of differing appraisals, coping that increases the risk of illness versus coping that decreases it, and the generality versus specificity issue, where particular attention was given to the distinction between positive and negative emotions. These distinctions and issues must be explored if we are to understand the ways in which psychological stress affects health, illness, morale, and social functioning.

It would be both simplistic and misleading, however, to consider each of these areas separately when in reality they are interdependent. For example, emotion is a response to cognitive appraisal; feelings of fear, guilt, excitement, or exhilaration each follow different cognitive appraisals. Appraisal and emotion, in turn, affect coping by influencing the choice of coping strategy and the effectiveness with which it is utilized. Finally, the feedback about the success of coping influences further appraisals, stimulating the entire process again. When we consider appraisals, emotions, and coping and their relationship to outcomes, we are in fact speaking of a complex and interrelated set of ongoing processes; these processes must be examined if we are to understand the ways in which psychological factors mediate the relationship between person and environment, and between stress and adaptational outcomes. Such psychodynamic research requires certain approaches in measurement and design, which are addressed in the next section.

RESEARCH DESIGN AND MEASUREMENT

Several important implications for research design and measurement emerge clearly from the theoretical issues raised above concerning the roles of mediating cognitions, different kinds of emotion, and coping processes in adaptation (see also Lazarus and Cohen, 1976; Lazarus, 1978). These implications stem especially from two features of the way we look at stress. First, we treat stress as a *relational concept* that refers to transactions between person and environment which are characterized by harm-loss, threat, or challenge. Second, to understand stress relationships and their adaptational consequences in people requires that we consider the role of two related mediational psychological processes, namely, cognitive appraisal and coping, which shape the flow of each transaction and the adaptational outcome. Below we shall discuss briefly some of the main methodological implications of our theoretical perspective and of the substantive issues we have raised.

Laboratory versus Naturalistic Field Study

Although laboratory studies are useful in evaluating the relationship between stressors and short-range physiological responses such as elevated blood pressure (Obrist et al., 1977; Lazarus, in press), for many reasons they fail to tell us enough of what we need to know about the psychological, social, and physiological mechanisms underlying longer-range disease processes and other adaptational outcomes. There are at least three serious limitations of laboratory research. First, adaptational outcome measures such as changes in physical health, social functioning, and morale usually take time to evolve; experiments with humans cannot put us in touch with this long developmental process, or with the concurrent social and psychological processes affecting it. Second, it is not possible ethically or practically to produce in the laboratory levels of stress and disease comparable to those brought about by serious life crises and chronic, everyday stress-inducing hassles (see also Lazarus and Cohen, 1976). Nor is the laboratory well suited to create the rich variety of positive and distressing emotions we spoke about earlier that are so much a part of normal living, or to permit the person to utilize the full range and pattern of coping normally available in real life stress. Third, we cannot discover in the laboratory the ordinary sources of stress, and the coping patterns used by different kinds of persons and groups in their natural settings. If we depended only on the laboratory, we would remain ignorant of stress and coping processes throughout the course of human life. For these reasons, laboratory research on the substantive issues we have raised must be supplemented by field research centered on stress-related events and processes occurring naturally.

Levels of Analysis

In the past, stress research has been characterized either by restriction to a single level of analysis, say, physiological stress, social stress, or psychological stress, or by some form of reductionism resulting in confusion when processes at one level were taken automatically to stand for those at another. The three levels of stress analysis are to a degree independent, and they refer to different conditions, concepts, and mechanisms. If one level led automatically to another, we would not need coordinated interdisciplinary research, but could reduce stress to the lowest usable common denominator of explanation, the cellular or biochemical level, or perhaps ultimately the molecular or atomic level. However, the links between these levels are largely unexplored, tenuous, and complex, primarily because they have not been studied within the same research design.

Consider, for example, a form of social stress in which a social unit, say, the family, is undergoing disruption in functioning, as in divorce between the parents. Because of the divergent characteristics of individual members, this social stress may be psychologically and physiologically stressful for one member of the family but benign or stress-reducing for another. Therefore, one cannot take stress at the social level to stand automatically for stress at the individual psychological or tissue level. Or, to take another example, Mason and his colleagues (Mason et al., 1976), whose work we cited earlier, note that psychological stress is often confounded with physiological stress, and the effects attributed to the latter when in reality they are determined, at least in part, by the former. Only by measuring stress inputs and reactions at both levels within the same research framework can this source of confusion in understanding be eliminated.

The methodological implication of this, and of the fact that each level plays a crucial part in understanding the relationship of stress to adaptational outcome, is that the most thorough research must be designed to assess all three *concurrently* (Luborsky, Docherty, and Penick, 1973). Only then will the interrelationships be properly evaluated and understood; and research designs are needed to make such concurrent study possible. We believe that most of the important sources of stress in human life arise from the social context of living, from social arrangements based on shared meanings; in effect, they involve troubled interpersonal relationships. Social demands have their effects on any individual via cognitive appraisal and coping processes which determine how that individual views, reacts to, and handles them. In turn, outcomes are first noted through changes in psychological or social functioning, or through the operation of diverse physiological mechanisms in short-range physiological changes, and only later in long-range disease processes. These physiological effects can wax and wane as the social context changes, as psychological coping processes alter the troubled person–environment relationship, and as physiological mechanisms promote or hinder the development of more permanent disease processes.

Process and Flux

The essence of adaptation is change. That is, when confronted with a dangerous or demanding situation, a person copes, thus altering the stressful person–environment relationship and, in turn, the physiological disturbance or disease process. Person–environment relationships are always in flux: emotions are rising and falling and changing in quality, with attendant changes in tissue reactions. The way a person appraises what is happening is also constantly changing with changing circumstances and with his or her own cognitive and behavioral activity. Effective coping also requires that a person be attuned to the specific demands of the situation. The successfully adapted person does not do the same thing, or react in the same way, from one stressful encounter to another, though there are undoubtedly some things about his or her tendency to react that are comparatively stable. Research into the relationships between stress and adaptational outcomes must be designed to allow us to determine flux and change as well as stability. What is called for is a new type of assessment technology, namely, the measurement of process in contrast to most current practices of sampling traits or environmental conditions on a single occasion and assuming the data will be stable over time or across occasions.

Process measurement, which implies flux or change, can be illustrated briefly both for person traits and for environmental characteristics. A number of personality assessment scales are available to measure certain coping traits or styles. These scales emphasize how a person might usually respond psychologically, say, by vigilantly seeking information so as to permit order and control over events, or by avoiding or denying information that might be threatening. However, prediction from such trait measures as to how the person actually will cope with specific threat situations has been very poor (cf. Cohen and Lazarus, 1973). One can, alternatively, assess how an individual copes with diverse specific stress-ful encounters, in effect measuring the coping *process* as it occurs rather than seeking to measure a trait. In such a case we are in a position to determine how much coping changes with the nature of the encounter, and how stable any given coping pattern is for that individual.

Too often, particularly in laboratory or "trait" research, results observed are assumed to be typical of all such relationships. To take an obvious example, the pattern of physiological responses to a stressful circumstance among a group of college students should not necessarily be expected among a group of retired or ill persons. Similarly, patterns of appraisal, coping, and emotional response probably vary not only in different contexts, but also in different age, sex, and cultural subgroups. This concern with the issue of who is being studied is particularly critical in a research area as complex as the study of stress.

Similarly, we can measure the social network or support systems generally available to an individual. The usual assumption is that this will be a stable feature of the individual's life setting (a structural property), which may or may not be true. In fact, the social environment can change greatly from one period of life to another, or as a function of illness, divorce, or other forms of crisis. Even adaptational outcomes are change-able things, with morale, social functioning, and illness patterns differing from time to time, or from occasion to occasion. In short, to understand, at any or all levels of analysis, the mechanisms that are involved in adaptational outcomes such as health and illness, it is just as important to examine flux and change as it is to study stable structures.

The advantageous consequence of a process orientation is nicely illus-trated in a study of changes in blood pressure associated with job loss done by Kasl, Gore, and Cobb (1975). In this often-cited study, a group of men who were being laid off because of the closing of their factory were studied longitudinally and prospectively. The study began in the months preceding the closing of the factories, when the men were an-ticipating the loss of their jobs, and continued with repeated follow-ups at regular intervals up to two years later. A control group of men with stable employment showed no consistent changes in blood pressure over the same time. The men were studied with a variety of social-psychological and physiological measures, including blood pressure.

The findings of the study were that the laid-off men experienced a significant drop in diastolic blood pressure from the anticipatory phase to a period of 8 to 12 months after job loss. The magnitude of the change in diastolic blood pressure was correlated with subjective measures of disturbance and personality attributes such as ego resiliency, rather than with an objective measure of the actual length of unemployment. Kasl et al. did not include in their analysis men who failed to find work within 12 months after losing their jobs; it would be interesting to know what their blood pressure status was in comparison to those who did find jobs.

At any rate, we think this study serves as an excellent example of the kind of understanding which can be achieved when subjects are followed in such a way that longer-range consequences of a stressful life event can be understood in terms of the mechanisms which bring them about.

As noted earlier in this chapter, the mechanisms leading from a disturbed physiological state to enduring changes in function are unknown. Intuitively, highly stable or repetitive patterns of emotions, appraisals, or coping, whether related to a chronic stressful situation or simply characteristic of the person in many situations, might demonstrate such mechanisms as well as the sought-after connection between acute and chronic changes. This determination requires repeated and concurrent measurement of all these relevant variables across a period of time sufficient for such chronic changes to become manifest, or for changes such as exacerbation or remission to occur in those who already have disease.

Intraindividual Emphasis in Research Designs

All that we have said above concerning research design and measurement culminates in one major design contrast, namely, between within-individual and across-individual comparison (see also Lazarus and Cohen, 1976; Lazarus, 1978; Broverman, 1962; and Marceil, 1977). Most research, including epidemiological studies of social conditions or personality and morbidity or mortality as health outcomes, focuses on a single antecedent factor, measured once as a stable structure or trait, and some outcome factor, say, risk of illness or death, expressed in probability terms. This involves large samples and comparisons made strictly *across individuals*. Processes as they occur across occasions or time, that is, *within individuals*, cannot be examined in this type of research, since only one assessment of the antecedent, causal factor is made. Nor can the mechanisms, social, psychological, or physiological, be identified in this style of research, since what is happening when any individual gets sick, worsens, or improves cannot be known. What is needed to study such mechanisms, and to relate the divergent levels of analysis as we have proposed, is concurrent examination of social, psychological, and physiological processes in the same individuals across encounters or situations, and over time. Only in that way can we show how short-range physiological changes associated with stress, coping, and emotion can eventuate into disease or other negative adaptational outcomes in susceptible individuals.

SUMMARY

Although 20 years ago the field of psychosomatic medicine was rapidly becoming an obscure scientific discipline, recently it has been enjoying a resurgence of theoretical interest and research activity. Basic to this revival is the realization that the link between stress phenomena and disease needs to be examined in terms of three distinct but interrelated levels of analysis: social, psychological, and physiological. Consideration of all three levels is critical, since not only does each discipline have a unique contribution to make, but processes that are beneficial at one level can turn out to be detrimental at others, as when heavy drinking helps maintain psychological morale while severely impairing physical health and social functioning. Within this multidisciplinary paradigm, psychological stress theory emphasizes how mediating cognitions, emotions, and coping processes affect the adaptational outcomes of social functioning, psychological morale, and physical health.

This chapter has viewed stress, not as a result of an environmental stressor, but as dependent on whether a person *appraises* a situation as being benign, neutral, or stressful. Stressful appraisal takes three forms: harm-loss, threat, and challenge. We would expect that people who appraise a particular transaction with the environment as challenging would have higher morale, be less emotionally overwhelmed, and function better under pressure than those who construe the same transaction as threatening. From this standpoint, psychological stress is not, as is often argued, a demanding environmental condition (a stressor) or the body's generalized mobilization or defensive reaction to it (Selye, 1956, 1976; Holmes and Masuda, 1974), though it may have its origins in environmental events and produce bodily changes; rather, it depends on how a transaction is appraised or understood by the person.

Although currently in vogue, the generalist position, which admits of no necessary specific connection either between the stressor and the somatic response, or between the mediating cognitive or psychodynamic processes and that response, has been seriously challenged in recent years. Foremost among the challenges is the research of Lacey (1967), who has demonstrated specific somatic patterns of autonomic end-organ reactions to different types of person–environment relationships, and that of Mason (1975; Mason et al., 1976), who has found divergent patterns of hormonal response under several physical stressors. Further problems for the generalist position stem from the paucity of research correlating concurrent reactions during emotional arousal across *different* physiological response systems (e.g., adrenal medullary, adrenal cortical, autonomic, and other neuro-humoral systems) and the failure of existing research to find more than very modest correlations among different autonomic endorgan responses to the same stressor (Lazarus, Speisman, and Mordkoff, 1963). Thus, the concept of general arousal is left in considerable doubt.

A related question is how short-lived emotional episodes and stress reactions contribute to long-range disease processes. One possible link is through psychosocial factors, such as acculturation, socioeconomic status, and bereavement, which have been shown to affect rates of disease and overall mortality. Syme (1977b) has proposed that these risk factors create a general susceptibility to all disease—a generalist stance. However, this concept of general susceptibility leaves unexplained the *underlying mechanisms* through which psychosocial factors affect somatic health. A likely possibility is that stable psychological patterns of appraisal, emotion, and coping produce distinctive emotional and adaptational outcomes. The specifist position, favored in this chapter, is centered on such underlying mechanisms of given adaptational outcomes.

It is noteworthy that stress and adaptational outcomes are always mediated through coping processes that can either increase or decrease the risk of disease, low morale, and poor social functioning. Increases in the risk of disease occur through (1) direct tissue damage, (2) the mobilization required by coping, as is implied in Type A behavior, and (3) interference with adaptational behaviors, as when the refusal to face the danger of a suspicious breast lump delays or prevents medical treatment. On the other hand, evidence of decreases in risk of disease due to coping is also quite common, and appears in such diverse forms as the number of pregnancy complications, mortality rates in dislocated aged, length of postsurgical recovery, survival rates of patients suffering from advanced cancer, levels of stress hormone secretion, and hypertension. Coping is a powerful and complex mediating factor affecting disease outcome.

Cognitive appraisal, emotions, and coping are interdependent processes. For example, cognitive appraisal influences the quality and intensity of the emotional response, while appraisal and emotion together influence the choice of coping strategy and its effectiveness. Coming full circle, feedback about the success of coping can mold subsequent cognitive appraisals.

The study of these complex interrelationships has certain methodological implications, an important one being whether research into the relationship of stress to adaptational outcomes is best done in the laboratory or in a naturalistic field setting. Although the laboratory setting is sometimes useful in evaluating the relationship between stressors and short-range physiological response, it is also limited in a number of critical areas. First, monitoring long-term changes in physical health, morale, and social functioning is not feasible in the laboratory. Second, practical and ethical considerations make it impossible to produce in the laboratory the levels and diversity of stress and coping encountered in everyday life. Third, the laboratory is not suited to describing the ordinary sources of stress encountered in everyday life, or to the description of individual, group, and cultural differences in coping patterns found in naturalistic settings. For these reasons laboratory research must be supplemented by field studies in which social, psychological, and physiological patterns are examined concurrently.

Since appraisals, emotions, and coping patterns ebb and flow in a person's changing commerce with the environment, a new type of assessment is needed that measures process and variation within individuals and across situations, as well as structure and stability. For example, by assessing how a person copes in diverse transactions, it becomes possible to evaluate the sensitivity of an individual's coping pattern to changes in the environment, and its stability across such transactions. Only by doing longitudinal assessments of patterns of appraisals, emotions, and coping, at three levels of analysis concurrently, shall we be able to unravel the complex relationships involved in human adaptation to the stress of life.

References

Aldrich, C. K., and Mendkoff, E. Relocation of the aged and disabled: A mortality study. *Journal of the American Geriatric Society 11:* 185–194, 1963.

Alexander, F. G., and Selesnick, S. T. *The History of Psychiatry.* New York: Harper & Row, 1966.

Ax, A. F. The physiological differentiation between fear and anger in humans. *Psychosomatic Medicine 15:* 433–442, 1953.

Bolles, R. C. Cognition and motivation: Some historical trends. In Weiner, B. (ed.), *Cognitive Views of Human Motivation*. New York: Academic Press, 1974, pp. 1–20.

Bradburn, N. M., and Caplowitz, D. *Reports on Happiness: A Pilot Study of Behavior Related to Mental Health*. Chicago: Aldine, 1965.

Broverman, D. M. Normative and ipsative measurement in psychology. *Psychological Review 69:* 295–305, 1962.

Cassel, J. The contribution of the social environment to host resistance. *American Journal of Epidemiology 104:* 107–123, 1976.

Cohen, F., and Lazarus, R. S. Active coping processes, coping dispositions, and recovery from surgery. *Psychosomatic Medicine 35:* 375–389, 1973.

Cousins, N. Anatomy of an illness (as perceived by the patient). *New England Journal of Medicine 295:* 1458–1463, 1976.

Dember, W. N. Motivation and the cognitive revolution. *American Psychologist 29:* 161–168, 1974.

Duffy, E. *Activation and Behavior*. New York: Wiley, 1962.

Ellis, A. *Reason and Emotion in Psychotherapy*. New York: Lyle Stuart, 1962.

Elmadjian, F., Hope, J. M., and Lamson, E. T. Excretion of epinephrine and norepinephrine udner stress. *Recent Progress in Hormone Research 14:* 513–553, 1958.

Engel, B. T. Stimulus-response and individual response specificity. *Archives of General Psychiatry 2:* 305–313, 1960.

Engel, G. L. Memorial lecture: The psychosomatic approach to individual susceptibility to disease. *Gastroenterology 67:* 1085–1093, 1074.

Engel, G. L. The need for a new medical model: A challenge for biomedicine. *Science 196:* 129–136, 1977.

Engel, B. T., and Bickford, A. F. Response specificity. *Archives of General Psychiatry 3:* 478–489, 1961.

Fenichel, O. *The Psychoanalytic Theory of Neurosis*. New York: W. W. Norton, 1945.

Frankenhaeuser, M. The role of peripheral catecholamines in adaptation to understimulation and overstimulation. In Serban, G. (ed.), *Psychopathology of Human Adaptation*. New York: Plenum, 1976, pp. 173–191.

Funkenstein, D. H., King, S. H., and Drolette, M. E. *Mastery of Stress*. Cambridge: Harvard University Press, 1956.

Glass, D. C. *Behavior Patterns, Stress and Coronary Disease* (Complex Human Behavior Series). New York: Halstead Press (Wiley), 1977.

Goldfried, M., and Goldfried, A. P. Cognitive change methods. In Kanfer, F. H., and Goldstein, A. P. (eds.), *Helping People Change*. New York: Pergamon, 1975, pp. 89–116.

Graham, D. T. Some research on psychophysiologic specificity and its relation to psychosomatic disease. In Roessler, R., and Greenfield, N. S. (eds.), *Physiological Correlates of Psychological Disorder*. Madison, Wisconsin: University of Wisconsin Press, 1962, pp. 221–238.

Hackett, T. P., and Cassem, H. Psychological management of the myocardial infarction patient. *Journal of Human Stress 1:* 25–38, 1975.

Herd, J. A. Cardiovascular correlates of psychological stress. Paper presented at conference on The Crisis in Stress Research: A Critical Reappraisal of the Role of Stress in Hypertension, Gastrointestinal Illness, Female Reproductive Dysfunction. Boston University School of Medicine, Department of Psychosomatic Medicine, Boston, October 20–22, 1977.

Hofer, M. A., Wolff, C. T., Freidman, S. B., and Mason, J. W. A psychoendocrine study of bereavement. Parts I and II. *Psychosomatic Medicine 34:* 481–504, 1972.

Holmes, T. M., and Masuda, M. Life change and illness susceptibility. In Dohrenwend, B. S., and Dohrenwend, B. P. (eds.), *Stressful Life Events.* New York: Wiley, 1974, pp. 45–86.

Kanner, A. D., Kafry, D., and Pines, A. Conspicuous in its absence: The lack of positive conditions as a source of stress. Unpublished manuscript, 1977.

Kasl, S. V., Gore, S., and Cobb, S. The experience of losing a job: Reported changes in health, symptoms and illness behavior. *Psychosomatic Medicine 37:* 106–122, 1975.

Katz, J. L., Weiner, H., Gallagher, T. G., and Hellman, L. Stress, distress, and ego defenses. *Archives of General Psychiatry 23:* 131–142, 1970.

Kemper, T. *A Social Interaction Theory of Emotions.* New York: Wiley, 1978.

Lacey, J. I. Somatic response patterning and stress: Some revisions of activation theory. In Appley, M. H., and Trumbull, R. (eds.), *Psychological Stress.* New York: Appleton-Century-Crofts, 1967, pp. 14–37.

Lazarus, R. S. *Psychological Stress and the Coping Process.* New York: McGraw-Hill, 1966.

Lazarus, R. S. Emotions and adaptation: Conceptual and empirical relations. In Arnold, W. J. (ed.), *Nebraska Symposium on Motivation.* Lincoln: University of Nebraska Press, 1968, pp. 175–265.

Lazarus, R. S. Psychological stress and coping in adaptation and illness. In Lipowski, Z. J., Lipsitt, D. R., and Whybrow, P. C. (eds.), *Psychosomatic Medicine: Current Trends and Clinical Applications.* New York: Oxford University Press, 1977, pp. 14–26.

Lazarus, R. S. A strategy for research on psychological and social factors in hypertension. *Journal of Human Stress 4:* 35–40, 1978.

Lazarus, R. S., and Averill, J. R. Emotion and cognition: With special reference to anxiety. In Spielberger, C. D. (ed.), *Anxiety: Current Trends in Theory and Research,* Vol. II. New York: Academic Press, 1972, pp. 242–283.

Lazarus, R. S., Averill, J. R., and Opton, E. M., Jr. Toward a cognitive theory of emotion. In Arnold, M. (ed.), *Feelings and Emotion.* New York: Academic Press, 1970, pp. 207–232.

Lazarus, R. S., and Cohen, J. B. Theory and method in the study of stress and coping in aging individuals. Paper presented at the Fifth WHO Conference on Society, Stress and Disease: Aging and Old Age, Stockholm, Sweden, June 14–19, 1976.

Lazarus, R. S., and Launier, R. Stress-related transactions between person and environment. In Pervin, L. A., and Lewis, M. (eds.), *Perspectives in Interactional Psychology,* New York: Plenum, 1978.

Lazarus, R. S., Speisman, J. C., and Mordkoff, A. M. The relationship between autonomic indicators of psychological stress: Heart rate and skin conductance. *Psychosomatic Medicine 25:* 19–30, 1963.

Levi, L., and Kagan, A. Adaptation of the psychological environment to man's abilities and needs. In Levi, L. (ed.), *Society, Stress and Disease,* Vol. I. London: Oxford University Press, 1971, pp. 395–404.

Lindsley, D. B. Emotions. In Stevens, S. S. (ed.), *Handbook of Experimental Psychology*. New York: Wiley, 1951, pp. 473–516.

Lipowski, Z. J. Psychosomatic medicine in the seventies: An overview. *American Journal of Psychiatry 134:* 233–244, 1977.

Luborsky, L., Docherty, J. P., and Penick, S. Onset conditions for psychosomatic symptoms: A comparative review of immediate observation with retrospective research. *Psychosomatic Medicine 35:* 187–204, 1973.

Malmo, R. B. Activation: A neuropsychological dimension. *Psychological Review 66:* 367–386, 1959.

Mandler, G. *Mind and Emotion.* New York: Wiley, 1975.

Marceil, J. C. Implicit dimensions of idiography and nomothesis: A reformulation. *American Psychologist 32:* 1046–1055, 1977.

Marmot, M. G., and Syme, S. L. Acculturation and coronary heart disease in Japanese Americans. *American Journal of Epidemiology 104:* 225–247, 1976.

Mason, J. W. Emotion as reflected in patterns of endocrine regulation. In Levi, L. (ed.), *Emotions: Their Parameters and Measurement.* New York: Raven Press, 1975, pp. 143–181.

Mason, J. W., Maher, J. T., Hartley, L. H., Mougey, E., Perlow, M. J., and Jones, L. G. Selectivity of corticosteroid and catecholamine response to various natural stimuli. In Serban, G. (ed.), *Psychopathology of Human Adaptation.* New York: Plenum, 1976, pp. 147–171.

Meichenbaum, D. *Cognitive-Behavior Modification.* New York: Plenum, 1977.

Nuckolls, K. B., Cassel, J., and Kaplan, B. H. Psychosocial assets, life crisis, and the prognosis of pregnancy. *American Journal of Epidemiology 95:* 431–441, 1972.

Obrist, P. A., Langer, A. W., Grignolo, A., Stutterer, J. R., Light, K. C., and McCubbin, J. A. Blood pressure control mechanisms and stress: Implications for the etiology of hypertension. Paper read at Hahnemann College's Fifth International Symposium on Hypertension, San Juan, Puerto Rico, January 9–12, 1977.

Orden, S. R., and Bradburn, N. Dimensions of marriage happiness. *American Journal of Sociology 73:* 715–731, 1968.

Ostfeld, A. M. The interaction of biological and social variables in cardiovascular disease. *Milbank Memorial Fund Quarterly 45:* 13–18, 1967.

Parkes, C. M., Benjamin, B., and Fitzgerald, R. G. Broken heart: A statistical study of increased mortality among widowers. *British Medical Journal 11:* 740–743, 1969.

Rosenman, R. H., Brand, R. J., Sholtz, R. I., and Friedman, M. Multivariate prediction of coronary heart disease during 8.5 year follow-up in the Western Collaborative Group Study. *American Journal of Cardiology 37:* 903–910, 1976.

Sapira, J. D., Scheib, E. T., Moriarty, R., and Shapiro, A. P. Differences in perception between hypertensive and normotensive populations. *Psychosomatic Medicine 33:* 239–250, 1971.

Schachter, J. Pain, fear, and anger in hypertensives and normotensives. *Psychosomatic Medicine 19:* 17–29, 1957.

Schachter, S. The interaction of cognitive and physiological determinants of emotional state. In Spielberger, C. D. (ed.), *Anxiety and Behavior.* New York: Academic Press, 1966, pp. 193–224.

Schachter, S., and Singer, J. E. Cognitive, social and physiological determinants of emotional state. *Psychological Review 69:* 379–399, 1962.

Schwartz, G. E., and Weiss, S. M. What is behavioral medicine? *Psychosomatic Medicine 39:* 377–381, 1977.

Selye, H. *Stress without Distress.* Philadelphia: J. B. Lippincott, 1974.

Selye, H. *The Stress of Life.* New York: McGraw-Hill, 1956. Revised ed., 1976.

Shapiro, D., Tursky, B., and Schwartz, G. E. Differentiation of heart rate and blood pressure in man by operant conditioning. *Psychosomatic Medicine 32:* 417–423, 1970.

Singer, M. T. Presidential Address—Engagement-involvement: A central phenomenon in psychophysiological research. *Psychosomatic Medicine 36:* 1–17, 1974.

Stahl, S. M., Grim, C. E., Donald, S., and Neikirk, H. J. A model for the social sciences and medicine: The case for hypertension. *Social Science and Medicine 9:* 31–38, 1975.

Syme, S. L. Psychosocial determinants of hypertension. Paper presented at Hahnemann College's Fifth International Symposium on Hypertension, San Juan, Puerto Rico, January 9–12, 1977 (a).

Syme, S. L. Epidemiologic research in hypertension: A critical appraisal. Paper presented at the Conference on the Crisis in Stress Research, Boston University School of Medicine, Boston, Massachusetts, October 20–21, 1977 (b).

Syme, S. L., and Berkman, L. F. Social class, susceptibility and sickness. *American Journal of Epidemiology 104:* 1–8, 1976.

Von Kugelgen, E. Psychological determinants of the delay in decision to seek aid in cases of myocardial infarction. Unpublished doctoral dissertation, University of California, Berkeley, 1975.

Weiner, H. *Psychobiology and Human Disease.* New York: Elsevier, 1977.

Weiner, H., Singer, M. T., and Reiser, M. F. Cardiovascular responses and their psychological correlates. I. A study in healthy young adults and patients with peptic ulcer and hypertension. *Psychosomatic Medicine 24:* 477–498, 1962.

Weisman, A. D., and Worden, J. W. Psychosocial analysis of cancer deaths. *Omega: Journal of Death and Dying 6:* 61–75, 1975.

Wolff, C. T., Friedman, S. B., Hofer, M. A., and Mason, J. W. Relationship between psychological defenses and mean urinary 17-hydroxycorticosteroid excretion rates: I. A predictive study of parents of fatally ill children. *Psychosomatic Medicine 26:* 576–591, 1964.

6

Psychosocially-Induced Stress and Disease—Problems, Research Strategies, and Results

Lennart Levi and Aubrey Kagan

Laboratory for Clinical Stress Research/WHO, Psychosocial Center, Karolinska institutet, Fack, S-10401 Stockholm, Sweden

1. PSYCHOSOCIAL FACTORS AND HEALTH

The evidence that environmental physical stimuli may cause disease—in the sense that exposure to them or avoidance or manipulation of them, increases, decreases, or removes the chance of becoming ill, or reverses ill health when it occurs—is established for a large number of factors and diseases.

The role of extrinsic, *psychosocial* stimuli is not so clear. It should be noted, however, that the participants of the 27th World Health Assembly Technical Discussions of May 16, 1974 called attention to "three agreed bases" from which to consider the role of psychosocial factors: (a) the importance of all aspects of the human environment, including the psychosocial and socioeconomic factors, for human health and man's well-being; (b) the increasing awareness that psychosocial factors can precipi-

The studies reported in this paper have been supported by, inter alia, the Swedish Medical Research Council, the Swedish Work Environment Fund, the Swedish Delegation for Applied Medical Defence Research, the Swedish Delegation for Social Research, the Bank of Sweden Tercentenary Fund and the Folksam Insurance Group, Stockholm.

tate or counteract physical and mental ill health, profoundly modify the outcome of health action, and influence the quality of human life; (c) the resulting need for a holistic and ecological approach in social and health action and for a corresponding reorientation of medical and paramedical education and training (9).

Briefly, then, the major assumptions in the general area of research on psychosocial factors and health are that such factors can:

Precipitate or counteract ill health,
Influence well-being, and
Modify the provision, acceptance, use, and outcome of health action.

Although these assumptions may be well supported in *general* terms, much research is needed to demonstrate which psychosocial factors are pathogenic, to whom, how much, and under which circumstances.

2. RESEARCH GOALS

It follows that our major research goals must be to *identify,* and wherever possible or necessary, find ways therapeutically and/or preventively, to modify:

Structures and processes in the total *environment* that can elicit pathogenic psychosocial stimuli (e.g., rapid social change, disruption of cultural patterns), i.e., *high-risk situations:*
Individual determinants of the propensity of human beings to react to such stimuli (e.g., personality, customs, attitudes), i.e., *high-risk groups;*
Psychosocially induced physiological, psychological, and social *mechanisms* leading to disease (e.g., neuroendocrine dysfunction, anxiety, self-destructive behavior), i.e., *high-risk reactions;*
Psychosocially-induced mental and physical *disease;* and decrease in well-being (quality of life).

To this end, attention must be focused on *characteristics* of, and *discrepancies* between, man's abilities, needs, and expectations on the one hand, and environmental demands and opportunities and the perceived outcome on the other. We are further interested in problems created by *conflicts* between various human roles, e.g., at work and outside work.

3. CHOICE OF VARIABLES AND PROBLEM AREAS

Discrepancies—subjective, objective, or both—occur, person–environment fit becomes unsatisfactory, and man reacts.

Some of the potentially pathogenic reactions are primarily of a *subjective,* emotional nature. Man may experience anxiety, depression, frustration, or alienation. Feelings such as these, though considered trivial in some quarters, may be clearly detrimental to health and well-being, and very effectively make our lives miserable.

Some potentially pathogenic reactions are best described in *behavioral* terms. Examples of potentially pathogenic or even lethal behavior are: abuse of drugs, alcohol, or tobacco; taking unnecessary risks in traffic or at work; and destructive behavior such as criminality or suicide.

On a third level, descriptions can be made in *physiological* terms. It is well known that a variety of environmental psychosocial stimuli, e.g., "life change," (cf. Rahe, 1972 [55]), elicit specific physiological reactions and as well, a set of nonspecific ones. The latter—the "stress" reaction (Selye) is characterized inter alia by enhanced sympathoadrenomedullary activity and, concomitantly, by increased lipolysis, under certain circumstances contributing to a hyperlipoproteinemia. These and other phylogenetically old adaptational reactions, usually rather obsolete in today's psychosocial environment, prepare the organism for a physical activity that is infrequently performed. Simultaneously with this prolonged state of physical "preparedness," the "rate of wear and tear" in the organism is hypothesized to increase, as are eventually morbidity and mortality.

Accordingly, our studies focus on various situations suspected to represent high risk for various groups believed to be particularly vulnerable, and on high-risk reactions of the three types described above.

High-risk situations that we are currently studying include, for example, (a) abrupt changes in work which conflict with the circadian rhythm of various bodily functions, (b) simultaneous exposure to demanding full-time work and care of family and children, (c) abrupt reduction in environmental demands and the quality of life, in connection with periretirement, and (d) occurrence of breast cancer.

High-risk groups comprise, for example, people who are exposed to shift-work and whose circadian rhythms are difficult to adapt; or people who are exposed to changes that demand adaptation but are unable to cope.

High-risk reactions are studied partly in real-life settings and partly in laboratory experiments. These studies are concerned with adrenocortical, adrenomedullary, and thyroid activity; immunological reactions; and feelings and behavior.

4. RESEARCH STRATEGIES AND TACTICS

Our research strategies combine:

Key hypothesis-testing (basic research)
Evaluation of health actions (applied research), and
Collection of quantified information on the interrelationships of various elements of the man–environment ecosystem (data bank).

Accordingly, our research projects are usually carried out in three consecutive steps:

Problem identification with survey techniques;
Longitudinal, multidisciplinary intensive studies of the intersection of high-risk situations and high-risk groups as compared with controls;
Controlled intervention, including laboratory experiments as well as therapeutic and/or preventive interventions in real-life settings (e.g., natural experiments).

5. SOME RESULTS

5.1 General Approach

Laboratory disciplines of careful measurement and rigorous control (34) have been applied to human studies both in the laboratory under conditions approximating real life (16, 23, 25, 32) and under real-life conditions (21, 22, 35, 47, 51, 52) for periods of from a few hours to six months, in a manner that is scientifically productive and socially acceptable.
Studies have focused on the relationships between

Psychosocial stimuli and potentially pathogenic physiological mechanisms;

Psychosocial stimuli and morbidity;
Potentially pathogenic physiological mechanisms and morbidity;
. Psychobiological characteristics (''programming'') of the organism, and potentially pathogenic physiological mechanisms in its response to psychosocial stimuli;
Interacting variables and the potentially pathogenic chain of events mentioned above.

5.2 Specific Studies

These studies have resulted in the demonstration that:

1. Pleasant psychosocial stimuli as well as unpleasant ones produce increased adrenaline excretion (1)—a U-shaped adrenaline excretion curve representing the relation to the pleasant-unpleasant experience continuum (8, 24, 30, 31, 33).

2. Exposure to a wide variety of everyday psychological stimuli provokes a pronounced increase in adrenaline excretion, in a number of individuals equivalent to the rises seen in pheochromocytoma (27-29).

3. There is a significant, positive relationship under habitual conditions of life between life change score and adrenaline excretion (45).

4. Males react more strongly to visual psychosexual stimulation than females, subjectively and by adrenaline excretion (30).

5. Caffeine ingestion increases adrenaline excretion; this effect is modified by cognitive factors (10, 11, 26).

6. Alcohol ingestion leads to increased excretion of adrenal cortical and medullary hormones for as much as one week after the ingestion (2).

7. Psychosocial stimuli cause an increase in plasma triglycerides which is prevented by nicotinic acid treatment without affecting sympathoadrenomedullary reactions (4, 5).

8. Adrenaline excretion exhibits pronounced circadian variation even under conditions of constant activity and environment (13-15, 17, 18, 50). The adrenaline circadian pattern is much less dependent on external synchronization than the noradrenaline circadian pattern (12, 51).

9. Psychophysiological relationships between subjective reactions and catecholamine excretion are of two different types, one linked to circadian rhythm, the other to duration of exposure to environmental stressors (32).

10. Adaptation of the circadian rhythms of adrenaline excretion and of alertness to shift change of work from day to night, is still incomplete after three weeks (12, 47, 51). It is accompanied by increased plasma

levels of glucose, potassium, cholesterol, and uric acid and by a decrease in plasma gastrin (47, 52). Return of the latter to initial values after return to day work takes longer in subjects with higher neuroticism scores (52):

11. Exposure to a stressful three-day vigil causes a pronounced decrease in serum iron to levels below normal (25, 32).

12. In response to a stressful three-day vigil, blood lymphocyte interferon-producing capacity increases (43), whereas phagocytosis decreases after the first day, and then increases during the rest of the vigil and for several days afterward (42).

13. Exposure to a stressful three-day vigil results in a significant decrease in blood coagulation factors V, VIII, IX, and fibrinogen (44).

14. The same long-term exposure increases erythrocyte sedimentation rate and protein-bound iodine without a change in hematocrit level (25, 32).

15. Complete food deprivation for a 10-day period in subjects of normal weight (22) results in a marked decrease in lymphocyte synthesis of DNA in response to stimulation with pokeweed mitogen, and in complement factor C_3 in serum. Thyroid activity is influenced as reflected in decreases in T_3 and T_4 and an increase in reverse T_3. Adrenaline excretion increases markedly; cortisol exhibits a slight progressive increase, and human growth hormone increases transiently.

5.3 Holistic Approach

The psycho- and pharmacologico-socially-determined changes in biological function outlined above, have been linked (36) with other work showing associations between such changes and high risk for a variety of disease conditions on the one hand (19, 33, 36) and associations between such social determinants and disease conditions on the other (3, 6, 19, 27, 28, 39–41, 46, 48).

5.4 A Model of the "Psychosocial Stress Health System" and Its Uses

On the basis of this work and that of others, a model of the "psychosocial factors–pathogenic mechanisms–health" system has been proposed (see Figure 6.1), its elements have been defined (19), and knowledge of some interrelationships of these elements has been increased (21, 33, 36, 38, 51, 52).

Key hypotheses have been identified. A strategy for community re-

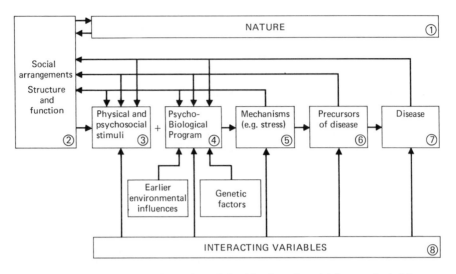

Figure 6.1. A theoretical model for the interrelationship of psychosocial factors, physical factors, and disease. The organism is exposed to nature (1). This exposure is often modified by social arrangements (2). The resulting influence might be mediated through ''higher nervous processes,'' in which case the stimuli are psychosocial (3). The organism's propensity to react depends on earlier environmental influences and genetic factors, conditioning its ''psychobiological program'' (4). Some of the reactions—psychological, behavioral, physiological—may be of significance as mechanisms (5) in apathogenic process. Some of the latter are nonspecific—''stress (Selye),'' while others are specific. Both may lead to precursors of disease (6) and to disease (7). This sequence of events can be promoted or counteracted by interacting variables (8). The entire process is dynamic with continuous feedback.

search has been put forth (7, 19, 20, 34, 37, 38, 49, 53) which combines in an efficient and effective way the simultaneous objectives of testing fundamental hypotheses, evaluating health actions of prime importance to the community studied, and obtaining additional data that may later be of value to investigators and administrators. This has been applied successfully to three-year-old children in day care centers (21). A program of work of this type has been outlined, and preliminary work has shown that the strategy can now be applied to problems of working mothers in heavy industry, of shift work, and of periretirement.

6. INTERNATIONAL PROGRAM

In 1973 the World Health Organization designated the laboratory a WHO Collaborating Centre for Research and Training in Psychosocial Factors and Health. Its functions were to:

Carry out research on health effects of psychosocial factors to provide a more comprehensive basis for health action.

Train scientists from various countries for this purpose and to facilitate transcultural studies.

Coordinate, document, and advise on research elsewhere.

Cooperate with other institutions in carrying out studies.

Carry out methodological developments.

Develop procedures for disseminating information on public health measures.

7. SUMMARY OF RECENT ACTIVITIES

1. WHO: Consultation and cooperation on WHO Programme on Psychosocial Factors and Health; proposal of a research program; development of an information system. Organization of a workshop with senior health administrators from developing and developed countries on "Psychosocial Factors and Health and Health Care."

2. Cooperation with IFIAS and WHO, and Human Ecological Society and WHO.

3. Cooperation with ILO in preparing a report on "Application of Ergonomics to Prevention of Mental Stress."

4. Nordic Council of Ministers—Occupational Mental Health: In a unanimous recommendation taken at its 22nd Session, the Nordic Council (joint organization of the parliaments of the five Nordic countries) recommended to the Nordic Council of Ministers (joint organization of the corresponding governments) initiation of a program on psychosocial aspects of the work environment with the eventual aim of reducing stress in working life. This program is currently being implemented, focusing on work environment and health in elementary school teachers. Our Laboratory/Centre has been entrusted with coordinating this program, in collaboration with researchers and labor unions in the Nordic countries.

5. International, Interdisciplinary Symposia: The fifth symposium in our series "Society, Stress and Disease" was held in Stockholm in June 1976; it focused on psychosocial and health problems occurring toward the end of the human life cycle. This symposium was jointly sponsored by the World Health Organization and the University of Uppsala, and was made possible through the generosity of the Trygg-Hansa Insurance Group. The proceedings of the entire series will be published by the Oxford University Press; those of the first three symposia of this series are

already available (27, 39, 54). The fourth volume is presently being edited and is focusing on "Society, Stress and Disease: Working Life." It will be in print in 1979.

6. Consultation and cooperation with organizations in other countries on problems related to psychosocial factors and health—Denmark, W. Germany, Mexico, Spain, Switzerland, USSR.

7. Sweden—Mental Health Protection and Promotion: The Swedish Parliament has commissioned the Swedish government to prepare an official report on problems, needs, and possibilities in the area of "mental health protection and promotion." This work is being carried out by a commission within the National Health and Welfare Board, with our Laboratory serving as the Secretariat. Its final report was made public in 1978 (National Health and Welfare Board, 1978) (56).

8. Research Projects: Our present studies focus on:

Day care nurseries, elementary schools, and child health.
Environment and health of working mothers.
Environment and health of shift-workers, with special attention to chronobiological aspects.
Periretirement, health, and well-being.
Psychosocially-induced stress reactions: endocrine and immunological aspects.
Stress and hypertension: psychosocial factors in etiology and pathogenesis.
Stress of breast cancer.

9. Fellowships—Long-term Visiting Scientists: one from Brazil, two from Costa Rica, one from Israel.

References

1. Andersson, B., Hovmöller, S., Karlsson, C.-G., and Svensson, S. Analysis of urinary catecholamines: An improved autoanalyzer fluorescence method. *Clin. Chim. Acta 51:* 13–28, 1974.
2. Brohult, J., Levi, L., and Reichard, H. Urinary excretion of adrenal cortical and medullary hormones in man during and after one single massive dose of ethanol, and their modification by chlormethiazole. *Acta Med. Scand. 188:* 5–13, 1970.
3. Carlestam, G., and Levi, L. Urban conglomerates as psychosocial human stressors. General aspects, Swedish trends, and psychological and medical implications. A contribution to the United Nations Conference on the Human Environment. Royal Ministries for Foreign Affairs and Agriculture, Stockholm, 1971, 74 pp.

4. Carlson, L. A., Levi, L., and Orö, L. Plasma lipids and urinary excretion of catecholamines in man during experimentally induced emotional stress, and their modification by nicotinic acid. *J. Clin. Invest. 47:* 1795–1805, 1968.

5. Carlson, L. A., Levi, L., and Orö, L. Stressor-induced changes in plasma lipids, and urinary excretion of catecholamines, and their modification by nicotinic acid. In Levi, L. (ed.), *Stress and Distress in Response to Psychosocial Stimuli.* Laboratory and real life studies on sympathoadrenomedullary and related reactions. *Acta Med. Scand.* Suppl. *528:* 91–105, 1972. Also published by Pergamon Press, Oxford (International series of monographs in experimental psychology, Vol. 17), 1972.

6. Cleary, P. J. Life events and disease: A review of methodology and findings. Report No. 37 from the Laboratory for Clinical Stress Research, Stockholm, November, 1974.

7. Eisenberg, L., and Levi, L. Possibilities for WHO-supported research in mental disorders at cellular, individual and social levels. Background paper for the advisory committee on medical research, World Health Organization, Geneva, 1974.

8. Euler, U. S. v, Gemzell, C. A., Levi, L., and Ström, G. Cortical and medullary adrenal activity in emotional stress. *Acta Endocrin., Kbh. 30:* 567–573, 1959.

9. Evang, K., Hassler, F., Levi, L., Myer, E. E., Sainsbury, P., and Weeratunge, C. E. S. Promoting health in the human environment. World Health Organization, Geneva, 1975, 69 pp.

10. Fröberg, J., Karlsson, C.-G., Levi, L., Linde, L., and Seeman, K. Test performance and subjective feelings as modified by caffeine-containing and caffeine-free coffee. In Heim, F., and Ammon, H. P. T. (eds.), *Caffein und andere Methylxanthine.* Stuttgart-New York: Schattauer-Verlag, 1969, pp. 15–20.

11. Fröberg, J., Carlson, L. A., Karlsson, C.-G., Levi, L., and Seeman, K. Effects of coffee on catecholamine excretion and plasma lipids. In Heim, F., and Ammon, H. P. T. (eds.), *Coffein und andere Methylxanthine.* Stuttgart-New York: Schattauer-Verlag, 1969, pp. 65–73.

12. Fröberg, J., Karlsson, C.-G., and Levi, L. Shift work: A study of catecholamine excretion, self-ratings, and attitudes. Paper presented at Second International Symposium on night and shift work, Slanchev Bryag, Bulgaria, September 1971. *Studia Laboris et Salutis* No. *11:* 10–20, 1972.

13. Fröberg, J., Karlsson, C.-G., Levi, L., and Lidberg, L. Circadian variations in performance, psychological ratings, catecholamine excretion and urine flow during prolonged sleep deprivation. In Colquhoun, W. P. (ed.), *Aspects of Human Efficiency. Diurnal Rhythm and Loss of Sleep.* London: English Universities Press, 1972, pp. 247–260.

14. Fröberg, J., Karlsson, C.-G., Levi, L., and Lidberg, L. Circadian variations in performance, psychological ratings, catecholamine excretion, and urine flow during prolonged sleep deprivation. *Int. J. Psychobiology 2:* 23–36, 1972.

15. Fröberg, J. E. Circadian rhythms in catecholamine excretion, performance and self-ratings. Report No. 36 from the Laboratory for Clinical Stress Research, Stockholm, April, 1974.

16. Fröberg, J., Karlsson, C.-G., Lennquist, S., Levi, L., Mathé, A. and Theorell, T. Renal and adrenal function: A comparison between responses to cold and to psychosocial stressors in human subjects. Report No. 40 from the Laboratory for Clinical Stress Research, Stockholm, November, 1974.

17. Fröberg, J., Karlsson, C.-G., Levi, L., and Lidberg, L. Circadian rhythms of catecholamine excretion, shooting range performance and self-ratings of fatigue during sleep deprivation. *Biological Psychology 2:* 175–188, 1975.
18. Fröberg, J., Karlsson, C.-G., Levi, L., and Lidberg, L. Psychobiological circadian rhythms during a 72-hour vigil. *Försvarsmedicin 11:* 192–201, 1975.
19. Kagan, A. R., and Levi, L. Health and environment—Psychosocial stimuli. A review. *Soc. Sci. Med. 8:* 225–241, 1974.
20. Kagan, A. R. A community research strategy applicable to psychosocial factors and lth. In Levi, L. (ed.), *Society, Stress and Disease: Working Life.* London, New York, Toronto: Oxford University Press, in press.
21. Kagan, A. R., Cederblad, M., Höök, B. and Levi, L. Evaluation of the Effect of Increasing the Number of Nurses on Health and Behavior of 3 Year Old Children in Day Care, Satisfaction of their Parents, and Health and Satisfaction of their Nurses. Report No. 89 from the Laboratory for Clinical Stress Research, Stockholm, 1978.
22. Kjellberg, J., Levi, L., Palmblad, J., Paulsson, L., Teorell, T., and Yensen, R. Acute energy deprivation in man—Methodological problems and possibilities. *Acta Med. Scand. 201:* 9–13, 1977.
23. Levi, L. A new stress tolerance test with simultaneous study of physiological and psychological variables. *Acta Endocrin., Kbh. 37:* 38–44, 1961.
24. Levi, L. The urinary output of adrenaline and noradrenaline during different experimentally induced pleasant and unpleasant emotional states. *Psychosom. Med. 27:* 80–85, 1965.
25. Levi, L. Physical and mental stress reactions during experimental conditions simulating combat. *Försvarsmedicin 2:* 3–8, 1966.
26. Levi, L. The effect of coffee on the function of the sympathoadrenomedullary system in man. *Acta Med. Scand. 181:* 431–438, 1967.
27. Levi, L. (ed.). *Society, Stress and Disease,* Vol. I: *The Psychosocial Environment and Psychosomatic Diseases.* London, New York, Toronto: Oxford University Press, 1971, 485 pp.
28. Levi, L., and Kagan, A. R. A synopsis of ecology and psychiatry—Some theoretical and psychosomatic considerations, review of some studies and discussion of preventive aspects. *Excerpta Medica International Congress Series* No. *274:* 369–379, 1971.
29. Levi, L. *Stress and Distress in Response to Psychosocial Stimuli.* Laboratory and real life studies on sympathoadrenomedullary and related reactions. *Acta Med. Scand.* Suppl. No. *528,* 1972. Also published as Vol. 17 in the International series of monographs in experimental psychology, Oxford: Pergamon Press, 1972, 166 pp.
30. Levi, L. Sympathoadrenomedullary activity, diuresis and emotional reactions during visual sexual stimulation in females and males. In Levi, L. (ed.), *Stress and Distress in Response to Psychosocial Stimuli.* Laboratory and real life studies on sympathoadrenomedullary and related reactions. *Acta Med. Scand.* Suppl. *528:* 74–90, 1972. Also published by Pergamon Press, Oxford (International series of monographs in experimental psychology, Vol. 17), 1972.
31. Levi, L. Sympathoadrenomedullary responses to "pleasant" and "unpleasant" psychosocial stimuli. In Levi, L. (ed.), *Stress and Distress in Response to Psychosocial Stimuli.* Laboratory and real life studies on sympathoadrenomedullary and related reactions. *Acta Med. Scand.* Suppl. *528:* 55–73, 1972. Also published by Pergamon

Press, Oxford (International series of monographs in experimental psychology, Vol. 17), 1972.

32. Levi, L. Psychological and physiological reactions to and psychomotor performance during prolonged and complex stressor exposure. In Levi, L. (ed.), *Stress and Distress in Response to Psychosocial Stimuli*. Laboratory and real life studies on sympathoadrenomedullary and related reactions. *Acta Med. Scand*. Suppl. *528:* 119–142, 1972. Also published by Pergamon Press, Oxford (International series of monographs in experimental psychology, Vol. 17), 1972.

33. Levi, L. Psychosocial stimuli, psychophysiological reactions, and disease. In Levi, L. (ed.), *Stress and Distress in Response to Psychosocial Stimuli*. Laboratory and real life studies on sympathoadrenomedullary and related reactions. *Acta Med. Scand*. Suppl. *528:* 11–27, 1972. Also published by Pergamon Press, Oxford (International series of monographs in experimental psychology, Vol. 17), 1972.

34. Levi, L. Methodological considerations in psychoendocrine research. In Levi, L. (ed.), *Stress and Distress in Response to Psychosocial Stimuli*. Laboratory and real life studies on sympathoadrenomedullary and related reactions. *Acta Med. Scand*. Suppl. *528:* 28–54, 1972. Also published by Pergamon Press, Oxford (International series of monographs in experimental psychology, Vol. 17), 1972.

35. Levi, L. Conditions of work and sympathoadrenomedullary activity: Experimental manipulations in a real life setting. In Levi, L. (ed.) *Stress and Distress in Response to Psychosocial Stimuli*. Laboratory and real life studies on sympathoadrenomedullary and related reactions. *Acta Med. Scand*. Suppl. *528:* 106–118, 1972. Also published by Pergamon Press, Oxford (International series of monographs in experimental psychology, Vol. 17), 1972.

36. Levi, L. General discussion. In Levi, L. (ed.), *Stress and Distress in Response to Psychosocial Stimuli*. Laboratory and real life studies on sympathoadrenomedullary and related reactions. *Acta Med. Scand*. Suppl. *528:* 143–149, 1972. Also published by Pergamon Press, Oxford (International series of monographs in experimental psychology, Vol. 17), 1972.

37. Levi, L. Humanökologie-Psychosomatische Gesichtspunkte und Forschungsstrategien. *Psychosomatische Medizin 5:* 92–107, 1973.

38. Levi, L., and Andersson, L. Population, environment and quality of life. A contribution to the United Nations World Population Conference. Royal Ministry for Foreign Affairs, Stockholm, 1974. Expanded version *Psychosocial Stress—Population, Environment and Quality of Life* published by Spectrum Publications, Holliswood, New York, 1975, 142 pp.

39. Levi, L. (ed.). *Society, Stress and Disease*, Vol. II: *Childhood and Adolescence*. London, New York, Toronto: Oxford University Press, 1975, 550 pp.

40. Levi, L. Parameters of emotion: An evolutionary and ecological approach. In Levi, L. (ed.), *Emotions: Their Parameters and Measurement*. New York: Raven Press, 1975, pp. 705–711.

41. Levi, L. (ed.). *Emotions: Their Parameters and Measurement*. New York: Raven Press, 1975, 800 pp.

42. Palmblad, J., Fröberg, J., Granström, M., Karlsson, C.-G., Levi, L., and Unger, P. Stress and the human granulocyte: Phagocytosis and turnover. Report No. 34 from the Laboratory for Clinical Stress Research, Stockholm, December, 1973.

43. Palmblad, J., Cantell, K., Strander, H., Fröberg, J., Karlsson, C.-G., and Levi, L.

Stressor exposure and human interferon production. Report No. 35 from the Laboratory for Clinical Stress Research, Stockholm, April, 1974.

44. Palmblad, J., Blombäck, M., Egberg, N., Fröberg, J., Karlsson, C.-G., and Levi, L. Experimentally-induced stress in man: Effects on blood coagulation and fibrinolysis. *J. Psychosom. Res. 21:* 87–92, 1977.

45. Theorell, T., Lind, E., Fröberg, J., Karlsson, C.-G., and Levi, L. A longitudinal study of 21 subjects with coronary heart disease—Life changes, catecholamine excretion and related biochemical reactions. *Psychosom. Med. 34:* 505–516, 1972.

46. Theorell, T., Lind, E., and Flodérus, B. The relationship of disturbing life-changes and emotions to the early development of myocardial infarction and other serious illnesses. *Int. Journal of Epidemiology 4:4:* 281–293, 1975.

47. Theorell, T., and Åkerstedt, T. Day and night work: Changes in cholesterol, uric acid, glucose and potassium in serum, and in circadian patterns of urinary catecholamine excretion—A longitudinal cross-over study of railroad repairmen. *Acta Med. Scand. 200:* 47–53, 1976.

48. Theorell, T. Selected illnesses and somatic factors in relation to two psychosocial stress indices—A prospective study on middle-aged construction building workers. *J. Psychosom. Res. 20:* 7–20, 1976.

49. WHO: Psychosocial factors and health. Report of the Director-General, EB57/22, World Health Organization, Geneva, November 1975.

50. Åkerstedt, T., and Fröberg, J. E. Work hours and 24h temporal patterns in sympathetic-adrenal medullary activity and self-rated activation. In Colquhoun, P., Folkard, S., Knauth, P., and Rutenfranz, J. (eds.), *Experimental Studies of Shiftwork.* Opladen: Westdeutscher Verlag, 1975.

51. Åkerstedt, T., Patkai, P., and Dahlgren, K. Field studies of shiftwork. II. Temporal patterns in psychophysiological activation in workers alternating between night and day work. *Ergonomics 20: 6:* 621–631, 1977.

52. Åkerstedt, T., and Torsvall, T. Exposure to night work: Serum gastrin reactions, psychosomatic complaints and personality variables. *J. Psychosom. Res. 20:* 479–484, 1976.

53. Kagan, A. R., and Levi, L. Psychosocial factors, health and well-being. Paper presented at stress symposium, Sociedad Mexicana de Psiquiatría Biológica, Mexico City, in press.

54. Levi, L. (ed.). *Society, Stress and Disease,* Vol. III: *Female and Male Roles and Relationships.* London: Oxford University Press, 1978, 300 pp.

55. Rahe, R. H. Subjects' recent life changes and their near-future illness susceptibility. *Adv. Psychosom. Med. 8:* 2–19, 1972.

56. National Health and Welfare Board: Psykisk hälsovård—forskning, social rapportering, dokumentation och information (Mental Health Protection and Promotion—Research, Monitoring, Documentation and Information). Liber: Stockholm, 1978.

7

ects of Learning on Physical Symptoms Produced by Psychological Stress

Neal E. Miller
The Rockefeller University

f Body

stress to produce physical symptoms and the rapy to relieve such symptoms are based on ictions of the brain. One of the important to maintain that regulated level of the internal meostasis, one of the essential conditions for the e brain regulates vital functions such as breathing, heart w, blood pressure, body temperature, energy balance, and electro. alance; controls the relase of adrenaline into the blood; and controls the function of that master gland, the pituitary, which in turn controls the hormones essential to growth, sex, and reproduction, and the ACTH and corticosteroids released during stress, which have multiple effects throughout the body. The brain is also the source of emotions and drives such as love, anger, fear, hunger, and thirst, and contains the mechanisms for perception, learning, voluntary responses, and the highest mental processes: thought, reasoning, and artistic and scientific creativity.

Because the brain is the supreme organ of integration in the body, all the foregoing functions are closely interrelated (Miller, 1964). Reasoning and foresight leading to a judgment of danger—"The boat carrying my child may sink in this storm''—can elicit an emotion of fear. In turn, strong fear can distract from thinking and affect the vital functions of digestion, breathing, heart rate, blood flow, and blood pressure. These interrelated functions of the brain, the mechanisms for which neuroscientists are beginning to understand better, are the basis for the effects of psychological stress on bodily health. And they are the basis for the development of an important new field—behavioral medicine.

This chapter will concentrate, but not exclusively, on the effects of on type of higher brain function, namely learning, on one type of stressf emotion, namely fear, or anxiety as it is called when its source is vagu defined or ubiquitous. Fear is an important type of psychological st that has been studied extensively in both the clinic and the laborat This chapter will describe experiments on how learning can affec intensity and duration of strong fear and hence the effects of that f the body. It will also describe experiments on how fear can affect ing.

Fear as a Learnable Drive

One of the reasons that fear is so important is that it can be rapi. as a response to a new stimulus situation. Another reason is learned, it can serve as a strong drive to motivate further le performance. These properties of fear may be illustrated experiment (Miller, 1948). When rats are dropped into the l of the apparatus illustrated in Figure 7.1 with the door bet compartments open, they explore aimlessly back and fortl two compartments. If they are given a few trials during dropped into the left-hand compartment and receive a moderately strong electric shock there, they rapidly learn to run through the open door to the right-hand side where they escape from the electric shock.

If the shock is then permanently turned off, the rats will continue running for many trials. In order to demonstrate that this is more than the automatic persistence of a mere motor habit, the door between the two compartments is then closed but can be opened by rotating a little wheel above it. When the escape of the rat is prevented, he shows considerable agitation and other signs of fear such as urinating and defecating. He also performs a great variety of other responses, pushing, biting, scrabbling, until he finally happens to rotate the wheel which causes the door to drop so that he can escape into the safe compartment. During a number of

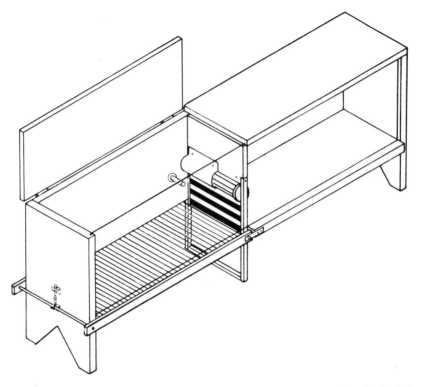

Figure 7.1. Apparatus for demonstrating that fear functions as a learned drive and a reduction in fear as a reward. (From Miller, 1948.)

trials, the rat rapidly learns to eliminate useless responses and to rotate the wheel promptly and vigorously.

As the animal becomes skilled at performing the response (called a coping response) that enables him to escape from the dangerous side of the apparatus, the signs of strong fear are greatly reduced; he no longer urinates or defecates, and eventually rotates the wheel in a relaxed, casual manner. A stranger coming in to observe the experiment at this point for the first time would have no clear indication that the wheel-turning was motivated by fear. But if a switch is thrown so that rotating the wheel no longer causes the door to drop, the rat becomes agitated; he rotates the wheel frantically, and urinates and defecates. Thus, it becomes clear that the successful coping response had inhibited the fear instead of eliminating the potentiality for it.

As the response of wheel-turning fails to open the door, the rat gradually abandons it and starts to perform other responses. When eventually he happens to press a lever that causes the door to drop and allows him to escape, he rapidly learns and continues to perform this new response. The learning of the two coping responses shows that fear has all the properties of a drive such as hunger or thirst, and that escape from fear has all the properties of a reward such as food for a hungry animal.*

The properties of fear illustrated in this experiment help us to understand it better. Fear can motivate the learning and performance of maladaptive behavior such as avoiding going to the dentist or failing to have a physical examination to locate a cancer in time to have it removed. But it can also motivate adaptive behavior such as buying insurance, being alert and driving carefully, taking prescribed medicine, or adopting a healthier lifestyle. The most important thing is not how afraid one is but what fear motivates one to do.

Innate Sources of Fear Induction and Reduction

Most experimental studies of fear have used pain as the unconditioned stimulus. For example, in the experiment just described, a mildly painful electric shock was the unconditioned (i.e., innate) source of the fear learned as a response to the left-hand side of the apparatus. A study by Fuller (1967), however, is an instructive exception. He found that if puppies were reared in a barren isolation chamber and then suddenly plunged into the normal complex environment, they showed signs of extreme fear which produced a long-lasting inhibition of normal canine behavior; they were extremely abnormal dogs. If, however, they were allowed to expose themselves gradually at their own pace through a small door that was opened between the barren and normal environments, they poked their noses out a little way and then retreated, poked them out a little farther and then retreated; and they soon showed fairly normal behavior. Apparently, a sudden exposure to a complex, unfamiliar environment can act as a traumatic, fear-inducing event, perhaps by producing a severe informational overload and/or by the complete removal of familiar stimuli for security.

Clinical evidence indicates many other sources of fear, such as sudden, intense, and unexpected stimuli; weird situations; threats of aggression;

---

*A similar experiment containing additional controls is described on page vii of Miller (1971) and in Delgado, Roberts, and Miller (1954).

social disapproval; the prospect of loss of love, loss of money, injury, illness, loneliness, helplessness, or death.

Miller (1951) has suggested that some objects or situations may have an innate, latent tendency to elicit fear. Clinical observations indicate that people are much more likely to acquire phobias of snakes, high places, or animals than of flowers, jewels, or butterflies. And experimental studies have shown that it is much easier to condition fear to pictures of potentially phobic objects such as snakes, and harder to extinguish fear of them than of pictures of neutral objects such as houses (Öhman, 1979; Öhman, Eriksson, and Olofsson, 1975).

Conversely, some situations seem to have a special ability to counteract fear. For example, Tinklepaugh and Hartman (1932) found that it was much harder to frighten baby monkeys if they were clinging to their mother than if they were separated from her. And Harlow and Zimmerman (1959) found that a soft terry-cloth mother surrogate could serve somewhat the same role. When frightened, human children cling to their parents and seem to be reassured by the ability to do so. Watson and Rayner (1920) could not use a loud sound to condition fear of an animal unless they took the child Albert off his mother's lap and, interestingly enough, prevented him from sucking his thumb. The role in combating stress of a wide variety of social supports and of belonging to a cohesive group has been emphasized by Wolf and Goodell (1976) and by Bruhn, Philips, and Wolf (1972). Bandura (1969) has demonstrated that imitating a fearless model can help to reduce fear. In some, but not in all cases, training in relaxation can reduce fear (Miller, 1978). More research is needed on ways of eliciting responses that are incompatible with fear.

One way of reducing the fear of a specific stimulus is to expose the subject to that stimulus immediately followed by a stimulus that elicits responses incompatible with fear. This is called counterconditioning. A less efficient way of reducing fear is repeatedly to expose the subject to the fear-inducing stimulus without any fear-inducing consequences. But if the subject promptly avoids the fear-inducing stimulus, this procedure can be extremely inefficient.

Fear in Combat

Studies of combat show that strong fear, or conflicts induced by it, can produce virtually all of the major symptoms of neurosis, psychosis, and psychosomatic illness. Some of these effects are a pounding heart and rapid pulse, dryness of the throat and mouth, strong feeling of muscular tension, trembling and exaggerated startle, sinking feeling of the stomach, perspiration, frequent need to urinate, irritability, aggression, overpowering urge to cry, run, or hide, confusion, feelings of unreality, feeling faint, nausea, fatigue, depression, slowing down of movements and thoughts, restlessness, loss of appetite, insomnia, nightmares, interference with speech, use of meaningless gestures, maintenance of peculiar postures, and (sometimes) stuttering, mutism, amnesia, and paralysis (Miller, 1951).

At first, these symptoms may come and go in a kaleidoscopic variety of patterns. But if any one of them is reinforced by a fear-reducing hope of escape from combat, that one will become learned (Dollard and Miller, 1950; Miller, 1975). The narrowing down of the kaleidoscopic array of symptoms resembles the trial-and-error learning of the rat to rotate the wheel in the experiment just described. Furthermore, the development of an effective symptom is usually associated with a reduction in the expressions of fear; the patient exhibits "la belle indifférence."

The power of the strong hope of escape from combat is shown by the fact that it can cause soldiers to be complacent or even elated after having received severe physical injuries that would cause extreme distress under civilian circumstances. The meaning of the physical injury—life-saving escape from combat or life-constricting burden under civilian circumstances—is a powerful psychological factor in determining how stressful it is.

To return to our earlier theme, even in combat fear can motivate adaptive behavior. In a study designed by the author, 37% of pilots reported flying better formation when they were strongly afraid, and 50% better when they were mildly afraid (Wickert, 1947).

Shift from Physical to Psychological Stress

In relatively recent times, our increased scientific understanding of nature has led to technological progress that, in the developed countries, protects all but the poor from the physical stresses of attacks from predatory animals, back-breaking manual labor, hunger, cold, and the dread plagues of infectious illnesses. As physical sources of stress become progressively less important, psychological sources become relatively more important. Furthermore, the same rapidly accelerating progress that has freed man from the worst physical stresses is increasing certain psychological stresses by forcing him to deal with rapid social changes.

Epidemiological and Life-Change Studies

Epidemiological studies have investigated conditions that produce psychological stress by requiring the learning of difficult adjustments. Among these conditions are immigration to a radically different social or physical environment and rapid social changes in the same environment. (Remember Fuller's dogs switched suddenly from the barren to the complex environment.) Other conditions are social disorganization, loss of social supports, and membership in groups with conflicting mores or markedly different social status. Such conditions have been found to increase the risk of mental disorders and also of psychosomatic symptoms such as ulcers, hypertension, myocardial infarction, and sudden cardiac death (Cassel, 1973; Jenkins, 1977). For example, Cassel (1970) cites 22 studies finding that natives living under apparently placid, socially well-integrated, primitive conditions had low blood pressure which did not increase with age. When members of the same racial stock moved to cities, they were found to have higher blood pressure which did increase with age.

The social conditions that have just been described as increasing psychological stress are associated not only with increases in the traditional psychosomatic diseases, but also with increased risks of other medical consequences such as tuberculosis, diabetes, leukemia, multiple sclerosis, and a wide range of minor complaints. Furthermore, prospective studies of individual cases indicate that the more numerous and drastic the life changes (e.g., losing a spouse) that have occurred within the last two years, the greater the risk of any one of a wide variety of mental or physical disorders (Kraus and Lilienfeld, 1959; Jacobs, Spilken, and Norman, 1969; Rahe, 1972; Wolf and Goodell, 1976; Klerman and Izen, 1977).

Although some of the foregoing investigations have used ingenious controls such as studying the effect of immigration to a place with better diet and sanitation, it is difficult entirely to rule out confounding factors such as exposure to pollution and increased amounts of saturated fats in the diet (Kasl, 1977; Ostfeld and D'Atri, 1977). However, the foregoing highly suggestive epidemiological and clinical studies are supported by a number of rigorously controlled experiments, most of which have had to be performed on animals. The general agreement of these two lines of evidence is impressive, but much more experimental work is needed to illuminate the details of the relationships among variables and of the mechanisms involved. The rest of the chapter will be concerned with experimental studies.

Effects on Immune System

Experiments from a number of different laboratories show that stress produced in a variety of different ways can affect the immune system (Stein, Schiavi, and Camerino, 1976). One of the ways of producing stress in animals has been to require them to perform an avoidance task over long periods of time. In one type of task, mice were placed in a compartment separated into two parts by a hurdle. The floor of each part was a grid of bars through which an electric shock could be delivered. A signal such as a tone came on a few seconds before the shock. If the mouse crossed to the other side quickly enough, he avoided the shock; if he did not respond quickly enough, the shock came on, and he had to escape from it by running to the other side. On the next trial, the mouse had to shuttle back in the opposite direction in order to avoid or escape the shock. Exposures to stresses to this type have been shown to increase the susceptibility to experimental infections and to hasten the time of death after implantation of a tumor (Rasmussen, 1969).

The foregoing effects would be expected from the immunosuppressant effects of corticosteroids released by the adrenal cortex during stress. But since some immunosuppressant effects have been produced in animals whose adrenals have been surgically removed, the corticosteroids cannot be the only mechanism involved (Stein, Schiavi, and Camerino, 1976).

That we need to learn more about these effects of stress on the immune system and the mechanisms through which these effects are produced is suggested by a minority of studies that have produced results opposite to those described. For example, in a study by Palmblad et al. (1976), eight healthy human volunteers were subjected to a three-day vigil without sleep or rest, during which they were exposed to loud noises and a task of shooting with an electronic rifle at small targets. In this study, a measure of interferon production (important in defense against viruses) was elevated during the stress and still higher five days afterward. In this same study, a test of phagocytosis, the ability of white blood cells to ingest heat-killed bacteria, was lowered during the stress period, but rose after a five-day rest period to a level higher than that preceding the stress. This result suggests that it may be important to investigate in more detail the time course of the effects of stress on the immune response. That it will be desirable also to investigate the effects of different degrees of stress is shown by a study indicating that in mice low doses of adrenaline caused an increase in interferon response, whereas high doses caused a decrease (Jensen, 1969).

It is obvious that any effects of stress on the immune system are likely to have a wide range of medically significant consequences. With the availability of improved techniques for measuring effects on the immune system and, as will be described later, improved techniques also for producing psychological stress, further investigations of the effects of stress on the immune system and of the mechanisms involved should be most fruitful.

Sudden Cardiac Death

Clinical observations suggest that if a patient has a damaged heart, a severe emotional stress can kill him. These observations have been confirmed by carefully controlled experiments in the laboratory. In an early suggestive study, Richter (1957) found that wild rats disoriented by having their whiskers clipped off and forced to swim in cold water suffered sudden death by cardiovascular arrest. But, if such rats were allowed to escape from the water quickly once, they would continue to swim for many hours—an apparent demonstration of the powerful effect of the psychological factor of "hope."

In another study, Lown and Wolf (1971) produced experimental infarcts in the hearts of dogs by tying off a branch of the coronary artery. After this damage (analogous to that involved in a heart attack) they found that stimulating the stellate ganglion of the sympathetic nervous system, producing an effect like that which might be produced by strong fear, caused the damaged hearts to fibrillate. In fibrillation, instead of contracting simultaneously, the various muscle fibers contract at different times so that the heart quivers instead of pumping blood. This, of course, ordinarily would produce sudden death except for the fact that these investigators had equipment handy to defibrillate the heart immediately and enable it to beat normally again.

In a second experiment, Lown, Verrier, and Corbalan (1973) used a chronically implanted electrode in the ventricle of the heart to produce an extra beat called a premature ventricular contraction (PVC). PVCs frequently occur in a damaged heart. This group found that, if they stimulated strongly enough, instead of inducing a single PVC they induced a series of them. Any stimulation stronger than this induced fatal fibrillation. In order to spare the dogs from fibrillation and defibrillation, they used the stage of repeated PVCs just short of fatal fibrillation. The dogs were tested sometimes in a room where they previously had received electric shocks, and at other times in a room where they had been petted, fed, and never received electric shocks. The investigators found that the threshold for repeated PVCs (a symptom just short of sudden death) was considerably lower in the room where the dogs had previously received electric shocks than in the room where they had not. Since no physical stimulus of electric shock was delivered during the tests, the difference must have been produced by the purely psychological stress of having learned to fear that room. These experimentally controlled results confirm the clinical observation that a strong emotional stress sometimes can suddenly kill a person who has a malfunctioning heart.

Effects of Learning a Discrimination

The general paradigm of the last experiment and of those that I am going to describe next is illustrated in Figure 7.2. In a danger situation, learning affects the intensity or duration of the fear, which has a number of innate physiological effects, some of which produce physical pathology such as fibrillation of the heart or lesions in the stomach.

Observations in combat have indicated that one way of reducing fear is to learn to know what to expect or, in other words, to learn the discrimination between what is dangerous and what is safe (Miller, 1959, pp. 267–268). Instead of being continuously afraid, learning such a discrimi-

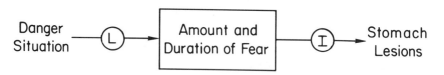

Figure 7.2. How learning (L) may affect the amount and duration of an emotional response such as fear, which in turn may have a direct innate (I) tendency to produce a psychosomatic effect such as increased stomach lesions.

nation allows the combatant to be afraid only when there actually is danger.

Figure 7.3 illustrates the apparatus in which Dr. Jay Weiss, one of the young scientists in my laboratory, studied the effects of learning such a discrimination on erosions in the stomachs of rats. These erosions presumably are an early stage in the formation of an ulcer. Each rat is semirestrained—he can move around somewhat but not much. Each restraining device is in a separate soundproof compartment not shown in the diagram. All rats have electrodes taped to their tails. The electrodes on

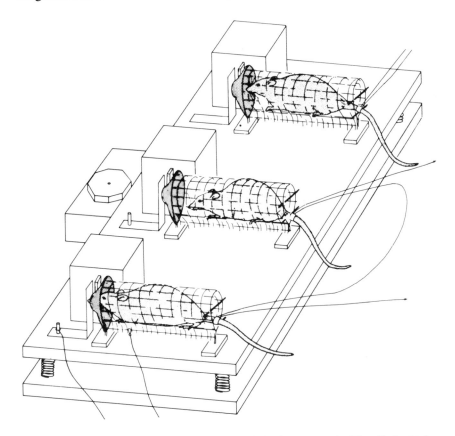

Figure 7.3. Apparatus for studying the effect of a discrimination on strength of fear. Each rat is in a separate, soundproof compartment not shown in the diagram. For the first rat, a tone signals occurrence of electric shock. The second rat receives exactly the same shocks because electrodes on his tail are wired in series with those on the tail of the first rat, but for him the tones come at a different time unrelated to the shocks. The third rat is a control receiving no shock. (From Weiss, Stone, and Harrell, 1970.)

the first two rats are wired in series so that they receive identical electric shocks. The only difference between these two rats is that for the first rat a tone always precedes the electric shock so that he can learn the discrimination of when it is dangerous and when it is safe. The second rat hears the same kind of tone but it comes at random times not associated with the shock, so that he cannot learn the discrimination. For the first rat, the shocks are predictable; for the second, they are unpredictable. The lucky third rat has the same electrodes on his tail, but is a control animal which receives no shock.

Figure 7.4 shows averaged results on groups of rats given these types of treatment. You can see that the rats subjected to unpredictable shocks had six times as much stomach damage as those that received the predict-

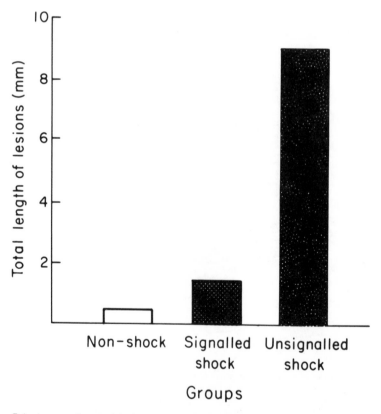

Figure 7.4. Amount of stomach lesions produced by shocks that are signaled so that rats can learn a discrimination, compared with those that are unsignaled so that no discrimination is possible. (From Weiss, 1970.)

able shocks. Since the physical strengths of the electric shocks delivered to both groups of animals were identical, the sixfold difference was the result of a purely psychological variable, the ability to learn a discrimination.

The results on gastric erosions are paralleled by those using other indices of fear. In an earlier experiment in my laboratory, Dr. Arlo Myers (1956) had shown more generalized fear of the stimulus situation as measured by more interference with drinking in rats that received unpredictable shocks and hence could not learn a discrimination. In the experiment just described, Weiss (1970) found the highest levels of plasma corticosterone, a hormone released during stress, in the rats that received the unpredictable shocks and lower levels in those receiving predictable shocks.

The results of the foregoing experiments confirm the observations in combat; they also confirm the importance of teaching discriminations in the course of psychotherapy (Dollard and Miller, 1950; Miller, 1975).

Disadvantage of Drugs

While drugs can be useful in temporarily reducing levels of fear that are too high, their disadvantage is that one cannot expect a drug to discriminate between a realistic and an unrealistic fear. Thus, the person who uses alcohol to reduce his fear of expressing himself normally and entering into the fun at a party runs a danger of reducing the realistic fear that restrains him from telling his boss what he really thinks about him or of driving dangerously on the way home.

Furthermore, the reduction in fear reinforces the habit of taking the drug, as was demonstrated in experiments by Davis and Miller (1963) and by Davis, Lulenski, and Miller (1968). One would expect the effect to produce psychological dependence.

Effects of Learning a Coping Response

Observations in combat have indicated that another way of reducing fear is learning a coping response—in other words, learning what to do to reduce the danger (Miller, 1959, pp. 267–268). You will remember in the first experiment described that, after the rat became skilled at the coping response of rotating the wheel to escape from a dangerous compartment into a safe one, his overt signs of fear were greatly reduced in the danger-

ous compartment but were increased when he was prevented from performing the coping response (Miller, 1951, p. 451).

Figure 7.5 shows the apparatus that Dr. Weiss (1972) used to secure
carefully controlled, quantitative information on the effects of being able
to learn a coping response. Again, the rats were semirestrained in devices
placed in separate sound proof compartments. The rat on the extreme left
can learn to escape the shock whenever it occurs by rotating the little
wheel connected to the device that turns off the shock. If he rotates the

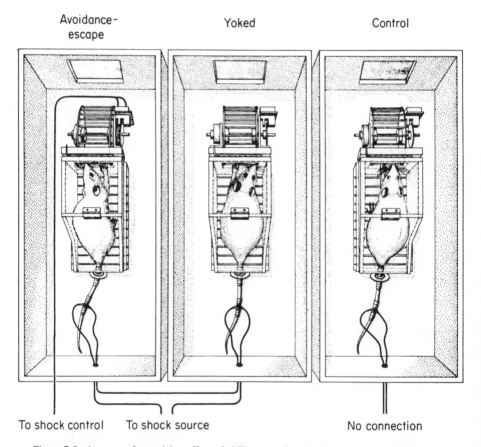

Figure 7.5. Apparatus for studying effect of ability to perform coping response on stress-induced
psychosomatic effects. The left-hand rat can turn off and/or avoid the shocks by rotating the wheel.
The center (yoked) rat receives exactly the same shocks because electrodes on his tail are wired in
series with those of his partner to the left, but his wheel has no control over the shocks. The
right-hand rat is a nonshock control. (Modified from Weiss, 1972.)

wheel promptly after a signal comes on, he can avoid the shock al-
together. Electrodes on the tail of this rat are wired in series with those on
the tail of the center rat so that both receive exactly the same electric
shocks. The center rat also has access to a wheel, but this wheel does not
have any control over the electric shocks, so that he is completely at the
mercy of his "stupid" partner. Such a rat is called a yoked control.
Again, the third rat is the control for the effects of being confined in the
apparatus without food; he has the same kind of electrodes on his tail but
receives no shock.

The results are shown in Figure 7.6. You can see that being able to
learn a simple coping response that controls the shock reduces considerably the amount of gastric lesions. Similar results have been secured in
experiments using interference with eating (the CER) as a measure of

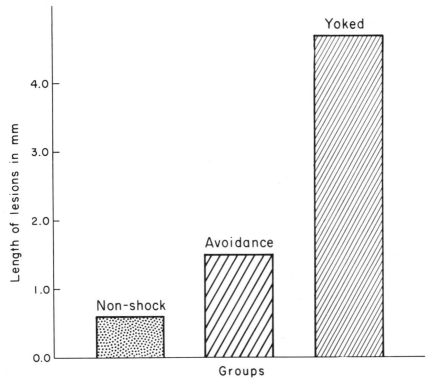

Figure 7.6. Effect of being able to perform an avoidance, coping response on the amount of stomach
lesions. Each yoked rat received exactly the same electric shocks as his avoidance partner because the
electrodes on their tails were wired in series. (From data in Weiss, 1968.)

fear. The animals able to learn the coping response also had lower levels of plasma corticosterone (Weiss, 1971a). Since the physical factor of shock received was equal for the two groups of rats, the reductions in gastric erosion, interference with eating, and level of plasma corticosterone must have been due to the purely psychological factor of being able to learn and perform a coping response.

Psychotherapists have found that it is extremely valuable to teach their patients more effective responses for coping with fear and with other emotional problems (Dollard and Miller, 1950; Hunt, 1975; Miller, 1975). Incidentally, the fear-reducing ability of a coping response may be one of the factors responsible for the powerful placebo effect that can be produced by taking a sugar pill or receiving a treatment that has no specific, direct, physical effect (Miller, 1975). On the other hand, if the coping response is too difficult or involves too much conflict, learning to perform it can increase the amount of stomach lesions (Weiss, 1971b).

Some Suggestions for Dealing with Fear

The experiments that have just been described suggest several practical measures to use in dealing with fear. Often fear exists as a vague, free-floating anxiety; its source is not clear; one tends to avoid thinking of the possible dangers. This is quite natural because, when thoughts of danger arouse fear, one way of escaping the fear is to put those thoughts out of mind, a tendency that is reinforced by the reduction in the strength of the fear. But to the extent that the thoughts are put out of one's mind, or in other words repressed, one loses the effectiveness of thinking as a means of solving the problem (Dollard and Miller, 1950). Thus, a first step in controlling fear is to resist the "ostrich-like" tendency to suppress or repress it; one must try to transform free-floating anxiety into fears of specific dangers. This is necessary because one cannot deal with a danger if one has not located it and thought about it.

Sometimes, when the dangers are scrutinized, it is found that they are not as bad as was thought. The dreaded possibilities turn out to be highly improbable or imaginary, or it is discovered that the fears were generalized from another situation that was quite different from the current one. Often, discriminating the realistic from the unrealistic fears can make one feel much better.

After the dangers have been located (but only after that), it is possible to plan and to carry out coping actions to reduce the ones that are realistic. Thus, the second step is to transmute worries into plans and actions. As we have seen, a coping response can powerfully reduce fear.

After doing all that he reasonably can, then and only then can one turn his attention to something else and stop thinking about the possible dangers.

Role of Conflict

In the last experiment described, the coping response was simple and effective. But there are other possibilities. One of these is illustrated by another experiment by Dr. Weiss (1971b). In this experiment, the apparatus was wired so that, whenever the animal on the extreme left, the one who could perform the coping response, rotated the little wheel he gave himself and his partner a brief pulse of electric shock. Thus, he had to give himself a shock in order to escape and/or avoid a longer train of shocks. The coping rat was in an avoidance-avoidance conflict or, in other words, between the devil and the deep blue sea.

Figure 7.7 shows the results. The left-hand side is a repetition of a previous experiment in which the coping response was simple because turning the wheel did not produce any additional electric shock to produce conflict. The results on the right-hand side, where the coping response was punished as well as rewarded, are dramatically different. Instead of having far fewer stomach lesions, the animals who could perform the coping response had far more. Since both rats received equal shocks, this result is yet another example of the power of a purely psychological factor—in this case, probably conflict.

A somewhat similar experiment has shown that if a coping response is the easy one of pressing a bar once, the coping rats have fewer stomach lesions than their yoked partners, but if the response is the difficult one of having to press the bar many times in order to avoid or escape the shock, the coping rats have more stomach lesions than their yoked partners (Tsuda and Hirai, 1975).

These experiments illustrate the importance of trying to find simple, effective coping responses that do not involve any conflict. They also indicate that the problem we have been discussing is a complicated one that could benefit from a considerable amount of additional experimental analysis. However, it should be noted that the experiments on the effects

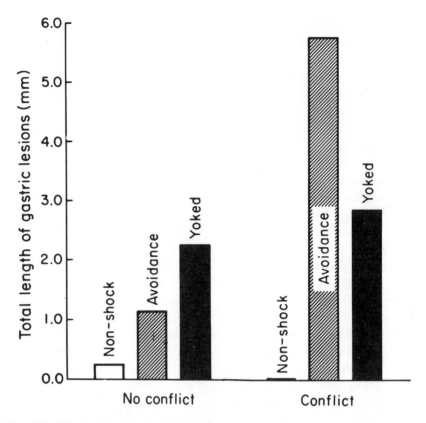

Figure 7.7. Being the "executive" rat that learns the avoidance, coping task reduces the amount of stomach lesions when the task is simple and clear-cut, but increases them when the task involves conflict. (From Weiss, 1971b.)

of a simple discrimination and of a simple coping response have been confirmed by experiments in a considerable number of other laboratories (Weiss, 1977).

Effects of Coping versus Helplessness on Brain Norepinephrine

Returning to the situation in which there is a simple coping response that does not induce conflict, Weiss, Stone, and Harrell (1970) in my laboratory found that the level of brain norepinephrine was increased in animals that could perform a simple coping response and decreased in their yoked partners who were helpless. These results are presented in Figure 7.8.

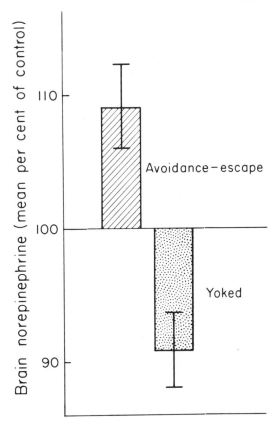

Figure 7.8. Compared with nonshock control rats, those that are able to perform an avoidance-escape response have an increased level of norepinephrine in their brain, while their helpless, yoked partners, who have no coping response available, have a decreased level of brain norepinephrine. (From Weiss, Stone, and Harrell, 1970.)

This difference in brain norepinephrine conceivably could have been produced by the greater muscular activity of the animals that were rewarded for rotating the wheel as opposed to those for whom this response was of no avail. As a control for muscular activity, Weiss and I performed another experiment. Each rat was semirestrained in a device on the top of a wheel 36 cm in diameter, the 14-cm wide screen-mesh top of which formed the floor under the device. Thus, the rat could run in place with the wheel rotating under him. Electric shocks were delivered via electrodes fastened to the tail of the rat. When a tone came on as a signal for shock, the rats in one group could avoid or escape the shock by actively running on the wheel. For the other group, the coping response was the opposite, passive one of remaining motionless on the wheel. Each rat in the active and the passive groups had a yoked partner in a similar device on another wheel. The electrodes on the tails of the two partners were wired in series so that they received exactly the same electric shocks, but only the coping member of the pair controlled the shocks; the yoked partner had no control over the shocks.

The results are presented in Figure 7.9. Looking at the lower part of the figure, you can see that the yoked partners represented by the solid bars displayed an intermediate and approximately equal amount of running,

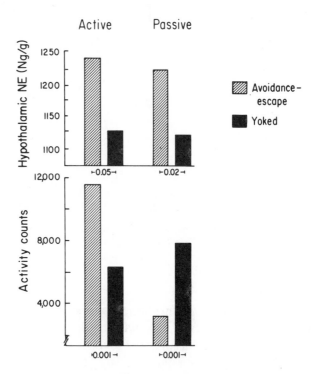

Figure 7.9. The level of norepinephrine in the brain is determined primarily by the availability of a simple coping response rather than by the level of physical activity. Rats trained in an active avoidance-escape coping response of running show more activity than their yoked partners, while those trained in a passive coping response of not moving show less activity than their yoked partners. But both avoidance-escape rats show higher levels of brain norepinephrine than their yoked partners. (From Weiss, Glazer, and Phorecky, 1976.)

but, as would be expected, the rats with the active coping response ran much more than their partners, while the ones with the passive coping response ran much less. If the physical activity of running were the main factor affecting the level of brain norepinephrine, we would expect the active group to show higher levels than their partners and the passive group to show lower levels than their partners. On the other hand, if the availability of a coping response were the main factor involved, we would expect both coping groups to show higher levels of brain norepinephrine than their yoked partners. The upper part of Figure 7.9 shows that the results were clearly in line with this latter expectation. Therefore, it is the ability to perform a coping response, rather than the level of physical activity, that is responsible for the difference in the level of brain norepinephrine.

The foregoing results are especially interesting because the drugs that can induce or deepen a depression if given to the wrong people are the ones that deplete norepinephrine (and other monoamines) in the brain, whereas the drugs that are useful in treating depression are those that increase the level of norepinephrine or its effectiveness as a neurotransmitter at the synapse (Schildkraut, 1969). Situations like the death of a loved one, in which there is no available coping response, are known to produce temporary depressions in people. Thus it appears that a lowered level (or effectiveness) of norepinephrine at the synapse may be involved in both drug-induced and situationally-induced depressions.

On the other hand, returning to Figure 7.8 it is interesting to note that successfully performing a coping response can raise the level of norepinephrine—which, in turn, might be expected to elevate the emotional mood. One might even speculate that meeting and overcoming a certain number of difficulties may be desirable from the point of view of happiness and mental health (Miller, 1972).

The foregoing mechanisms may have evolved because of their adaptive value. The depressive effects of a lower level of brain norepinephrine induced by failure and helplessness might have the value of saving the individual from wasting energy by continual striving in a hopeless situation. The opposite, elating effects of a higher level of brain norepinephrine might have the value of increasing activity in a situation where it is successful. But perhaps the biochemical overactivity of the depletion-depressive mechanism and/or an unusually severe situation in which coping responses are not available might in some cases lead to a depletion of norepinephrine, producing an emotional depression that reduces the probability of successful coping, leading to further failure and depletion of norepinephrine, and so on in a vicious circle.

Effects of Norepinephrine on Performance

The vicious-circle hypothesis that has just been stated assumes that a lowered level of norepinephrine will interfere with successful learning and performance of a coping response. Weiss and Glazer (1975) performed experiments to test this hypothesis. In one apparatus they exposed rats to the stress of a series of unpredictable and uncontrollable electric shocks, a situation in which the animals could not learn any coping responses. As we have seen, this situation produces a depletion of brain norepinephrine.

The immediate aftereffects of this treatment were tested in another apparatus consisting of two compartments with a grid floor separated by a hurdle 5 cm high. The task of these rats was to learn to respond to a danger signal by climbing over the hurdle to the other side. If they did this within 5 seconds, they avoided any shock. If they did not respond quickly enough, they received the shock and had to climb over the hurdle to the opposite side to escape from it. On alternate trials they had to shuttle back to the original side. This learning task is called shuttle avoidance.

The results were that the rats that had been exposed to the uncontrollable shock were much poorer in their performance in the shuttle avoidance apparatus. That this result was not specifically limited to prior treatment by electric shocks was shown by another experiment in which the prior stress was swimming in cold water, a stress also known to deplete brain norepinephrine. Similar results were secured in this experiment. That the rats were not so debilitated that it was impossible for them to climb over the hurdle, was shown by the fact that they could do so to escape the shock once it was turned on; but they did not learn to respond to the danger signal in order to avoid the shock. That the rats were not merely made stupid was shown by the fact that they could learn to perform the less effortful response of poking their nose into a hole to avoid the shock. Apparently, the rats could learn and could climb over the hurdle, but could not muster the activation to perform an effortful response to the danger signal. An influenza-like illness sometimes leaves me in a similar condition; I can prepare and give a lecture that is scheduled for that day (jump over the hurdle when the shock is on), but I cannot muster the ambition to prepare in advance for lectures that must be delivered soon.

If the common element in the foregoing experiments was indeed the depletion of brain norepinephrine, one might expect the effects to be counteracted by an antidepressant drug known to counteract the depletion of brain norepinephrine, and also other brain monoamines. Conversely, one might expect the effects of a drug known to deplete brain norepinephrine to be able to substitute for the prior stresses of electric shock or cold swim. And indeed, both of these expectations were verified. A dose of pargyline (100 mg/kg) was found to counteract the effects of prior exposure to the stress of unavoidable, unpredictable shocks, and pretreatment by a monoamine depleter, tetrabenazine (2 mg/kg), was found to produce aftereffects indistinguishable from those of pretreatment by the stress of the electric shock or cold swim (Glazer et al., 1975).

Habituation to Effects of Stress on Norepinephrine and on Behavior

If the effects of a single acute stress are indeed achieved via depletion of norepinephrine (and possibly other monoamines), one might expect that repeated exposures to the stress could increase the activity of the enzyme that synthesizes norepinephrine; for example, by releasing it from the effects of end-product inhibition. In this case, rats that had been toughened by a series of daily stresses might show less depletion of norepinephrine when exposed to one more acute stress than would rats that were exposed to the stress for the first time. Then, if the effects of stress on behavior are indeed mediated by its effects on norepinephrine, we also would expect the animals that had been toughened up to be more resistant to the deleterious behavioral aftereffects of the acute stress than those that have not had the previous exposure.

In order to test for the preceding possibilities, one group of rats was exposed to the acute stress of electric shocks once a day for 14 days while another group of rats received no such toughening-up treatments. After this, the first group was given a fifteenth day of exposure to the acute shock stress while the second group was given its first day of acute stress. As a control, a third group was never subjected to any acute stress. Then all groups were sacrificed, and the effects on norepinephrine metabolism in the brain were determined.

Exactly as expected, the group that had been exposed to a prior series of shocks was found to have a higher level of activity of tyrosine hydroxylase, the enzyme that synthesizes norepinephrine, than both the group that had not been given the prior exposure to shock and the control group that received no shock at all (Weiss et al., 1975). As would be expected from this increased synthesis, the group with prior exposures showed less depletion of norepinephrine than did the group that had not had the prior exposure; in fact, the former group showed the same level of norepinephrine as the controls. Finally, the group with prior exposures showed much less uptake of labeled norepinephrine (presumably, at the presynaptic terminals) than did either the rats without previous exposure or the nonshock controls. All of these effects would be expected to increase the effectiveness of norepinephrine as a transmitter at the synapse in the toughened rats. In addition, an unpredicted effect was found. The rats toughened by prior exposure showed much less elevation of corticosterone, a hormone released under stress.

Then a similar experiment was performed with the behavioral measure of performance in the shuttle avoidance task being substituted for the test of brain metabolism of norepinephrine. As would be predicted from the results of the pharmacological test, the toughening-up procedure was found to protect the rats from the deleterious immediate aftereffects of exposure to acute stress on the learning in the shuttle avoidance task.

In yet other sets of behavioral experiments, it was found that the tolerance produced by prior exposure to stress was not stress-specific. Prior exposure to cold swim reduced the deleterious aftereffects of a single exposure to traumatic shocks, and prior exposure to traumatic shocks reduced the deleterious aftereffects of a single exposure to cold swim.

Tests for cross-tolerance effects on the metabolism of brain norepinephrine were not quite so comprehensive and involved only the effects of prior exposure to cold swim on the immediate aftereffects of traumatic electric shocks. Here the only significant difference was that the prior exposure to cold swim reduced the uptake of norepinephrine after exposure to the different type of stress of electric shock. This result suggests that the change in uptake of norepinephrine played the most significant role in producing the behavioral effects of toughening-up.

Selye (1961) has found similar cross-tolerance effects, and also cross-sensitization effects, in his studies of the effects of prior exposure to one type of physical stress on the physical aftereffects of subsequent exposure to a different type of stressor.

Finally, if the repeated depletions of norepinephrine (and possibly other monoamines) produced by repeated prior exposure to stress did play a significant role in the toughening-up process, one would expect that a similar toughening-up effect could be produced by repeated doses of a drug, such as tetrabenazine, that produces a temporary depletion of norepinephrine. That this was indeed the case is shown in Figure 7.10. The top two curves show that the placebo pretreatment of 14 daily injec-

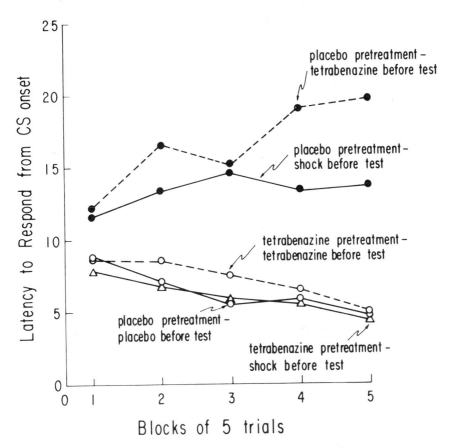

Figure 7.10. Effects of prior depletion of norepinephrine on subsequent resistance to stress. Exposure for the first time to either a norepinephrine-depleting drug, tetrabenazine, or to the stress of unpredictable, unavoidable electric shocks, has the aftereffect of causing rats in the top two curves to run slowly and fail to learn. Repeated prior exposures to tetrabenazine enable rats in the bottom two curves to resist the aftereffects of either tetrabenazine or the stress of unpredictable, unavoidable electric shocks; rats in these groups learn to run progressively faster and are no different from a control group never shocked. (From Glazer et al., 1975.)

tions of isotonic saline did not protect the rats from the aftereffects of either traumatic shocks or an injection of tetrabenazine before the shock shuttle-avoidance test. The animals in these groups took a long time to run and showed no improvement with repeated trials. The bottom curves show that the pretreatment of 14 daily injections of tetrabenazine protected the animals from the aftereffects of either an injection of tetrabenazine on the fifteenth day or traumatic shocks given for the first time on the fifteenth day. Both of these groups showed faster running and progressive improvement during a series of training trials; they were not reliably different from the control rats that had had a placebo pretreatment and only a placebo injection before the shuttle-avoidance test.

The conclusion from the foregoing experiments is that, under at least some circumstances, prior exposures to stress can build up one's physical and behavioral ability to tolerate the effects of stress. But the effects obviously need to be investigated further. For example, if the prior exposures come too closely together, their effects may be cumulative so that instead of toughening the individual up, the exposures have the effect of a more prolonged and perhaps completely overwhelming stress. Conversely, if the stresses are spaced too far apart, it is conceivable that any toughening-up value they have will be dissipated by the passage of time. Thus, there are still plenty of problems to investigate.

Learning to Resist Pain and Fear

In the preceding experiments, the results of the brain assays and the tests with various drugs demonstrated that the behavioral aftereffects of the single traumatic stressors and the toughening-up effects of prior exposures to similar stresses were achieved primarily via the effects of these treatments on the metabolism of brain norepinephrine and possibly on other brain monoamines. In other words, those effects were primarily unlearned. But Dollard and Miller (1950, p. 132) have suggested that a child's early experiences may cause it to learn either a general habit of responding actively to find a way out of a painful situation or a general habit of apathy and helplessness. In other words, Dollard and Miller suggest that under some circumstances, an ability to resist behavioral disruption produced by pain and fear can be the result primarily of learning.

In an experiment to test the possibility of learning to resist pain and fear, hungry rats were trained to run down a short alley in order to secure food (Miller, 1960). After having thoroughly learned, they were divided into two groups matched on speed of running. Each group was run five trials a day for a period of an additional 15 days. During this time, one group received gradually increasing shocks at the goal. During the weaker shocks the rats were rewarded for continuing to run and to eat in the presence of the cues of fear and pain. Thus it was expected that they would learn to run in the face of increasingly strong fear and pain. Furthermore, there was some reason to believe that the responses elicted by eating would be incompatible with those of fear so that the animals would tend to learn responses inhibiting fear, a procedure called counter-conditioning.

The other group received no such habituation to gradually increasing electric shocks but on the sixteenth day were suddenly introduced to the full strength of the shocks that the other group were receiving by that time. From then on, the strength of shocks remained constant for both groups.

The results are presented in Figure 7.11. It can be seen that, during the test trials, the group gradually exposed to shock ran more than twice as fast as the sudden group. To put the results in a different way, on the last day of testing, on only three out of 70 tests did the rats in the gradual group fail to reach the goal within the three minutes allowed. There were 43 such failures (i.e., 14 times as many) in the sudden group.

That the benefits of gradual exposure in this experiment were due to specific learning in the alley was shown by a control experiment which showed that a similar series of gradually increasing shocks given in a different situation outside the alley did not produce any appreciable beneficial effects. A characteristic of learning is that it is affected by the stimulus situation; if the result had been produced by enzyme induction or any other purely physiological effects on brain monoamines, one would have expected it to have been the same irrespective of the stimulus situation in which the shocks were delivered. Indeed, the shocks given in the preceding set of experiments were delivered outside the test situation. Those shocks were far stronger than the ones used in the present experiment, which is why they depleted brain monoamines. Presumably those in the present situation were too mild to have any appreciable depleting effect.

In the experiments that have been described, the two different mechanisms—building up physiological tolerance to stress and building up learned resistance to stress—were separated. Under many circumstances, one might expect these two mechanisms to be operating simultaneously.

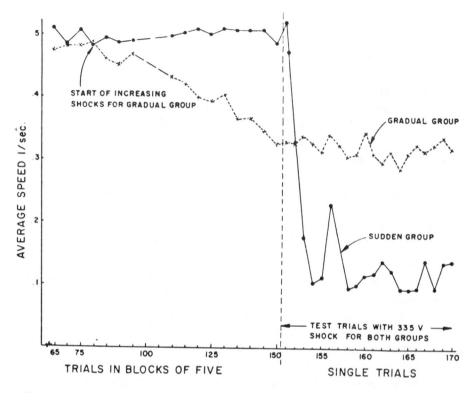

Figure 7.11. During a series of gradually increasing shocks at the goal, rats learn to resist the effects of pain and fear. Therefore, during a series of strong shocks, they run more than twice as fast as those suddenly introduced to shocks of this strength. (From Miller, 1960.)

A series of experiments by Seligman and his associates (see Seligman, 1975) has suggested that under appropriate circumstances both animals and people can learn to give up in the face of difficulties, a phenomenon which he has christened "learned helplessness." There is some controversy, however, about whether the animals are learning a general habit of helplessness or whether they are learning specific responses, such as crouching in a position that minimizes the painfulness of inescapable electric shocks, that interfere with their performance in the test situation (Weiss, Glazer, and Pohorecky, 1976; Glazer and Weiss, 1976a,b).

To date, the effects of learning to persist in the face of pain and fear on the physical consequences of stress have not been investigated. It seems plausible that under some circumstances subjects who have learned to persist in the face of pain and fear would subject themselves to more stress and hence suffer more physical consequences than those who have not learned to do so or who have learned to give up quickly. The approach-avoidance conflict theory predicts that subjects who approach nearer to a dangerous goal should experience more fear than those who remain so far away from it that they are not seriously tempted to approach (Miller, 1951, 1975).

Under other circumstances, however, clinical evidence suggests that patients who give up hope have a poorer prognosis. For example, there are some patients who, when told that they have inoperable cancer, will turn their face to the wall and soon die for no apparent physical reason (Lewis Thomas, personal communication).

We have seen that learning and other psychological factors can have an important effect on the physical effects produced by stress. It should be equally obvious that there still is a great deal left for us to learn about these important phenomena.

Acute versus Chronic Fear

One of the variables that needs to be investigated further is the difference between the effects of acute and chronic fear. For example, Cannon (1929) found that acute fear inhibits the secretion of hydrochloric acid in the stomach. On the other hand, in a series of experiments on dogs, monkeys, and even a patient in psychoanalysis, Mahl found that chronic fear could have the opposite effect of increasing the secretion of hydrochloric acid in the stomach (Mahl, 1949, 1952; Mahl and Karpe, 1953). A further indication of the need to study temporal factors in more detail comes from an experiment in which Polish et al. (1962) found that monkeys that had a high baseline fasting level of secretion of hydrochloric acid reduced the secretion during a six-hour period of avoidance training but rebounded to a level far above their initial baseline during a postavoidance test. Monkeys with a lower baseline level showed similar reduced secretion during avoidance training but did not rebound above their baseline level during a postavoidance test. This last result shows the importance of individual differences. There is considerable evidence that the effects of stress can depend on constitutional factors as well as on learning.

Learned Visceral Responses

Thus far, we have been discussing primarily how learning can affect the strength and duration of a stressful emotion such as fear, which, in turn, has an innate physiological tendency to produce physical effects such as stomach lesions. This type of effect was illustrated in Figure 7.2. A different way in which learning may produce a physical effect is illustrated in Figure 7.12. This figure illustrates a theoretical possibility that learning can affect not only the strength and duration of an emotion such as fear but also the type of visceral response—increased or decreased heart rate—elicited by that drive. One way that learning can affect the type of visceral response elicited is indirectly, as when the natural tendency for a frightened patient to breathe more rapidly reduces the level of carbon dioxide in the blood and hence causes the heart to beat more rapidly. If the rapid heart rate attracts medical attention that achieves some goal for the patient such as being relieved of responsibility by being diagnosed as sick, one would expect the rapid breathing to be rewarded and learned. And indeed there is evidence that this sort of thing does occur (Pickering, 1974).

There is ample evidence from experiments on both animals and people that learning can in one way or another affect visceral responses (Miller, 1978). For example, both rats (DiCara and Miller, 1969) and monkeys (Engel and Gottlieb, 1970) have been trained to increase their heart rate when they are rewarded for that response by avoidance and/or escape from electric shock; they have also been trained to produce the opposite response of decreasing their heart rate when they are rewarded for that

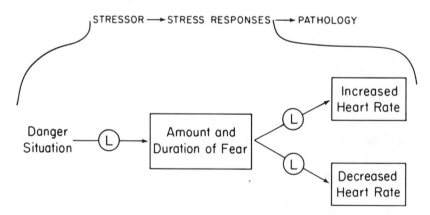

Figure 7.12. Two different ways in which learning (L) may affect a psychosomatic symptom: (1) it may affect the amount and duration of an emotional response such as fear, which, in turn, may have an innate, direct tendency to produce psychosomatic change, as was the case in Figure 7.2; and (2) it may affect the type and amount of viseral change that is elicited in response to a given emotional stimulus. (From Miller, 1972.)

response. People have been trained to produce both increases and decreases in heart rate, cardiac arrhythmias (skipped beats), blood pressure, blood flow to the skin, the galvanic skin response, and salivation (Kimmel, 1974; Miller, 1978). The therapeutic effects of such training, commonly called biofeedback, have been greatly exaggerated by the public media and by some overenthusiastic clinicians—something that unfortunately is quite common with almost any new approach. The therapeutic effectiveness of such training has not yet been definitely proved. But for a number of applications the preliminary results are encouraging enough to merit the further rigorous testing that will be necessary to evaluate them (Miller, 1978).

As far as therapeutic applications are concerned, it is not necessarily important whether the results are achieved by direct control over the visceral function or indirectly as in the case of the hysterical patient who learns to cause the heart to beat far too rapidly by overbreathing. Scientifically, however, and probably in the long run also practically, this is an important problem. The complexities are discussed elsewhere (Dworkin and Miller, 1977; Miller, 1978). Recent work on patients extensively paralyzed by polio, muscular dystrophy, or lesions interrupting the spinal cord strongly suggests that direct control may be possible (Pickering et al., 1977; Miller and Brucker, 1979). If this is correct, visceral learning may play an important role in maintaining normal homeostasis in the face of challenges by stressors and also in the shaping of psychosomatic responses to stress (Miller and Dworkin, 1979).

SUMMARY

The brain controls vital functions such as body temperature and blood pressure; it controls hormones, emotions, learning, and higher cognitive processes. Its role in controlling and integrating all of these functions provides a basis for the ability of psychological stress to produce physical symptoms and of psychological factors to relieve them. One of the important types of psychological stress is fear, or anxiety as it is called when its source is vague or ubiquitous. Fear can be learned as a response to new stimuli. It also can function as a drive to motivate the learning and performance of new responses; a reduction in fear can serve as a reward to reinforce those responses. Thus, how one has learned to respond to a fear is frequently far more important than how afraid one is.

In virtually all experimental work, pain has been used as the unconditioned stimulus innately to elicit fear. But clinical observations suggest that there are many other potential sources of fear. Furthermore, it is easier to condition fear to certain types of stimuli than to others. Certain stimuli (for example, for an infant, being near to its mother) can reduce fear.

Intense fear can elicit virtually all the symptoms of neurosis and even of psychosis. It also can elicit a kaleidoscopic array of psychosomatic effects. Symptoms that are reinforced by a reduction in fear are likely to be learned.

Epidemiological and life-change studies suggest that fear and other stresses can produce a wide range of medically adverse effects such as cardiovascular diseases, diabetes, gastrointestinal disturbances including ulcers, and increased susceptibility to malignancies and to infectious diseases. But in these studies it is difficult to rule out the effects of confounding factors such as exposure to conditions that produce disease, and changes in habits of eating, smoking, and drinking. However, these epidemiological and clinical observations are confirmed by a number of experimental studies in which it is possible to exert much better control over such confounding factors. Experimental studies indicate that fear can have a significant effect on the immune system, which, in turn, would be expected to produce a broad array of medically significant consequences. Experiments also show that in animals with damaged hearts fear can increase the likelihood of sudden cardiac death, and that strong chronic fear can increase the secretion of hydrochloric acid and can produce lesions in the stomach.

Observations in psychotherapy and in combat indicate that two important factors in reducing fear are learning to discriminate between when it is dangerous and when it is safe, and learning a coping response to reduce the danger. Rigorously controlled experimental studies confirm those observations. They show that learning a discrimination can reduce the level of chronic fear and its psychosomatic consequences such as stomach lesions, elevated levels of corticosterone, and depletion in brain norepinephrine. Furthermore, animals who learn a simple coping response to control a painful electric shock show less fear as measured by interference with eating, levels of plasma corticosterone, and stomach lesions than do those who receive exactly the same electric shocks without being able to control them. But if the coping response involves enough conflict, having to perform it can increase the amount of stomach lesions. One of the first steps in controlling fear is learning to locate the source of the danger and to discriminate real from imaginary dangers. The next step is to devise plans and carry out coping actions to reduce the danger.

Performing a simple, effective coping response can increase the level of brain norepinephrine, an effect analogous to that produced by drugs that combat psychological depression and induce euphoria. Inability to do anything about pain or fear can reduce the level of brain norepinephrine, an effect analogous to that of drugs that induce a psychological depression. Depression of brain norepinephrine interferes with the subsequent ability to perform effortful coping responses. Other brain monoamines also may be involved.

Repeated exposure to stress can increase the activity of the enzymes that synthesize norepinephrine in the brain and also increase its effectiveness as a neurotransmitter in the synapse by retarding its rate of reabsorption into presynaptic terminals. As might be expected from these effects, prior exposure to stress can reduce its depressive aftereffects on behavior. In addition to the foregoing physiological effects, it is possible to learn to resist the effects of pain and fear. It also may be possible to learn to change the visceral responses elicited by fear.

ACKNOWLEDGMENTS

Work reported from the author's laboratory was supported by U.S. Public Health Service research grants MH 19991, MH 269B0, and HL 21532, and by a grant from the Alfred P. Sloan Foundation.

References

Bandura, A. *Principles of Behavior Modification*. New York: Holt, Rinehart, and Winston, 1969.

Bruhn, J. G., Philips, B. U., and Wolf, S. Social readjustment and illness patterns: Comparison between first, second and third generation Italian-Americans living in the same community. *J. Psychosom. Res. 16:* 387–394, 1972.

Cannon, W. B. *Bodily Changes in Pain, Hunger, Fear and Rage*. New York: Appleton, 1929.

Cassel, J. Physical illness in response to stress. In Levine, S., and Scotch, N. (eds.), *Social Stress*. Chicago: Aldine, 1970, pp. 189–209.

Cassel, J. The relation of the urban environment to health: Implications for prevention. *Mt. Sinai J. Med. 40:* 539–550, 1973.

Davis, J. D., and Miller, N. E. Fear and pain: Their effect on self-injection of amobarbital sodium by rats. *Science 141:* 1286–1287, 1963.

Davis, J. D., Lulenski, G. C., and Miller, N. E. Comparative studies of barbiturate self-administration. *Int. J. Addictions 3:* 207–214, 1968.

Delgado, J. M. R., Roberts, W. W., and Miller, N. E. Learning motivated by electrical stimulation of the brain. *Am. J. Physiol. 179:* 587–593, 1954.

DiCara, L. V., and Miller, N. E. Heart-rate learning in the noncurarized state, transfer to the curarized state, and subsequent retraining in the noncurarized state. *Physiol. Behav. 4:* 621–624, 1969.

Dollard, J., and Miller, N. E. *Personality and Psychotherapy.* New York: McGraw-Hill, 1950.

Dworkin, B. R., and Miller, N. E. Visceral learning in the curarized rat. In Schwartz, G. E., and Beatty, J. (eds.), *Biofeedback: Theory and Research.* New York: Academic Press, 1977, pp. 221–242.

Engel, B. T. and Gottlieb, S. H. Differential operant conditioning of heart rate in the restrained monkey. *J. Comp. Physiol. Psychol. 73:* 217–225, 1970.

Fuller, J. L. Experiential deprivation and later behavior. *Science 158:* 1645–1652, 1967.

Glazer, H. I., and Weiss, J. M. Long-term and transitory interference effects. *J. Exp. Psychol.: Animal Behav. Processes 2:* 191–201, 1976a.

Glazer, H. I., and Weiss, J. M. Long-term interference effect: An alternative to "learned helplessness." *J. Exp. Psychol.: Animal Behav. Processes 2:* 202–213, 1976b.

Glazer, H. I., Weiss, J. M., Pohorecky, L. A., and Miller, N. E. Monoamines as mediators of avoidance-escape behavior. *Psychosom. Med. 37:* 535–543, 1975.

Harlow, H. F., and Zimmerman, R. R. Affectional responses in the infant monkey. *Science 130:* 421–432, 1959.

Hunt, H. F. Behavior therapy for adults. In Freedman, D. X., and Dyrud, J. E. (eds.), *American Handbook of Psychiatry,* 2nd ed., Vol. 5: *Treatment.* New York: Basic Books, 1975, pp. 290–318.

Jacobs, M. A., Spilken, A., and Norman, M. Relationship of life change, maladaptive aggression, and upper respiratory infection in male college students. *Psychosom. Med. 31:* 31–44, 1969.

Jenkins, C. D. Epidemiological studies of the psychosomatic aspects of coronary heart disease. *Adv. Psychosom. Med. 9:* 1–19, 1977.

Jensen, M. M. The influence of vasocative amines on interferon production in mice. *Proc. Soc. Exp. Biol. Med. 130:* 34–39, 1969.

Kasl, S. V. Contributions of social epidemiology to studies in psychosomatic medicine. *Adv. Psychosom. Med. 9:* 160–223, 1977.

Kimmel, H. D. Instrumental conditioning of autonomically mediated responses in human beings. *Am. Psychol. 29:* 325–335, 1974.

Klerman, G. L., and Izen, J. E. The effects of bereavement and grief on physical health and general well-being. *Adv. Psychosom. Med. 9:* 63–104, 1977.

Kraus, A. S., and Lilienfeld, A. M. Some epidemiologic aspects of the high mortality rate in the young widowed group. *J. Chronic Dis. 10:* 207–217, 1959.

Lown, B., and Wolf, M. Approaches to sudden death from coronary heart disease. *Circulation 44:* 130–132, 1971.

Lown, B., Verrier, R., and Corbalan, R. Psychologic stress and threshold for repetitive ventricular response. *Science 182:* 834–836, 1973.

Mahl, G. F. Effect of chronic fear on the gastric secretion of HCl in dogs. *Psychosom. Med. 11:* 30–44, 1949.

Mahl, G. F. Relationship between acute and chronic fear and the gastric acidity and blood-sugar levels in *Macaca mulatta* monkeys. *Psychosom. Med. 14:* 182–210, 1952.

Mahl, G. F., and Karpe, R. Emotions and hydrochloric acid secretion during psychoanalytic hours. *Psychosom. Med. 15:* 312–327, 1953.

Miller, N. E. Studies of fear as an acquirable drive: I. Fear as motivation and fear reduction as reinforcement in the learning of new responses. *J. Exp. Psychol. 38:* 89–101, 1948.

Miller, N. E. Learnable drives and rewards. In Stevens, S. S., (ed.), *Handbook of Experimental Psychology.* New York: Wiley, 1951, pp. 435–472.

Miller, N. E. Liberalization of basic S-R concepts: Extensions to conflict behavior, motivation and social learning. In Koch, S. (ed.), *Psychology: A Study of a Science,* Study 1, Vol. 2. New York: McGraw-Hill, 1959, pp. 196–292.

Miller, N. E. Learning resistance to pain and fear: Effects of overlearning, exposure and rewarded exposure in context. *J. Exp. Psychol. 60:* 137–145, 1960.

Miller, N. E. Physiological and cultural determinants of behavior. In *The Scientific Endeavor.* New York: The Rockefeller Institute Press, 1964, pp. 251–265. Also *Proc. Nat. Acad. Sci. USA 51:* 941–954, 1964.

Miller, N. E. *Neal E. Miller: Selected Papers.* Chicago: Aldine-Atherton, 1971.

Miller, N. E. Interactions between learned and physical factors in mental illness. *Semin. Psychiat. 4:* 239–254, 1972.

Miller, N. E. Applications of learning and biofeedback to psychiatry and medicine. In Freedman, A. M., Kaplan, H. I., and Sadock, B. J. (eds.), *Comprehensive Textbook of Psychiatry,* 2nd ed. Baltimore: Williams & Wilkins, 1975, pp. 349–365.

Miller, N. E. Biofeedback and visceral learning. *Annu. Rev. Psychol. 29:* 373–404, 1978.

Miller, N. E., and Brucker, B. S. Learned large increases in blood pressure apparently independent of skeletal responses in patients paralyzed by spinal lesions. In Birbaumer, N., and Kimmel, H. D. (eds.), *Biofeedback and Self-Regulation.* Hillside, N.J.: Lawrence Erlbaum Associates, in press.

Miller, N. E., and Dworkin, B. R. Homeostasis as goal-directed learned behavior. In Thompson, R. F. (ed.), *Neurophysiological Mechanisms of Goal-Directed Behavior and Learning.* In press.

Myers, A. K. The effects of predictable vs. unpredictable punishment in the albino rat. Ph.D. Thesis, Yale University, 1956.

Öhman, A. Fear relevance, autonomic conditioning, and phobias: A laboratory model. In Bates, S., Dockens, W. S., Grestam, K.-G., Melin, L., and Sjödén, P.-O. (eds.), *Trends in Behavior Therapy.* New York: Academic Press, in press.

Öhman, A., Eriksson, A., and Olofsson, C. One-trial learning and superior resistance to extinction of autonomic responses conditioned to potentially phobic stimuli. *J. Comp. Physiol. Psychol. 88:* 619–627, 1975.

Ostfeld, A. M., and D'Atri, D. A. Rapid sociocultural change and high blood pressure. *Adv. Psychosom. Med. 9:* 20–37, 1977.

Palmblad, J., Cantell, K., Strander, H., Fröberg, J., Karlsson, C.-G., Levi, L.,

Grantström, M., and Unger, P. Stressor exposure and immunological response in man: Interferon-producing capacity and phagocytosis. *J. Psychosom. Res. 20:* 193–199, 1976.

Pickering, G. W. *Creative Malady.* New York: Oxford University Press, 1974.

Pickering, T. G., Brucker, B., Frankel, H. L., Mathias, C. J., Dworkin, B. R., and Miller, N. E. Mechanisms of learned voluntary control of blood pressure in patients with generalised bodily paralysis. In Beatty, J., and Legewie, H. (eds.), *Biofeedback and Behavior.* New York: Plenum Press, 1977, pp. 225–234.

Polish, E., Brady, J. V., Mason, J. W., Thach, J. S., and Niemack, W. Gastric contents and the occurrence of duodenal lesions in the rhesus monkey during avoidance behavior. *Gastroenterology 43:* 193–201, 1962.

Rahe, R. H. Subjects' recent life changes and their near-future illness susceptibility. *Adv. Psychosom. Med. 8:* 2–19, 1972.

Rasmussen, A. F., Jr. Emotions and immunity. *Ann. N.Y. Acad. Sci. 164:* 458–461, 1969.

Richter, C. On the phenomenon of sudden death in animals and man. *Psychosom. Med. 19:* 191–198, 1957.

Schildkraut, J. J. *Neuropsychopharmacology and the Affective Disorders.* Boston: Little, Brown, 1969.

Seligman, M. E. P. *Helplessness on Depression, Development, and Death.* San Francisco: W. H. Freeman, 1975.

Selye, H. Nonspecific resistance. *Ergebn. allg. Pathol. pathol. Anat. 41:* 208–241, 1961.

Stein, M., Schiavi, R. C., and Camerino, M. Influence of brain and behavior on the immune system. *Science 191:* 435–440, 1976.

Tinklepaugh, D. L., and Hartman, C. G. Behavior and maternal care of the newborn monkey (*Macaca mulatta*—"*M. rhesus*"). *J. Genet. Psychol. 40:* 257–286, 1932.

Tsuda, A., and Hirai, H. Effects of the amount of required coping response tasks on gastrointestinal lesions in rats. *Jap. Psychol. Res. 17:* 119–132, 1975.

Watson, J. B., and Rayner, R. Conditioned emotional reactions. *J. Exp. Psychol. 3:* 1–14, 1920.

Weiss, J. M. Effects of coping responses on stress. *J. Comp. Physiol. Psychol. 65:* 251–260, 1968.

Weiss, J. M. Somatic effects of predictable and unpredictable shock. *Psychosom. Med. 32:* 397–408, 1970.

Weiss, J. M. Effects of coping behavior in different warning signal conditions on stress pathology in rats. *J. Comp. Physiol. Psychol. 77:* 1–13, 1971a.

Weiss, J. M. Effects of punishing the coping response (conflict) on stress pathology in rats. *J. Comp. Physiol. Psychol. 77:* 14–21, 1971b.

Weiss, J. M. Psychological factors in stress and disease. *Scient. Am. 226* (No. 6): 104–113, 1972.

Weiss, J. M. Psychological and behavioral influences on gastrointestinal lesions in animal models. In Maser, J. D., and Seligman, M. E. P. (eds.), *Psychopathology: Experimental Models.* San Francisco: W. H. Freeman, 1977, pp. 232–269.

Weiss, J. M., and Glazer, H. I. Effects of acute exposure to stressors on subsequent avoidance-escape behavior. *Psychosom. Med. 37:* 499–521, 1975.

Weiss, J. M., Glazer, H. I., Pohorecky, L. A., Brick, J., and Miller, N. E. Effects of chronic exposure to stressors on avoidance-escape behavior and on brain norepinephrine. *Psychosom. Med. 37:* 522–534, 1975.

Weiss, J. M., Glazer, H. I., and Pohorecky, L. A. Coping behavior and neurochemical changes: An alternative explanation for the original "learned helplessness" experiments. In Serban, G., and Kling, A. (eds.), *Animal Models in Human Psychobiology.* New York: Plenum Press, 1976, pp. 141–173.

Weiss, J. M., Stone, E. A., and Harrell, N. Coping behavior and brain norepinephrine level in rats. *J. Comp. Physiol. Psychol. 72:* 153–160, 1970.

Wickert, F. (ed.). *Psychological Research on Problems of Redistribution.* Army Air Force Aviation Psychology Program, Research Report No. 14. Washington, D.C.: U.S. Government Printing Office, 1947.

Wolf, S. G., and Goodell, H. *Behavioral Science in Clinical Medicine.* Springfield, Illinois: Charles C Thomas, 1976.

8.

The Auto-Pharmacology* of Stress: An open letter to Dr. Hans Selye

M. Rocha e Silva**

*Department of Pharmacology, Faculty of Medicine, U.S.P., Ribeiraõ Preto, Saõ Paulo, Brazil****

Dear Selye:

I have your letter of March 30, 1977, with the kind invitation to write a chapter for your forthcoming book *A Guide to Stress Research* as a contribution to the International Institute of Stress (IIS) to which you deservedly act as President. The chapter would deal with my work on *stressology*, and I have long meditated about the dilemma: How could I contribute to a book on a subject that I do not consider my specialty, and yet not let down the call from a friend, my association with whom I have considered one of my prides since 1941, when I first met you at the Federation Meeting in Chicago?

By that time, I was in my first stay in the U.S., as a Guggenheim Fellow from Brazil for the period 1940–42, i.e., some 36 years ago. Ever since, I have always been associated with you, and have a picture hanging on my wall at the Biological Institute, in São Paulo, showing you as a young celebrity looking at the microscope, possibly on some aspects of

---

*Auto-pharmacology is understood here in the sense given to it by Sir Henry H. Dale and his associates, in Refs. 1–5.
**Written while in tenure of a Fogarty International Center Scholarship-in-Residence, at the NIH, Bethesda, maryland.
***Permanent address.

your then recently described general adaptation syndrome (G.A.S.). In 1946, on my way to England as a Fellow of the British Council, after stopping in Toronto to work with Jaques, Scroggie, and Fidlar (1947) (Ref. 6), on the release of histamine by peptone, I visited your laboratory (then your Institute of Experimental Medicine, now expanded into the IIS), as I recall, as your first nominee to a Claude Bernard Scholarship, to give one or two conferences to your group of distinguished scientists, including Dr. G. Masson, with whom I had more contact.

By that time (1946–47) I had two associates of mine, Drs. J. Leal Prado and Eline S. Prado, working in your laboratory. Together with Leal Prado, I decided to test the newly introduced synthetic antihistamine Benadryl (diphenhydramine) against your "stressing symptom" observed after the injection of egg white in rats, which then became known as the "egg white edema," of the paws and snout of the rat. And it worked!

The edema was strongly reduced by a proper injection of Benadryl. Since I was only in your laboratory for a few days, I handed the performance of further experiments over to Leal Prado, and was later surprised to know that Leal Prado, with his extraordinary sense of goodwill, or maternal instincts, handed it over to one of your youngest associates, Jacques Leger, who proceeded with the study of that phenomenon in relation to the action of antihistamines, with Dr. G. Masson. Incidentally, the name of Leal Prado was included in two papers (Leger, Masson, and Prado, 1947a,b). Thereafter, Leger continued with Masson to study some aspects of the phenomenon (Leger and Masson, 1947–48) and made it the object of his doctoral thesis. Later on, this action of antihistamines was studied by Halpern (1960) and many others, and I think that it is still an interesting subject for research. (See Refs. 7–11.)

I don't want to raise any personal issues in relation to this historical event that, if nothing else, would illustrate a frequent happening in experimental biology, but I would like to *stress* the fact, which will contribute to an understanding of the meaning of this letter, of our different ways of thinking. To you, such a symptom was of the kind that you would *see* as a manifestation of your general adaptation syndrome (G.A.S.), though to me it appeared as the manifestation of an *autopharmacological phenomenon,* as defined by Sir Henry H. Dale in the ideas of the twenties and early thirties (Refs. 1–5). The similarity of the "egg white edema" to the manifestations of anaphylaxis, in which I had been chiefly interested since my stay in Chicago (1940–41), with Carl Dragstedt, had suggested to me that the main mediator of such a symptom as the edema of the paws and snout of the rat, could be histamine—released from its stores in the tissues (at that time mast-cells were not yet known to be reservoirs of histamine and heparin), according to the experiments by Bartosch, Feldberg, and Nagel (1932), Dragstedt and Gebauer-Fuelnegg (1932), Schild (1936), Code (1937, 1939), Katz (1940, 1942), and so many others who had shown that histamine is released in dog's, guinea pig's and rabbit's anaphylaxis (Refs. 12–17). Much later came the story that histamine and heparin are confined to mast-cells (Riley and West, 1953, 1959; see Mota, 1966, and your book on mast-cells: Selye, 1965), and therefore anaphylaxis, egg white, peptone, and many similar agents might be working through disruption of mast-cells. For the mechanism of these reactions and a complete review of the subject, see the *Handbook of Exp. Pharmacology,* Vol. XVIII, Parts 1 and 2 (M. Rocha e Silva, ed., 1966 and 1977), and especially the chapters by Goth (1977), Uvnäs (1977), and Charkravarty (1977). (See Refs. 18–26).

But, in 1946, only histamine was known to produce such a generalized vascular reaction, with increase in "capillary permeability," using the nomenclature of that time (only in 1961, Majno and collaborators called attention to the fact that mediators such as histamine, serotonin, and bradykinin act upon the microvasculature at more calibrated sites [60 μ diameter] than common capillaries, suggesting the name "increased vascular permeability" to denote the increased passage of carbon particles through the walls of the small vessels; Refs. 27, 28). Then came 5-HT (serotonin), following the publication by Rowley and Benditt (1956) (Ref. 29) showing that serotonin in the rat skin was 200 times more potent than histamine, when assayed by the "blue test." Later on, it was shown that only in rodents could serotonin be a serious competitor for histamine and bradykinin.

In the meantime, bradykinin (Bk) was discovered in our laboratory at the Biological Institute of São Paulo (Rocha e Silva, Beraldo, and Rosenfeld, 1949). For a personal account of "The Bradykinin Story," see Rocha e Silva (1977) in the interesting publication *Discovery Processes in Modern Biology* (Klemm, ed., 1977), to which you yourself contributed the history of stress ("Biological Adaptation to Stress"), presenting your ideas about the ways of an investigator, wherefrom I got the inspiration to write this personal letter. (See Refs. 30–32.)

In later years, the prostaglandins, discovered in 1934 by von Euler (see von Euler, 1934, 1936) (Refs. 33–34) came to be regarded as the most important mediator of the acute inflammatory reactions (Vane, 1971,

1973). Again, we are going to show how vain it is to try to accumulate so many honors on a single factor, in this case, prostaglandins (PGs), actually representing a bunch of 20 or so different factors, such as PGE_1, PGE_2, PGE_3 ... $PGF_{1\alpha}$, $PGF_{2\alpha}$, $PGF_{3\alpha}$ ... A and B, and so forth, including precursors (arachidonic acid, thromboxanes, and so forth). For a review, see a number of papers appearing in many periodicals, and in the specialized one *Prostaglandins*, and also Refs. 35–37.

As I said elsewhere (Rocha e Silva, 1973; Ref. 38): "It was difficult to fight so many warriors (PGs) with a single one (Bk)" even if we may consider the number of derivatives (Lys-Bk, Met-Lys-Bk, and bradykininogen, Bkg, itself). The advantage of bradykinin was that, being a polypeptide, actually the first strongly hypotensive one described in the literature, it became important by itself and especially as a product resulting from incomplete or partial hydrolysis of a protein (proteolysis), having been the object of at least 12 international symposia: in Montreal (1953), London (1959), New York (1964), Florence (1965), Ribeirão Preto (1966), Fiesole (1969), Florence (1971), San Francisco (1972), Ribeirão Preto (1974), Reston, Virginia (1974), Fiesole (1975), and Rio de Janeiro (1976); and each year now we are having Kinin Symposia (Kinin 75, Kinin 76, Kinin 77), the next announced to be in Tokyo (Kinin 78). IN Fiesole, in 1969, the Academia Kininensis Fiesolana was founded, which already held three international meetings, under the direction of Sicuteri and his colleagues in Florence. (See Refs. 38–40 and also Refs. 47, 52, 53, 78, 83.)

However, I have to *stress* again that for a certain time the prostaglandins appeared to obscure the role of the kinins, since about everything that had been demonstrated for bradykinin appeared to be mediated by one or the other PGE or PGF, or PGA or PGB. But the difference had always been that what had been shown with sweat and tears to be produced by Bk or one of its derivatives in the course of 20 hard years, was shown to be produced by PGs just like that, sometimes in a single paper or abstract. However, in later years, or months, or weeks, things are slowly changing, and the fate of PGs appears to be entangled with that of Bk. But now we are jumping to more modern times or even to the future, which I was intending to leave to the end of this letter.

It is enough to say that the theme in many such symposia has been the "Mechanism of the Inflammatory Reactions." If one assumes that inflammation is certainly a basic component of your GAS, a typical manifestation of *stressology*, we are inclined to include such a symptom, or syndrome as that exemplified by the "rat's egg white edema" in the field of inflammation, and study it as a multimediated reaction, in which many endogenous principles or factors may play a significant role: histamine, 5-HT (serotonin), the kinins (bradykinin, Lys-Bk, Met-Lys-Bk, and possibly other high-molecular-weight peptides derived from bradykininogen, such as Gly-Arg-Met-Lys-Bk, the so-called *pachykinins;* we feel that even proteins containing as a terminal sequence that of Bk, such as kininogens themselves, might possibly act as vascular permeability factors; see Refs. 41–43)$_>$ prostaglandins, as well as their precursors and analogues, the slow-reacting substances (SRA-S), substance-P$_>$ and the many permeability factors still waiting for a proper chemical identification. For details see Rocha e Silva (1970), Rocha e Silva and Garcia-Leme (1972) (Ref. 44), (Ref. 45), and the forthcoming Vol. XVIII/2 of the Heffter's handbook on *Histamine and Anti-histaminics,* and Vol. 50 of the same handbook on *Inflammation,* edited by Vane and Ferreira (1978).

When I came back to your laboratory, on the occasion of the XIX International Congress of Physiological Sciences held in Montreal, 1953, we had, by your invitation, a symposium on the "Mechanism of Inflammation," held in your home, for a general discussion with many distinguished physiologists, pharmacologists, biochemists, and pathologists. In that meeting, edited later on by your group (Ref. 47), there was a magnificent discussion on all aspects of inflammation, and I recall that there were many clashes between pharmacologists and pathologists, and biochemists, and stressologists, and I heard many nasty names in low voices exchanged between the participants. As regards my work, I had a reasonably civilized struggle with Menkin, whom I recall being designated the "No. 1 Public Enemy" of histamine. Actually, by that time our criticism of Menkin's *leukotaxine* ended a discussion between Menkin and my associate Oto Bier, that started at the 1st International Congress of Microbiology held in New York, in 1939 (Bier and Rocha e Silva, 1939; Ref. 50). By that time I was strongly in favor of histamine, as the main mediator of inflammation, under the influence of the classical work by Th. Lewis and the English school of pharmacology, and strongly against leucotaxine, which we considered, Bier and myself, as not well identified in the inflammatory exudates. In a certain sense, we may now assume that Menkin was right, looking for a new principle in the exudates after application of turpentine to the pleura of rabbits and guinea pigs. Only by that time we thought that his experiments would not exclude histamine: in the first place, histamine was there in the exudates obtained by injecting turpentine to the pleural cavity of such animals; in the second place, his testing method, by using the "blue test" in the guinea pig's and rabbit's skin, would not exclude the participation of histamine because histamine was also there, in the guinea pig's and rabbit's skin. To exclude histamine release by his tests was not in Menkin's plans. However, it became the concern of a fine group of investigators at the Lister Institute in London, under the guidance of Miles and Miles (1952). We now know that what was missing in Menkin's experiments, and only much later discovered, was the kinin system, of which bradykinin became the most prominent member. I have, however, to remind us that by the time Menkin (1938, 1940) published his experiments, he showed an essay in which "leukotaxine" had no effect on the isolated guinea pig ileum, thus excluding the kinins, and possibly also the prostaglandins. But the main drawback of Menkin's experiments was that he used almost solely the mentioned trypan or Evans "blue test" upon the rabbit's skin, and this method has been considered a highly unspecific one according to our experiments (Bier and Rocha e Silva, 1939; Rocha e Silva and Dragstedt, 1941), since all reagents that Menkin used for extraction and "crystallization" of his principle (Menkin, 1940) could produce a strong positive blue test in the animal skin (rabbits, guinea pigs, and rats). What was needed in such a case, would be to have a parallel biological assay, as was done with bradykinin a few years later (from 1948 on). (See Refs. 46 to 52.)

But, from a historical point of view, a strange coincidence that was never taken into consideration was that, at the International Physiological Congress in Montreal, in 1953, on the same day as your symposium on the "Mechanism of Inflammation" (Ref. 47), there was another symposium organized by Ulf von Euler and myself and presided over by Gaddum (1955) (Ref. 53) in which for the first time it was shown, by us and by van Arman, that the purified preparations of bradykinin had the property of increasing vascular permeability parallel to the degree of purity (see Rocha e Silva, 1953; van Arman, 1953: in Gaddum, ed., 1955; Refs. 53–55). As I remember, I came late to your symposium because at the same time I had to give a paper on bradykin at the other symposium, the first one on "Biologically Active Peptides." It was obvious by then that we were in the process of changing "paradigmas," in the sense of Kuhn (1971: *The Structure of Scientific Revolutions*, Ref. 56), and by that time bradykinin was forcing its entrance into the picture as a possible mediator of the increased vascular permeability in inflammation, and now we may say, in *stressology*. Later on, Vane (1973), on the basis of his discovery that aspirin and indomethacin inhibit synthesis of PGs, being at the same time good or potent anti-inflammatory agents, attempted or suggested another change of "paradigma": "Each substance, as its involvement is proposed or demonstrated, has been regarded as the most important inflammatory mediator, only to be supplanted after a few years by the last pharmacological fashion. . . . During the past few years we have passed from the bradykinin phase into the prostaglandin phase" (Vane, 1973; Ref. 36). This is a good example of how misleading Kuhn's ideas about the structure of scientific revolutions can be. In a recent symposium on kinins and inflammation held in Rio de Janeiro, I presented a paper on "Bradykinin or Prostaglandins, a Doctor's Dilemma," in which I tried to show how wrong it is to assume that in the course of time, histamine gave way to bradykinin, and bradykinin to prostaglandins: "It is a known historical fact that the discovery of any new factor or scientific event, instead of closing doors, opens up new lanes, to which the old ones converge, amplifying views and landscapes to the future of scientific achievement" (*Agents and Actions,* Vol. 8/1, 1978). Happily, the solution of the dilemma came from Vane's laboratory, with the contribution of our associate Sergio H. Ferreira. In a series of papers with Vane and Moncada (Ferreira, Moncada, and Vane, 1974; Moncada, Ferreira, and Vane, 1974; Refs. 57 and 58), it was shown that in many cases of participation of PGs and Bk in inflammatory reactions, the first (PGs) act as a potentiator of bradykinin and, what is more interesting, that bradykinin activates the system of enzymes in charge of the synthesis of PGE; and since the latter may potentiate Bk, a double feedback mechanism, which seems to be important for the autopharmacology of pain and increase of vascular permeability, was established.

However, as in most feedback systems there may be a tendency to exaggerate one direction of the loop, assuming that in any case in which bradykinin was acting, prostaglandins may take the part of the lion, to explain most of the actions produced by Bk. This became apparent in the recent contribution by Needleman (1976) on the synthesis and function of prostaglandins in the heart, in which it is assumed that the effect of bradykinin on the heart, as described a long time ago in our laboratory (Antonio and Rocha e Silva, 1962), producing increased coronary flow and positive inotopic effect, would result from the synthesis of prostaglandins stimulated by bradykinin. Since this aspect is important and directly connected with your stress concept, I reproduce here the scheme of Needleman (Figure 8.1) to indicate that the phenomenon of relationship between mediators of *stress* can be very complicated. However, I think that the scheme proposed by Needleman is not complicated enough, since we have shown, with a graduate student of mine, Marco Morato, in collaboration with Abilio Antonio, in our laboratory that the scheme by Needleman cannot be as simple as that (Figure 8.1). With the isolated guinea pig heart (Langendorff's preparation) we have shown that under certain circumstances in which prostaglandins would not work, bradykinin continued to produce its coronary vasodilating and inotropic effects. This was particularly true if the perfused heart was submitted to the action of vasopressin (VP). By a pretreatment with VP (ADH), the beats and coronary flow would drop to levels incompatible with the continued work and vitality of the isolated guinea-pig heart preparation; if prostaglandin (PGE) was then injected, the situation was not very much changed, though if a sufficient dose of Bk (a few μg) was injected, there was an immediate change of the preparation with a normalization of the beat and perfusion flow (Refs. 59 to 62). The assumption that Bk works solely by promoting the synthesis of prostaglandins, can be completely excluded, in my opinion. Another possibility that has arisen by our experiments

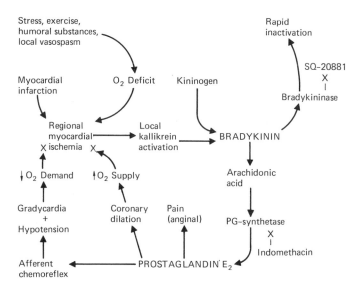

Figure 8.1. Hypothetical scheme for the interrelationship between bradykinin and prostaglandin in the isolated heart. According to Needleman (1976).

with the isolated heart of the guinea pig, is that PGs may release or activate the kinin system, which would strongly complicate the scheme presented in Figure 8.1. In other situations, as in pain production and increased vascular permeability in the rat's paw submitted to the action of phlogogenic agents, it has been repeatedly shown that even if prostaglandins are released or synthesized by bradykinin and at the same time potentiate its effect (on pain production, for instance), they (PGs) are presumably devoid of any algogenic activity and have rather trivial effects on vascular permeability. (See Refs. 57, 58.)

I cannot go too far in this synopsis of the autopharmacological aspects of the inflammatory reaction as a multimediated phenomenon, but would still like to *stress* the relationships between the release of Bk as a complex enzymatic phenomenon, and the no less complex phenomenon of blood clotting through the mediation of at least 15 factors, among which are the Hageman Factor (Factor XII), the Fletcher Factor, fibrinogen, and the activation of the plasminogen system into plasmin. All that became so involved with the kinin system that I refer to the scheme of Figure 8.2 and

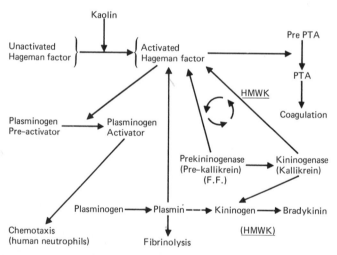

Figure 8.2. Interrelations between activation of bradykinin releasing enzymes (kininogenage or plasma kallikrein), plasmin, and the coagulation factors: Hageman Factor (Factor XII), plasma thromboplastin antecedent (PTA), Fletcher Factor (F.F.) = plasma pre-kininogenase or pre-kallikrein. The encircling arrows indicate a possible feedback loop, to which HMWK (high molecular weight kininogen) functions as a co-factor. According to Wuepper (1973), and Weiss, Gallin, and Kaplan (1974) and Meier et al. (1977) (Refs. 65, 66, 67).

to the current experiments by Kaplan, Movat, Greenbaum, Austen, Cochrane, and Wuepper, abundantly mentioned in the literature (Refs. 63 to 67). Those working on the chemistry of kininogen, in the United States, Canada, Japan, Germany, and Brazil, are also working on the biochemistry and the pharmacology of the phenomenon of activation of the kinin system and, therefore, are engaged in disentangling the phenomenon of stress, contributing to *stressology.* (See Refs. 72 to 89.)

I take the liberty of reminding you that there are always at least two ways to look at the world. We have been dealing up to now with pure pharmacological events, but somehow, by a closed circuit we came back to phenomena pertaining to *stress,* and I wish to analyze some general aspects of the difference in outlook of your school of thought and those who stick more to the analysis of the phenomena. You may have noticed that I did not mention the endocrinological aspects that are more in your line (Selye, 1971; Ref. 68), but rather those aspects that are studied by pharmacologists or biochemical pharmacologists. Though the biochemists do not like to be called pharmacologists, they are all doing some kind of biochemical pharmacology. We may notice that at the gigantic Biochemical Congresses, like the one held in Tokyo, in 1967, a considerable part of the program was filled with papers that intended to clarify some aspects of the mechanism of action of drugs. I would not, therefore, divide the world into a biochemical and a pharmacological one because they are the same. But there is another way to look at the world, and to those who have time, that is, the not-too-busy scientists, I would recommend the books by Castenada (2976) (Ref. 69) in which he describes the teachings of a Mexican sorcerer (brujo), Don Juan, of Sonora. There is a moment in which we don't know whether the author is really reporting his observations, or is playing a trick on us; but I was surprised to find in one of the books, the definition, or better the difference in "seeing" things or "looking at them," in agreement with what you said in your autobiographical sketch in the book edited by Klemm)1977) on *Discovery Processes in Modern Biology* (Ref. 70): "Looking and not seeing: There are two ways of detecting something that nobody can see: one is to aim at the finest details by getting as close as possible with the best available analysing instruments; the other is merely to look at things from a new angle when they show hitherto unexpected facets. The former requires money and experience; the latter presupposes neither; indeed it is actually aided by simplicity, the lack of prejudice, and the absence of those established habits of thinking which do tend to come after years of work.... Remember that the G.A.S. could have been discovered during the middle ages, if not earlier..." (Selye, 1977; Ref. 70).

That is the rub. The G.A.S. might have been defined by any good observer of the mechanism of disease, such as Hippocrates, Galen, Paracelsus, Harvey, Malpighi, Claude Bernard, Pasteur, or any of the modern biologists with an acute capacity for "looking at things." However, the participation of ACTH, corticoids, histamine, 5-HT, kinins, prostaglandins, and so forth could not, because such agents had a time to be recognized, and all depended upon their discoveries. They are *things* that did not exist in the high antiquity, in the Middle Ages, and even in the last century, and started to appear in the beginning of this century, when histamine was discovered in 1907, by Windaus and Vogt. Therefore, the two ways of looking at the world are not coincident but would translate two aspects of our vision of the world, much the same as the *tonal* and the *nagual* of the Mexican "brujos," as described in the last books by Castaneda (1976), *Separate Reality* and *Tales of Power* (Ref. 69). If you don't get hurt, we are living in the *tonal,* though you are plunged into the *nagual,* which accounts for your flying in the serene atmosphere of *stressology.* In a certain sense, we who live on the firmer grounds of the *tonal* are terrified when we think of flying away in the free spaces of the *nagual.* This is not a criticism but a strong manifestation of envy for not being able to abandon concrete substances as those of autopharmacology and plunge into the generalization of the general adaptation syndrome. But the contrast is strong enough to send the "not-too-busy scientist" to browse over the last chapters of *Tales of Power,* by Castaneda (1976). (See Refs. 69, 70.)

There is another way to look at the world, and that would be by analyzing the evolution, or better the revolutions of scientific knowledge, according to Kuhn's ideas of the structure of scientific revolutions; or else, according to the conceptions of Popper (Ref. 71) on the demarcation of a theory as scientific by the possibility of showing that it can be "falsified" by new facts or discoveries. I understand that both ways (Kuhn's and Popper's) are historiographical rather than epistemological, at least as far as biological theories are concerned. Kuhn's ideas of changing of paradigma may be useful in understanding the history of physical theories, and Popper's ideas not even that. From this point of view, the theories about the mediation of the inflammatory reaction are highly illuminating. In the first case, that is Kuhn's paradigma, we can see that many of the views of the same phenomena can still be valid, though in many cases contradictory. I recall that the participation of anaphylatoxin in anaphylactic phenomena, as put forward by Friedemann, Friedberger, and Bordet in the second decade of this century, and denoted by "the humoral theory of anaphylaxis," was considered for many years incompatible with the "histamine theory of anaphylaxis," as put forward by Dale and his collaborators (Refs. 1 to 5), especially after the paper by Dale and Kellaway (1922), in which anaphylatoxin was considered a mere artifact. The histamine theory became the most acceptable after the mentioned works by Feldberg, Dragstedt, Schild, Code, and many others (see Rocha e Silva, 1966; Ref. 22) showing the release of histamine in different forms of anaphylactic shock. By that time I had entered the field and tried to show that the release of histamine results from the activation of proteolytic enzymes resulting in cytolysis of platelets and leucocytes in the dog's and rabbit's anaphylaxis or in peptone shock (Rocha e Silva et al., 1938, 1939, 1940; Refs. in 22). That idea, that proteolytic enzymes were the nodal center of any pathological phenomenon, not only of those inducing anaphylaxis and allergy, led us to discover bradykinin, by using a snake venom (of the *B. jararaca*) containing a protease, and trypsin. Ever since, bradykinin has been the prototype of a peptide released by the partial breakdown of a protein (bradykininogen). In short succession, we had found with Hamberg (Refs. 73, 74) that the specific bradykinin-forming protease had the specificity of enzymes like trypsin, namely splitting substrates such as BAME and TAME. What was significant enough was that the protease contained in the venom of *B. jararaca* had a more specific capacity of splitting the bond holding Bk to bradykininogen (Bkg), though trypsin, which was found from the beginning to release Bk from Bkg, would complete the hydrolysis of the substrate (Bkg), resulting in products that no longer precipitated with TCA (Hamberg and Rocha e Silva, 1956; Rocha e Silva and Garcia-Leme, 1972; Rocha e Silva, 1970) as represented in Figure 8.3. To my knowledge, that was the first observation showing the possibility of separating a small peptide, with strong pharmacological activity from a bulky protein, as that represented by Bkg, part of the α_2-globulin fraction of plasma, through the specific action of a protease, as that contained in the venom of *B. jararaca*. Formation of angiotensin I and II is another example of partial hydrolysis generating an active peptide, but the proteolytic nature of renin was still questioned by the time bradykinin was discovered. Figure 8.3 shows this historical event which later on became the prototype of similar

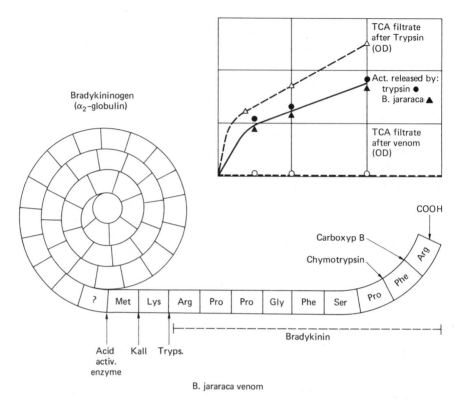

Figure 8.3. Nature of the linkages of bradykinin and related peptides to the globular protein molecule belonging to the α_2-complex of plasma globulins. In the *inset*, release of equivalents of Bk activity by the venom of *B. jararaca* and by trypsin. Note that for the same released activity, there was a total breakdown of the Bkg becoming soluble in 15% TCA, though with the venom, practically the whole substrate was still precipitable with TCA. This is a good example of partial hydrolysis, releasing a pharmacologically active agent from a high molecular weight protein (Hamberg and Rocha e Silva, 1957; Refs. 73, 74).

phenomena of partial hydrolysis of proteins, to study the release of active pharmacological principles. The whole field of the study of kallikreins (kininogenins) with Werle, Webster, Pierce, Pisano, Kaplan, Wuepper, Cochrane, Austen, Guimarães, and many others showed many important aspects of this phenomenon for biological and medical sciences. For reviews, see Erdös, 1970; Pisano, 1975; Pisano and Austin, 1976 (Refs. 45, 72, and 78).

But now, to finish this long letter, one last word to Kuhn's and Popper's views about the revolutions and falsifications of theories in biology and medicine. Even when a paradigma becomes exhausted or "falsified" by new facts or phenomena and transformed into a new one, the old paradigma can reappear like a phoenix from the ashes of the previous one. Along that line, we ended a recent review of the importance of kinins, to explain many aspects of inflammation and of physiological processes (Ref. 63) after being considered *démodé* (Ref. 36) by prostaglandins, in these words: "What we tried to demonstrate in this Minireview ('Present Trends of Kinin Research') is that the potentialities of the whole kinin field to penetrate deeper into important physiopathological phenomena are still great, and instead of being *démodé,* the bradykinin phase is still giving fruits in Auto-Pharmacology" (Rocha e Silva, 1974; Ref. 63).

Is that a different way to look at your "stress phenomenon" (*stressology*)? Maybe it is only complementary. It reminds me of those pictures made of fabrics produced by Indians of a certain island on the Panamanian coast, which they call *Mola,* with strange though beautiful figures of their folklore. To understand how they make them, we have to look at the *obverse* of the pictures and admire the network of different colored fabrics they used to make them.

To end this letter, I can see that after all I have been able to write a paper on "Stressology," which could fit your program for a *Guide to Stress Research.*

With my kindest personal regards, I am
Yours faithfully,
Prof. Mauricio Rocha e Silva
Fogarty International Center, NIH
Bethesda, Maryland 20014, U.S.A.

References

1. Dale, H. H. The Herter Lectures. I. Capillary poisons and shock. II. Anaphylaxis. III. Chemical structure and physiological actions. *Bull. Johns Hopkins Hosp. 31:* 257–265, 1920.
2. Dale, H. H. Progress in autopharmacology. *Bull. Johns Hopkins Hosp. 53:* 297–347, 1933.
3. Dale, H. H., and Laidlaw, P. P. The physiological action of β-iminazolylethylamine. *J. Physiol. (Lond.) 41:* 318–344, 1910.
4. Dale, H. H. Some chemical factors in the control of the circulation. Lecture III. Local vasodilator reactions. *Lancet 1:* 1285–1290, 1929.
5. Dale, H. H. and Kellaway, C. H. Anaphylaxis and anaphylatoxins. *Phil. Trans. B. 211:* 273–315, 1922.
6. Rocha e Silva, M., Scroggie, A. E., Fidlar, E., and Jaques, L. B. Liberation of

histamine and heparin by peptone from isolated dog's liver. *Proc. Soc. Exp. Biol. Med. 64:* 141–146, 1947.

7. Leger, J., and Masson, G. Effect of antihistamine substances on edema produced by egg white. *Am. J. Med. Sci. 214:* 305–307, 1947.

8. Leger, J. and Masson, G. Studies on egg white sensitivity in rat, influence of endocrine glands. *Ann. Allergy 6:* 131–143, 1948.

9. Leger, J., Masson, G. and Prado, J. L. Reaction oedemateuse chez le rat. Influence des substances anti-histaminiques. *Rev. Can. Biol. 6:* 359–361, 1947a.

10. Leger, J., Masson, G., and Prado, J. L. Hypersensitivity to egg white in rat. *Proc. Soc. Exp. Biol. Med. 64:* 306–370, 1947b.

11. Halpern, B. N. Substances histamino-libératrices et processus de libération de l'histamine endogène. *Actualités Pharmacologiques 13:* 109–129, 1960.

12. Bartosch, R., Feldberg, W., and Nagel, E. Das Freiwerden eines histaminähnlichen Stoffes bei der Anaphylaxie des Meerschweinchens. *Pflügers Archiv Ges. Physiol. 230:* 129–153, 1932.

13. Dragstedt, C. A. and Gebauer-Fuelnegg, E. Studies in anaphylaxis. I. The appearance of a physiologically active substance during anaphylactic shock. *Am. J. Physiol. 102:* 512–519, 1932.

14. Schild, H. O. Histamine release and anaphylactic shock in isolated lungs of guinea-pigs. *Quart. J. Exp. Physiol. 26:* 165–179, 1936.

15. Code, C. F. The histamine content of the blood of guinea pigs and dogs during anaphylactic shock. *Am. J. Physiol. 127:* 78–93, 1939.

16. Katz, G. Histamine release from blood cells in anaphylaxis *in vitro. Science 91:* 221, 1940.

17. Katz, G. Histamine release in the allergic skin reaction. *Proc. Soc. Exp. Biol. Med. 49:* 272–277, 1942.

18. Riley, J. F., and West, G. E. The presence of histamine in tissue mast-cells. *J. Physiol. 210:* 528–537, 1953.

19. Riley, J. F. *The Mast Cells.* Edinburgh: E. & S. Livingstone, 1959.

20. Mota, I. Release of histamine from mast cells. In *Handbook Exp. Pharmacol.* Vol. XVIII/I. Berlin, Heidelberg, New York: Springer-Verlag, 1966, pp. 569–636.

21. Selye, H. *The Mast Cells.* Washington, D.C.: Butterworths, 1965.

22. Rocha e Silva, M. (ed.). Histamine and antihistaminics. *Handbook Exp. Pharmakol.* Vol. XVIII/I: *Histamine.* Berlin, Heidelberg, New York: Springer-Verlag, 1966.

23. Rocha e Silva, M. (ed.). Histamine and ant.histaminics. *Handbook Exp. Pharmacol.,* Vol. XVIII/II. Berlin, Heidelberg, New York: Springer-Verlag, 1977.

24. Goth, A. On the general problem of histamine release. Ibid., 1977, pp. 57–74.

25. Uvnäs, B. The mechanism of histamine release from mast cells. Ibid., 1977, pp. 75–92.

26. Chakravarty, N. Metabolic changes in mast cells associated with histamine release. Ibid., 1977, pp. 93–108.

27. Majno, J., and Palade, G. E. Studies on inflammation. I. Effect of histamine and serotonin on vascular permeability. *J. Biophys. Biochem. Cytol. 11:* 571–605, 1961.

28. Majno, G., Palade, G. E., and Schoefl, G. I. Studies on Inflammation. II. The site of action of histamine and serotonin along the vascular tree. A topographic study. *J. Biophys. Biochem. Cytol. 11:* 607–626, 1961.

29. Rowley, D. A., and Benditt, E. P. 5-Hydroxytryptamine and histamine as mediators of the vascular injury produced by agents which damage mast cells. *J. Exp. Med. 103:* 399–412, 1956.

30. Rocha e Silva, M., Beraldo, W. T., and Rosenfeld, G. A new factor (bradykinin) released from plasma globulin by snake venom and trypsin. *Am. J. Physiol. 156:* 261–273, 1949.

31. Rocha e Silva, M. The bradykinin story. In Klemm (ed.), *Discovery Processes in Modern Biology.* Huntington, New York: R. E. Krieger, Publish. Co., 1977.

32. Selye, H. Biological adaptations to stress. Ibid., 1977, pp. 266–288.

33. Euler, U. S. von. Zur Kenntnis der pharmakologischen Wirkung von Nativsekreten und Extrakten männlicher accessorischer Geschlechtsdrüsen. *Arch. Exp. Pathol. Pharmakol. 175:* 78–84, 1934.

34. Euler, U. S. von. On the specific vasodilating substances from accessory genital glands in man and certain animals (prostaglandin and vesiglandin). *J. Physiol. (Lond.) 98:* 213–234, 1936.

35. Vane, J. R. Inhibition of prostaglandin synthesis as a mechanism of action for aspirin-like drugs. *Nature, New Biology 231:* 232–235, 1971.

36. Vane, J. R. Inflammatory substances. A book review. *Nature 214:* 141, 1973.

37. Vane, J. R. Prostaglandins and aspirin-like drugs. In *Proc. 5th Internat. Congr. Pharmacol.,* San Francisco, 1972. Basel: Karger, 1974, pp. 352–378.

38. Rocha e Silva, M. Opening remarks to a symposium on inflammation, Rib. Preto, 1973. *Agents and Actions 3:* 265–266, 1973.

39. Sicuteri, F., Rocha e Silva, M., and Back, N. (eds.). Bradykinin and related kinins. Cardiovascular, biochemical and neural actions. Symposium, Fiesole, 1969. *Advances Exp. Med. Biol.,* Vol. 8. New York: Plenum Press, 1970.

40. Back, N., and Sicuteri, F., (eds.). Vasopeptides: Chemistry, pharmacology and pathophysiology. Symposium Fiesole (1971). *Advances Exp. Med. Biol.,* Vol. 21. New York: Plenum Press, 1972.

41. Ryan, J. W., and Rocha e Silva, M. Release of kinins by acidified bovine pseudoglobulin. *Biochem. Pharmacol. 20:* 459–462, 1971.

42. Reis, M. L., Okino, L., and Rocha e Silva, M. Comparative pharmacological actions of bradykinin and related kinins of larger molecular weight. *Biochem. Pharmacol. 20:* 2935–2946, 1971.

43. Rocha e Silva, M. *Kinin Hormones. With special reference to bradykinin and related kinins.* Springfield, Illinois: Charles C Thomas, 1970.

44. Rocha e Silva, M., and Garcia-Leme, J. *Chemical Mediators of the Acute Inflammatory Reaction.* Oxford: Pergamon Press, 1972.

45. Erdös, E. G. (ed.). Bradykinin, kallidin and kallikrein. *Handbook Exp. Pharmacol.,* Vol. XXV. Berlin, Heidelberg, New York: Springer Verlag, 1970.

46. Rocha e Silva, M., and Dragstedt, C. A. Observations of trypan blue capillary permeability test in rabbits. *J. Pharmacol. Exp. Ther. 73:* 405–411, 1941.

47. Jasmin, G., and Robert, A. (eds.). *The Mechanism of Inflammation,* An International Symposium. Montreal: Acta Inc., 1953.

48. Menkin, V. The role of inflammation on immunity. *Physiol. Rev. 18:* 366–418, 1938.

49. Menkin, V. *Dynamics of Inflammation.* New York: Macmillan, 1940.

50. Bier, O. G., and Rocha e Silva, M. Untersuchungen über Entzündung. I. Mechanismus der Erhöhung der Capillarpermeabilität mit besonderer Berücksichtigung der Rolle des Histamins. *Virchow's Archiv Pathol. Anat. 303:* 325–336, 1939.
51. Miles, A. A., and Miles, E. M. Vascular reaction to histamine, histamine liberator (compound 48/80, phenylethylamine compounds) and leukotaxine in skin of guinea pigs. *J. Physiol. (Lond.) 118:* 228–257, 1952.
52. Rocha e Silva, M., and Rothschild, H. A. (eds.). *Symposium on Vasoactive Polypeptides: Bradykinin and Related Kinins.* Rib. Preto, 1966. Sao Paulo: Edart Edit., 1967.
53. Gaddum, J. H. (ed.). *Polypeptides which Stimulate Plain Muscles and Blood Vessels* (Symposium. Montreal, 1953). Edinburgh: E. & S. Livingstone, 1955.
54. Rocha e Silva, M. Bradykinin: Occurrence and properties. Ibid., 1953, pp. 45–47.
55. van Arman, C. G. Interrelationship among some peptide precursors. Ibid., 1953, pp. 103–114.
56. Kuhn, T. S. *The Structure of Scientific Revolutions.* Chicago: University of Chicago Press, 1971.
57. Ferreira, S. H., Moncada, S., and Vane, J. R. Potentiation by prostaglandins of the nociceptive activity of bradykinin in the dog knee joint. *Brit. J. Pharmacol. 50:* 461 P, 1974.
58. Moncada, S., Ferreira, S. H., and Vane, J. R. Sensitization of pain receptors of dog knee joint by prostaglandins. In Robinson, H. J., and Vane, J. R. (eds.), *Prostaglandin Synthetase Inhibitors.* New York: Raven Press, 1974.
59. Needleman, P., Key, S. L., Denny, P. C., Isakson, P. C., and Marshall, G. R. The mechanism and modification of bradykinin-induced coronary vasodilation. *Proc. Natl. Acad. Sci. USA 72:* 2060–2075, 1975.
60. Needleman, P. The synthesis and function of prostaglandins in the heart. *Fed. Proc. 35:* 2376–2381, 1976.
61. Antonio, A., and Rocha e Silva, M. Coronary vasodilation produced by bradykinin on the isolated mammalian heart. *Circul. Res. 11:* 910–915, 1962.
62. Rocha e Silva, M., Morato, M., Almeida, A. P., and Antonio, A. In Sicuteri, F., Back, N., and Haberland, G. L. (eds.), *Kinins,* Pharmacodynamics and biological roles, Symposium Fiesole (1975). *Advances Exp. Med. Biol.,* Vol. 70. New York: Plenum Press, 1976.
63. Rocha e Silva, M. Minireview. Present trends of kinin research. *Life Sciences 15:* 7–22, 1974.
64. Rocha e Silva, M. Kinin trail. Possible significance of bradykinin and related kinins to auto-pharmacology. *Proc. 5th Internat. Congr. Pharmacol.,* San Francisco, Basel: Karger, 5: 250–266, 1973.
65. Weiss, A. S., Gallin, J. I., and Kaplan, A. P. Fletcher factor deficiency. A diminished role of Hageman factor caused by absence of prekallikrein with abnormalities of coagulation, fibrinolytic, chemotactic activity and kinin generation. *J. Clin. Invest. 53:* 622–633, 1974. See also Meier, H. L., et al. Activation and function of human Hageman factor. *J. Clin. Invest. 60:* 18–31, 1977.
66. Wuepper, K. D., Lawrence, T. G., and Cochrane, C. G. Proenzyme components of the plasma-kinin system. (Abstr.) *J. Clin. Investig. 49:* 105a, 1970.

67. Wuepper, K. D. Prekallikrein deficiency in man. *J. Exp. Med. 138:* 1345–1355, 1973.
68. Selye, H. *Hormones and Resistance.* I and II. Berlin, Heidelberg, New York: Springer-Verlag, 1971.
69. Castaneda, C. *Separate Reality,* and *Tales of Power.* New York: Pocket Books Co., 1976.
70. Klemm, W. R. (ed.). *Discovery Processes in Modern Biology.* Huntington, New York: R. E. Krieger Publish. Co., 1977.
71. Popper, K. *Unended Quest: An Intellectual Autobiography.* London: Fontana Collins, 1976.
72. Pisano, J. J. Chemistry and biology of the kallikrein-kinin system. In *Proteases and Biological Control.* Cold Spring Harbor Library, 1975, pp. 199–222.
73. Hamberg, U., and Rocha e Silva, M. On the release of bradykinin by trypsin and snake venom. *Arch. Internat. Pharmacodynamie 110:* 222–238, 1957a.
74. Hamberg, U., and Rocha e Silva, M. Release of bradykinin as related to the esterase activity of trypsin and the venom of *Bothrops jararaca. Experientia 13:* 489–490, 1957b.
75. Guimarães, J. A., Borges, D. R., Prado, E. S., and Prado, J. L. Kinin-converting aminopeptidase from human serum. *Biochem. Pharmacol. 22:* 3157–3172, 1973.
76. Guimarães, J. A., Chen Lu, R., Webster, M., and Pierce, J. V. Multiple forms of human plasma kininogen. (Abstr.) *Fed. Proc. 33:* 641, 1974.
77. Prado, J. L. Proteolytic enzymes as kininogenases. In Erdös, E. G. (ed.), *Handbook Exp. Pharmacology,* Vol. XXV, pp. 156–192, 1970.
78. Pisano, J. J., and Austen, K. F. (eds.). *Chemistry and Biology of the Kallikrein-Kinin System in Health and Disease.* Symposium, Reston, Va., Fogarty Internat. Center (1974), Proc. no. 27. Washington, D.C.: U.S. Government Printing Office, 1976.
79. Haberland, G. L. and Rohen, J. W. Edits. *Kininogenases, Kallikrein.* New York: Publish. K. L. Schattauer, 1973.
80. Movat, H. Z., Steinberg, S. G., Habal, F. M., and Ranadive, N. Demonstration of a kinin-generating enzyme in the lysosomes of human polymorphonuclear leucocytes. *Lab. Invest. 29:* 669–684, 1973.
81. Oshima, G., Gecse, A., and Erdös, E. G. Angiotensin I converting enzyme of the kidney cortex. *Biochem. Biophys. Acta 350:* 26–37, 1974.
82. Oshima, G., Kato, J., and Erdos, E. G. Subunits of human plasma carboxypeptidase N (kininase I; anaphylatoxin mediator). *Biochem. Biophys. Acta 365:* 344–348, 1974.
83. Erdös, E. G., Back, N., and Sicuteri, F. (eds.). *Hypotensive Peptides.* Symposium, Florence, 1965. New York: Springer-Verlag, 1966.
84. Ryan, J. W., Roblero, J., and Stewart, J. M. Inactivation of bradykinin in the pulmonary circulation. *Biochem. J. 110:* 795–797, 1968.
85. Ferreira, S. H., Moncada, S., and Vane, J. R. Prostaglandins and the mechanism of analgesia produced by aspirin-like drugs. *Brit. J. Pharmacol. 49:* 86–97, 1973.
86. Diniz, C. R., and Carvalho, I. V. A micromethod for the determination of bradykininogen under several conditions. *Ann. N.Y. Acad. Sci. 104:* 77–89, 1963.

87. Jacobson, S., and Kritz, M. Some data on two purified kininogens from human plasma. *Brit. J. Pharmacol. 29:* 25–36, 1967.
88. Komiya, M., Kato, H., and Suzuki, T. Bovine plasma kininogens. I. Further purification of high molecular weight kininogen and its physicochemical properties (I, II, III). *J. Biochemistry 76:* 811–822, 823–832, and 833–845, 1974.
89. Lewis, G. P. Kinins in inflammation and tissue injury. In Erdös, E. G. (ed.), *Handbook Exp. Pharmacol.,* Vol. XXV, pp. 516–530, 1970.

9.
Endorphins and Stress

Jean Rossier,* Floyd E. Bloom, and Roger Guillemin
The Salk Institute, La Jolla, California

I. INTRODUCTION

In 1973, three different laboratories (55, 69, 71) simultaneously reported that brain membranes contain specific receptors for opiates. Using synaptosomal membrane preparations, opiates were bound in a stereospecific fashion. Such preparations were further able to differentiate between opiate agonists and antagonists. In the absence of sodium, both agonists and antagonists bind firmly to receptor sites; in the presence of sodium, agonists bind much less tightly than antagonists (56, 70). The importance of this discovery of opiate receptors was further enhanced when it was shown that opiate receptors were heavily concentrated in brain regions implicated in pain perception and also in the limbic system (38).

These observations stimulated many workers to search for possible endogenous ligands for these receptors. These ligands were characterized in the brain at the end of the year 1975 (36).

These endogenous opioid ligands, which have been extracted from brain and pituitary, have been called "endorphins" after the suggestion of E. Simon: *endo*genous m*orphine* substances. Despite their relatively brief recorded history, endorphins have already become a household word in neuropharmacology. Furthermore, our thoughts on how these peptides may function in brain and pituitary in conditions such as stress, and how the several individual peptides are related to each other, have undergone several phases of revision. At the time of the original molecular identifi-

*Chargé de Recherche INSERM.

cation of Met[5]-enkephalin (M-e) and Leu[5]-enkephalin (L-e) (36), the possibility of one or more other endorphins of pituitary origin had already been suggested (13, 26, 27, 59, 72). When sequencing studies of the purified M-e revealed it to be the N-terminal pentapeptide (36) of the erstwhile pituitary hormone β-lipotropin (B-LPH) (40, 41) (see the sequence in Figure 9.1), the possibility that B-LPH was the prohormone of at least pituitary M-e was temporarily viable. In fact, that possibility appeared to be strengthened by the subsequent isolation, purification, sequencing, and synthesis of α-endorphin (A-E) (30, 45, 46), β-endorphin (B-E) called also C-fragment (10, 14, 15, 28, 42–44, 47), γ-endorphin (G-E) (45–47), and δ-endorphin (D-E) called also C'-fragment (20, 29), all of which fragments of B-LPH were found to be extractable from brain adn pituitary, to exhibit some action as specific opioid agonists, and to contain M-e as their N-terminal pentapeptide (see Table 9.1 for structures). When subsequent tests in vitro (10, 14, 39) and in vivo (8, 9, 11, 28, 48) revealed that B-E was by far the most potent and longest-acting of the natural peptides, some workers concluded that the transient opioid actions of M-e and L-e indicated that these substances were merely weakly active breakdown products of the naturally active hormone, B-E (11, 23, 26, 68). Others interpreted the same data to mean that the natural "neuro-

β-LIPOTROPIN AND ITS NEUROTROPIC SUBUNITS

H·Glu-Leu-Ala-Gly-Ala-Pro-Pro-Glu-Pro-Ala-Arg-Asp-Pro-Glu-Ala-
  　　　　5　　　　　　　　　　　10　　　　　　　　　　15

Pro-Ala-Glu-Gly-Ala-Ala-Ala-Arg-Ala-Glu-Leu-Glu-Tyr-Gly-Leu-
  　　　20　　　　　　　　　　25　　　　　　　　　　30

Val-Ala-Glu-Ala-Gln-Ala-Ala-Glu-Lys-Lys-Asp-Glu-Gly-Pro-Tyr-
  　　　35　　　　　　　　　　40　　　　　　　　　　45

Lys-Met-Glu-His-Phe-Arg-Trp-Gly-Ser-Pro-Pro-Lys-Asp-Lys-Arg-
  　　　50　　　　　　　　　　55　　　　　　　　　　60

|Tyr-Gly-Gly-Phe-Met|Thr-Ser-Glu-Lys-Ser-Gln-Thr-Pro-Leu-Val-
61　　　　　　　65 **e**　　　　　　　70　　　　　　　　75

Thr|Leu|Phe-Lys-Asn-Ala-Ile-Val-Lys-Asn-Ala-His-Lys-Lys-Gly-
  α'　γ　　　　　80　　　　　　　85　　　　　　　90

porcine　　　　　　　　　　　　　　　　　　　　　Gln|OH
　　　　　　　　　　　　　　　　　　　　　　　　　　　β'

Figure 9.1. Amino acids sequence of β-LPH.

Table 9.1 Structure of the Opioid Peptides

	SEQUENCE	AUTHORS	
β-endorphin (B-E) or C-fragment	B-LPH$_{61-91}$	Bradbury et al., 1976	(9)
		Li et al., 1976	(43)
δ-endorphin (D-E) or C'-fragment	B-LPH$_{61-87}$	Bradbury et al., 1976	(9)
α-endorphin (A-E)	B-LPH$_{61-76}$	Guillemin et al., 1976	(30)
γ-endorphin (G-E)	B-LPH$_{61-77}$	Ling et al., 1976	(46)
Met^5-enkephalin (M-e)	B-LPH$_{61-65}$	Hughes et al., 1975	(36)
Leu^5-enkephalin (L-e)	Tyr-Gly-Gly-Phe-Leu	Hughes et al., 1975	(36)

transmitters'' opioid peptides were the succinctly acting M-e and L-e (66, 67), while the B-e was in their view to be regarded exclusively as a pituitary product whose longer duration of action was explicable by the protection from peptidic cleavage afforded by the greater length of the peptide chain. Curiously, this greater length did not improve the potency or duration of A-E, D-E, or G-E (8). Nevertheless, all workers seemed agreeable to the idea that opiate receptors in innervated tissues really represented the natural receptors to the endorphins and enkephalins.

Realistically, better definition of the roles and relations of these peptides was dependent upon the development of perfected methods for the optimal preservation and extraction (60) of the individual peptides and, equally as important, the development of specific antisera for radioimmunoassay (RIA) (31) and immunocytochemical localization of their storage sites in brain and pituitary (5, 6, 63). The results of such studies have just become known, and force the realization (1) that B-E-containing cells exist in both brain and pituitary (5, 6, 63); (2) that their regional distribution is different from that of the enkephalins in both brain (6, 7, 63) and pituitary (5, 63); and (3) that while B-E in brain and pituitary may be derived from B-LPH (27, 39) and be the source of A-E, G-E, and M-E (68), B-E and B-LPH cannot be the metabolic source of L-e. Finally, comparison of the actions of B-E with those of the enkephalins on central and peripheral receptors has led to the postulation there may not be simply a single, monolithic class of endorphin receptors which is acceptable to all the peptides, but rather that some receptors may be peptide-specific (49).

With these rapidly-evolving, revisionist views in mind, we have structured the present review chapter with the intention of surveying the relation of endorphins to stress.

II. NEURONS CONTAINING B-E EXIST SEPARATELY FROM THOSE CONTAINING ENKEPHALINS

Using specific radioimmunoassays we have shown that rat brain contains significant amounts of B-E (63). These B-E levels were unchanged in animals hypophysectomized for six to nine months (63). The regional distribution of B-E in rat brain shows no fixed relationship to radioimmunoassayable enkephalins (63), and many areas reported to be rich in enkephalin immunoreactivity (19, 33–35, 65, 74) are devoid of detectable B-E (see Table 9.2). We have also shown that immunocytochemical localization studies reveal B-E-containing neuronal perikarya and fiber tracts throughout the diencephalon, which can be clearly distinguished cytologically and immunologically from those cells and fibers observed to be enkephalin-containing neurons (19, 33–35, 65, 74).

B-E immunoreactive neuronal perikarya are localized in the basal tuberal hypothalamus (4). Varicose nerve fibers were distributed to the midline nuclear nucleus areas throughout the diencephalon and anterior pons (4).

Table 9.2 Distribution of Opioid Peptides in Brain and Pituitary Gland

	β-ENDORPHIN		ENKEPHALIN		
Pituitary	ng/mg tissue		mU-Enk/mg tissue		
whole	269 ± 20	(11)	72 ± 4		(6)
adenohypophysis	128 ± 9	(3)	3.7 ± 0.7		(3)
neurohypophysis and					
pars intermedia	1500 ± 600	(3)	740 ± 47		(3)
Pineal	ng/mg tissue		mU-Enk/mg tissue		
	4.8 ± 0.8	(10)	19 ± 2		(7)
Brain	ng/g tissue		U-Enk/g tissue		
whole	108 ± 8	(10)	25 ± 2		(6)
hypothalamus	490 ± 30	(5)	120 ± 7		(6)
septum	234 ± 34	(3)	85 ± 7		(6)
midbrain	207 ± 15	(5)	32 ± 1		(6)
medulla and pons	179 ± 5	(5)	30 ± 4		(6)
striatum	none	(5)	112 ± 11		(6)
globus pallidus			566 ± 23		(4)
hippocampus	none	(5)	13 ± 1		(6)
cortex	none	(5)	15 ± 2		(6)
cerebellum	none	(5)	5 ± 1		(6)

Means and standard error of the means; number of animals in parenthesis. One unit of immunoreactive enkephalin corresponds to 1 ng Leu⁵-enkephalin or 30 ng Met⁵-enkephalin.

Enkephalin fibers have a much broader distribution through the entire brain and spinal cord. Intense immunoreactivity with antisera to the enkephalin pentapeptides was visualized in the globus pallidus, central nucleus of the amygdala, and substantia gelatinosa. Sections of these enkephalin-rich regions showed no immunoreactivity when reacted with the anti-B-E sera. The diencephalon contains high amount of both enkephalin and B-E-immunoassayable material (see Table 9.2).

Serial section staining of diencephalic fields allowed direct comparison of fibers which were immunoreactive with the antisera to enkephalins and to B-E. A detailed, nucleus-by-nucleus analysis will be required for complete comparisons; however, in most cases the neuropil patterns and morphology of the reactive fibers permitted clear-cut separations. B-E reactive fibers could be traced for hundreds of micra within a given section, and they exhibited thick round varicosities of 3–5 μ. Enkephalin reactive fibers instead are 19, 33–35, 65, 74) isolated reactive dots, and these structures are much finer and rarely appeared to show connectedness for more than a hundred micra.

These recent observations indicate that B-E reactive neurons and nerve fibers exist within rat brain and are anatomically separable from those central neurons containing the enkephalin pentapeptides. These observations support the view (63) that enkephalins and B-E are contained within separate cellular systems in brain. Moreover, these observations suggest that the functional roles of these separate systems may be more diverse than the general term "opioid peptide" has been taken to imply until now.

III. BRAIN ENDORPHINS AND STRESS

Akil et al. (2) have shown that acute stress induced by inescapable electric foot shock promotes analgesia in rats and that this analgesic effect of stress was partially reversed by naloxone, a morphine antagonist. Simultaneously with that report, the explosion of observations began which characterized the endogenous brain peptides with opioid activity, enkephalins and endorphins. Therefore, it was tempting to seek correlations between the stress-induced analgesia and the levels of the brain opioid peptides. Madden et al. (50) reported that levels of opioid brain materials were increased after stress. That study, however, used radio–receptor displacement assays which cannot distinguish among the several endogenous peptides that share this biological property in vitro. Therefore, it was revealing when Fratta et al. (22), using a radioimmunoassay for M-e, were unable to detect any increase in brain immunoreactive material after stress. However, they proposed that another opioid peptide, B-E, could have been mobilized from the pituitary by stress to accumulate in brain tissue.

We have observed that when B-E is mobilized from the pituitary during stress and accumulates up to sixfold in plasma, the released B-E does not accumulate in brain (see section VI). On the contrary, hypothalamic levels of B-E are slightly, but significantly, reduced after the same 30-minute episode of electric foot-shock stress. (See Figure 9.2.) No change was observed in B-E immunoreactivity in other regions of the brain, the pineal, or the pituitary (61).

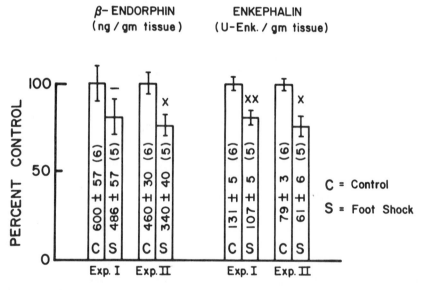

Figure 9.2. Hypothalamus content in opioid peptides after acute stress. Two stress protocols were used. In experiment 1 (Exp. I) animals were stressed for 1 h by inescapable electric footshocks (1 mA, 1 sec duration at random 12 per min) and killed after the last shock. In experiment II (Exp. II) the foot shocks were given for only 30 min, and after a delay of 15 min after the shocks the animals were killed. In both experiments, brains were quickly removed and dissected. The tissues were frozen on dry ice, weighed, and poured into 2 ml of 1 M aceic acid preheated to 98°C. After 15 min in the boiling bath, the tissues were homogenized (polytron, setting 6,10 s). After centrifugation (1,000g for 1 h) the supernatant was neutralized with 1 M NaOH and frozen before RIA. Results are expressed in ng per g of tissue for B-E and in units for L-e.

We have also observed that L-e levels in the hypothalamus were also decreased by around 20% after the same foot-shock stress. No change was observed in the other parts of the brain (cortex, thalamus, medulla, pons, hippocampus, cerebellum, and striatum), the pineal, or the pituitary (62).

Previously Fratta et al. (22) had observed that foot-shock-induced stress produced a 25% decrease of the hypothalamic content M-e immunoreactivity. However, as the difference between control and stressed groups was not statistically significant, Fratta et al. (22) had concluded that foot-shock-induced stress had no effect on the hypothalamic enkephalin levels.

Our results (Figure 9.2) show that in two different experimental conditions, foot-shock-induced stress produces a decrease of the hypothalamic L-e immunoreactivity. In both experimental protocols, the differences between controls and stressed animals were statistically significant. It can therefore be concluded that prolonged stress decreases the hypothalamic content of Leu^5-enkephalin immunoreactivity. We have also shown that B-E hypothalamic levels were decreased by such stress. Having demonstrated (4, 63) that B-E-containing neurons are different from those containing enkephalin, we propose that both sets of hypothalamic neurons are activated in response to this type of stress.

IV. B-E, B-LPH, and ACTH MAY BE SYNTHESIZED INTO A COMMON PRECURSOR IN THE PITUITARY

In the pituitary, our immunocytochemical and radioimmunoassay studies had indicated that B-E was found in every cell of the intermediate lobe and in isolated cells—corresponding to those reactive to antisera against ACTH—in the adenohypophysis (5). Previously, several groups of investigators had also found that ACTH and B-LPH were present in the same adenohypophyseal cells (17, 52, 54). Using an ACTH antiserum and serial sections to identify the corticotropic cells, they found that B-LPH immunoreactivity was also present in these cells. By electron microscopy it was also shown that both ACTH and B-LPH were present in only one cell type, which were found to be corticotrops on the basis of cytological criteria. In these cells both ACTH and B-LPH were mainly concentrated in secretory granules (54).

B-LPH contains the entire sequence of beta-MSH (B-LPH$_{41-58}$). It was shown by immunocytology that ACTH and B-MSH immunoreactivities are both present in the corticotropic adenohypophyseal cells of several species (16, 18, 53, 57). These observations suggest, therefore, that ACTH, B-LPH, and B-E and B-MSH are synthesized in the same hypophyseal cells.

For several years, the pituitary has been known to contain more than one molecular form of ACTH. The higher molecular weight forms of ACTH were called ''big ACTH.'' Recently, Mains, Eipper, and Ling (51) have identified in normal pituitaries several high molecular weight glycoprotein forms of ACTH with molecular weights of 31,000, 23,000, and 13,000 (designated 31k ACTH, 23k ACTH, and 13k ACTH, respectively). The molecular weight of ACTH$_{1-39}$ is 4,500 daltons.

Mains and co-workers (51) have used the ACTH-secreting mouse pituitary tumor cell line AtT-20 in order to study the kinetics of the ACTH synthesis. They found that the largest, 31k ACTH, is the precursor of the smaller forms of ACTH, and 23k ACTH is a biosynthetic intermediate. In the course of their experiments on the structure of 31k ACTH and 23k ACTH labeled with pulses of tritiated amino acids, analysis of tryptic peptides suggested that the fragments cleaved off during the conversion of 31k ACTH to 23k ACTH might be similar to B-LPH. Using well-characterized antisera to either ACTH or B-E, pulse-labeled cell products were indeed found to be immunoprecipitated. Peptide analysis of the immunoprecipitates showed that 31k ACTH contained peptide sequences similar to both ACTH and B-E, and therefore that ACTH and B-E had a common precursor.

Roberts and Herbert (58) have also characterized this common precursor to ACTH and B-LPH, using a cell-free system. When RNA messenger from cultures of the mouse pituitary tumor cells (AtT-20) is translated in a reticulocyte cell-free system, an immunoprecipitable ACTH peptide is synthesized with an apparent molecular weight of 28,500. The same-size-molecular-weight ACTH molecule is made when polysomes from AtT-20 cells direct the cell-free synthesis of protein. Using immunoprecipitation and tryptic peptides analysis, Roberts and Hubert (58) also demonstrated that the moleclar-weight-28,500 cell-free product contained the sequence of both ACTH and B-E.

The precursors characterized by Mains et al. (51) and by Roberts and Herbert (58) are slightly different in terms of their molecular weight, respectively 31,000 and 28,500. The difference appears to be due to the carbohydrate moieties which are incorporated in the 31k ACTH when the

AtT-20 cells are incubated. Posttranslation incorporation of carbohy-drates does not occur in the reticulocyte cell-free system used by Roberts and Herbert.

V. B-E AND ACTH ARE SECRETED CONCOMITANTLY BY THE PITUITARY GLAND

In the previous In the previous section it was shown that the two biologi-cally active polypeptides ACTH and B-E are part of a much larger precur-sor glycoprotein of 31,000 daltons. The common-precursor concept was supported by earlier data on immunocytochemistry of normal pituitary tissue; ACTH, B-LPH, the immediate B-E precursor, and the biologically active peptide B-E are all present in the anterior and intermediate lobes of the pituitary gland (5). These observations gave rise to the possibility that ACTH and B-E levels in the pituitary should vary in parallel if their synthesis was coupled.

Table 9.3 shows that ACTH and B-E immunoassayable levels in the pituitary and in blood do show close correlation. Long-term administra-tion of dexamethasone is known to decrease ACTH levels in blood and the pituitary. Such long-term treatment also decreased the B-E levels of blood and the pituitary. On the other hand adrenalectomy is known to increase ACTH levels in blood and the pituitary, and adrenalectomy also increased B-E levels in blood and the pituitary (32).

It is quite striking to note that even the absolute levels of ACTH and B-E are in any circumstances very close (i.e., molar equivalent) to each other. These recent data support the concept that B-E and ACTH are accumulated and secreted in an equimolar ratio (32).

Previously, a number of investigators noticed that ACTH and B-LPH were related peptides, in that B-LPH and B-MSH (B-LPH$_{41-58}$) and ACTH were secreted in response to the same stimuli (1, 3, 24). Abe et al. (1) were the first to develop a sensitive radioimmunoassay for human B-MSH. They showed that circulating levels of B-MSH immunoreactiv-ity closely parallel those of bioactive ACTH (1). Plasma levels were elevated in patients with Cushing's disease, with Addison's disease, and with ectopic tumors secreting ACTH (1). Both B-MSH and ACTH were elevated after surgical stress (laparotomy) (1). Levels of both peptides were decreased after dexamethasone treatment. On the other hand, both ACTH and B-MSH levels are increased after a metyrapone test (1). These

Table 9.3 Plasma and Pituitary Concentrations of Adrenocorticotropin (ACTH) and β-Endorphin, as Modified by Adrenalectomy and Administration of Dexamethasone, and, for Plasma Levels, as Modified by Hypophysectomy

TREATMENT	PLASMA (NG/ML)		WHOLE PITUITARY (μG/GLAND)		ADENOHYPOPHYSIS (μG/GLAND)	
	ACTH	β-ENDORPHIN	ACTH	β-ENDORPHIN	ACTH	β-ENDORPHIN
None (controls)	0.8 ± 0.2 (3)*	1.5 ± 0.2 (9)	4.8 ± 0.3 (3)	2.6 ± 0.2 (11)	2.7 ± 0.5 (3)	1.1 ± 0.2 (3)
Adrenalectomy	8.8 ± 1.6 (3)	8.8 ± 1.0 (6)†	9.9 ± 1.1 (3)†	10.8 ± 1.5 (3)†	8.3 ± 1.1 (3)†	5.4 ± 0.7 (3)†
Dexamethasone	< 0.2 (6)‡	< 1 (7)‡	2.1 ± 0.1 (6)§	1.2 ± 0.1 (7)†		
Hypophysectomy	< 0.2 (3)‡	< 1 (3)‡				

*Numbers in parentheses represent the number of replicates for that treatment; a total of 40 rats were used in three separate experiments, the results of which were pooled after demonstration of homogeneity of their variance (χ^2 test); results were studied by analysis of variance in a randomized (no block) design. †$P < .01$. ‡Indicates that the content of each (plasma) sample was at or below the lower limits of sensitivity of the assay. §$P = .05$ between experimental group and control group.

196

observations were confirmed by Gilkes et al. (24), who, in addition, have shown that in insulin-induced hypoglycemia both B-MSH and ACTH immunoreactivity were elevated. Gilkes et al. (24) suggested also that B-MSH immunoreactivity in human plasma was due to the presence of B-LPH rather than B-MSH. This suggestion was further substantiated by Bachelot, Wolfsen, and Odell (3), who demonstrated clearly by gel filtration experiments that B-MSH immunoreactivity in human plasma must be attributed to B-LPH or gamma-LPH (B-LPH$_{1-58}$). Bachelot et al. (3) also showed that B-LPH immunoreactivity and ACTH immunoreactivity varied in complete parallelism with each other. B-LPH and ACTH plasma levels were decreased following dexamethasone and increased following metyrapone. Values of plasma B-LPH immunoreactivity were elevated in Cushing's and Addison's diseases. In using a recently developed radioimmunoassay for human B-LPH whose characteristic is mainly an absence of cross-reactivity with B-MSH, Krieger, Liotta, and Li (37) showed that ACTH and B-LPH were elevated in Cushing's disease and Nelson's syndrome. They also found that plasma ACTH and B-LPH immunoreactivity rose in parallel in response to insulin-induced hypoglycemia.

Taken together, these studies and our recent one (see section VI) establish that immunoreactivity were secreted simultaneously in response to various stress and endocrine stimuli. More work must be done to characterize which molecular forms, ACTH, B-LPH, or B-E, are secreted. It is possible that in vivo, the pituitary secretes only the intact 31k ACTH precursor which contains ACTH, B-LPH, and B-E immunoreactivity. This precursor could then be subsequently cleaved by proteolytic enzymes, yielding ACTH, B-LPH, and finally B-E. This cleavage could be done in the bloodstream or more selectively by specific enzymes located close to the sites of action of these peptidic hormones. Anyway, more than 10 years afters its discovery, the peptide B-LPH may finally have found a physiological role as a precursor of the biologically active peptide B-E.

VI. PLASMA B-E AND ACTH AFTER STRESS

Since the early studies of Selye (64), ACTH has been recognized as the primary pituitary hormone secreted in response to acute stress in all the species studied. The teleological proposal has been to relate the acute secretion of ACTH to the corresponding immediate activation of the adrenal cortex for the secretion of glucocorticoids necessary for immediate increase of neoglucogenesis and the ensuing availability of energy-rich carbohydrates. In many, although not all, species, prolactin and growth hormone may also be released in similar conditions (12, 25). Growth hormone, ACTH, and prolactin are pituitary responses to stress, all affecting metabolism. Our recent results (see Figures 9.3 and 9.4) show that B-E is also released in equimolar ratio with ACTH in response to acute stress (32, 61).

Two methods were used to elicit acute stress. In one experiment (Figure 9.3) each rat had the right tibia-fibula broken instanteously, and trunk blood was collected at intervals ranging from 60 seconds to 30 minutes (32). The peak of ACTH and B-E secretion was found between 5 and 10 minutes after the stress. When this experiment was repeated using hypophysectomized rats, neither B-E nor ACTH was measurable in plasma after stress. This indicated that the B-E and ACTH measured in the normal animals after stress was of hypophyseal origin (32).

In another set of experiments (Figure 9.4) rats were stressed by exposure to inescapable electric foot shocks (1 mA, 1 second duration at random 12 per minute). Results show again a simultaneous release of B-E and ACTH. The peak of the secretion was found 10 minutes after the start of the electric shocks. This acute stress was quite successful in producing a high secretion of B-E. The 10-minute values were up to sixfold over the controls (61).

Currently we are investigating the role of this acute secretion of B-E. Is this secretion related to analgesia? At this stage, it is difficult to correlate our findings with the mechanisms involved in pain suppression. Although it has been reported that intravenous infusion of B-E induces analgesia in mice at doses of 9 mg/kg or more (73), and in cats at doses of 250 μg/kg (21), we find no analgesia in rats after even higher doses (up to 20 mg/kg). Furthermore, the blood concentrations reached by such doses would be more than three orders of magnitude higher than blood levels observed after stress. Further work is required to establish whether endocrine secretion of pituitary B-E and ACTH are causally related to the central analgesia produced by stress.

Stress is reported to induce analgesia which is in part reversed by naloxone (2). Our results indicate that while the analgesia may be concurrent with an increase of the secretion of B-E from the pituitary into blood, the brain content of B-E and enkephalin shows a decrease in the hypothalamus and no change elsewhere.

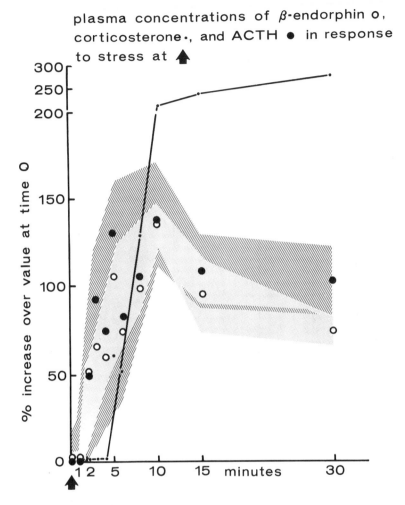

Figure 9.3. Plasma levels of ACTH (closed circles) and ^{b}-endorphin (open circles) measured by radioimmunoassays in trunk blood obtained from rats killed at times shown on the abscissa; acute stress (right tibia-fibula was broken) occurred at time zero. Solid line shows plasma levels of adrenal corticosterone measured by fluorometry. Shaded areas show confidence limits of the measurements. The correlation coefficient, p, between the two populations of ACTH and ^{b}-endorphin concentrations is 0.9708 for values of means (d.f. = 20) and 0.7785 for all individual values (d.f. = 64).

ACKNOWLEDGMENTS

This work was supported by grants DA-01785, HD 09690, AM 18811, and PHS International Fellowship TW 2323, as well as by grants from the W. R. Hearst Foundation and the Del Duca Foundation.

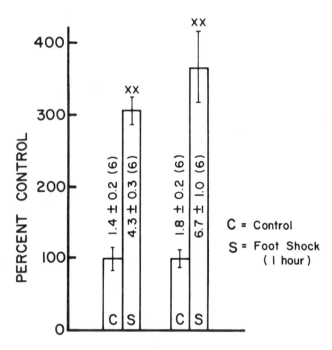

PLASMA LEVELS

β-ENDORPHIN   ACTH
(ng/ml)   (ng/ml)

Figure 9.4. *a,* Stress and plasma levels of ACTH and β-endorphin. Rats (Sprague Dawley, male 200 g) were stressed by exposure for 1 h to inescapable electric foot shocks (1 mA, 1 s duration, at random 12 per min). Directly after the end of the stress period, they were decapitated, and the trunk blood was collected on EDTA. After immediate centrifugation, the plasma was frozen until RIA. Randomized controls from the same lot of animals were killed at the same time (10 A.M.), directly after their removal from their cages. Their plasma samples were processed together with the samples of the stress animals, *b.* Time course study of blood levels for ACTH (x) and β-endorphin (·) after stress. A jugular cannula was implanted in the right jugular of a rat (Sprague Dawley, male 200 g). The cannula was flushed each day with a solution of heparin. Three days after the surgery, the stress experiment as described in part *a* was performed. The rat was placed in the experiment Perspex box 1 hr before the first electric foot shock. Blood samples were drawn 1 h and 1 min before the first shock and at the subsequent times indicated, and were processed as described above.

References

1. Abe, K., Nicholson, W. E., Liddle, G. W., Orth, D. N., and Island, D. P. Normal and abnormal regulation of β-MSH in man. *J. Clin. Invest. 48:* 1580–1585, 1969.
2. Akil, H., Madden, J., IV, Patrick, R. L., and Barchas, J. D. Stress induced increase in endogeneous opiate peptides: Concurrent analgesia and its partial research by

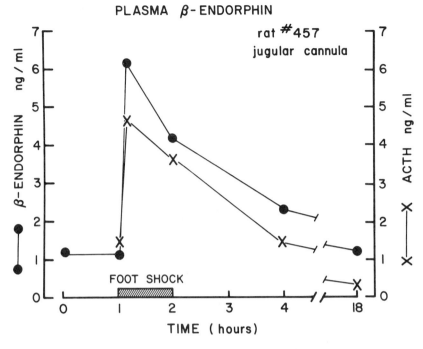

Figure 9.4. *b*

naloxone. In *Opiates and Endogenous Opioid Peptides*. Kosterlitz, H. W. (ed.), Amsterdam: Elsevier, North Holland, 1976, pp. 63–70.

3. Bachelot, I., Wolfsen, A. P., and Odell, W. D. Pituitary and plasma lipotropins: Demonstration of the artifactual nature of B-MSH. *J. Clin. Endocrinol. Metab. 44:* 939–946, 1977.

4. Bloom, F., Battenberg, E., Rossier, J., Ling, N., and Guillemin, R. Neurons containing β-endorphin in rat brain exist separately from those containing enkephalin: Immunocytochemical studies. *Proc. Natl. Acad. Sci. U.S.A. 75:* 1591–1595, 1978.

5. Bloom, F., Battenberg, E. Rossier, J., Ling, N., Leppaluoto, J., Vargo, T. M., and Guillemin, R. Endorphins are located in the intermediate and anterior lobes of the pituitary gland, not in the neurohypophysis. *Life Sci. 20:* 43–48, 1977.

6. Bloom, F. E., Rossier, J., Battenberg, E. L. F., Bayon, A., French, E., Henriksen, S., Siggins, G. R., Segal, D., Browne, R., Ling, N., and Guillemin, R. β-Endorphin: Cellular localization, electrophysiological and behavioral effects. In (ed)., Costa, E., and M. Trabucchi, *Advances in Biochemical Psychopharmacology. 18,* New York: Raven Press, 1978.

7. Bloom, F., Rossier, J. Battenberg, E., Vargo, T., Minick, S., Ling, N., and Guillemin, R. Regional distribution of β-endorphin and enkephalin in rat brain: A biochemical and cytochemical study. *Neuroscience Abstracts 3:* 286, Abstract No. 907, 1977.

8. Bloom, F. E., Segal, D., Ling, N., and Guillemin, R. Endorphin: Profound be-

havioral effects in rats suggest new etiological factors in mental illness. *Science 194:* 630–632, 1976.

9. Bradbury, A. F., Feldberg, W. F., Smyth, D. G., and Snell, C. R. Lipotropin C-fragment: An endogenous peptide with potent analgesic activity. In Kosterlitz, H. W. (ed.), *Opiates and Endogeneous Opioid Peptides.* Amsterdam: Elsevier, North Holland, 9–17, 1976.

10. Bradbury, A. F., Smyth, D. G., Snell, C. R., Birdsall, N. J. M., and Holme, E. C. C-fragment of lipotropin has a high affinity for brain opiate receptors. *Nature (Lond.) 260:* 793–795, 1976.

11. Bradbury, A. F., Smyth, D. G., Snell, C. R., Deakin, J. F. W., and Wendlandt, S. Comparison of the analgesic properties of lipotropin C-fragment and stabilized enkephalins in the rat. *Biochem. Biophys. Res. Commun. 74:* 748–754, 1977.

12. Bryant, G. D., Linzell, J. L., and Greenwood, F. D. Plasma prolactin in goats measured by radioimmunoassay: The effects of test stimulation, mating behavior, stress, fasting and of oxytocin, insulin and glucose injections. *Hormones 1:* 26–35, 1970.

13. Cox, B. M., Opheim, K. E., Teschemacher, H., and Goldstein, A. A peptide-like substance from pituitary that acts like morphine. *Life Sci. 16:* 1777–1782, 1975.

14. Doneen, B. A., Chung, D., Yamashiro, D., Law, P. Y., Loh, H. H., and Li, C. H. β-endorphin: structure activity relationships on the guinea pig ileum and opiate receptor binding assays. *Biochem. Biophys. Res. Commun. 74:* 656–662, 1977.

15. Dragon, N., Seidah, N. G., Lis, Mo. Routhier, R., and Chretien, M. Primary structure and morphine-like activity of human β-endorphin. *Can. J. Biochem. 55:* 666–670, 1977.

16. Dubois, M. P. Localisation cytologique par immunofluorescence des secretions corticotropes, [a] et [b] melanotropes au niveau de l'adenohypophyse des bovins, ovins et procins. *Z. Zellforsch 125:* 200–209, 1972.

17. Dubois, M. P. and Graf, L. Demonstration by immunofluorescence of the lipotrophic hormone LPH in bovine, ovine and porcine adenohypophysis. *Horm. Metab. Res. 5:* 229, 1973.

18. Dupoyy, J. P., and Dubois, M. P. Ontogenesis of the α-MSH, β-MSH and ACTH cells in the foetal hypophysis of the rat. Correlation with the growth of the adrenals and adrenocortical activity. *Cell Tiss. Res. 161:* 373–384, 1975.

19. Elde, R., Hokfelt, T., Johansson, O., and Terenius, L. Immunohistochemical studies using antibodies to leucine enkephalin: Initial observations on the neurons system of the rat. *Neuroscience 1:* 349–351, 1976.

20. Feldberg, W. S., and Smyth, D. G. The C-fragment of lipotropin a potent analgesic in cat. *J. Physiol. (Lond.) 260:* 30–31P, 1976.

21. Feldberg, W. J., and Smyth, D. G. Analgesia produced in cats by the C-fragment of lipotropin and by a synthetic pentapeptide. *J. Physiol. (Lond.) 265:* 25–27P, 1977.

22. Fratta, W., Yang, H.-Y. T., Hong, J., and Costa, E. Stability of Met[5]-enkephalin in brain structures of morphine-dependent or foot shock stressed rats. *Nature 268:* 452–453, 1977.

23. Geisow, M. J., Deakin, J. F. W., Dostrovsky, J. O., and Smyth, D. G. Analgesic activity of lipotropin C fragment depends on carboxyl terminal tetrapeptide. *Nature 269:* 167–168, 1977.

24. Gilkes, J. J. H., Bloomfield, G. A., Scott, A. P., Lowry, P. J., Ratcliffe, J. G.,

Landon, J., and Rees, L. H. Development and validation of a radioimmunoassay for peptides related to β-melanocyte-stimulating hormone in human plasma: The lipotropins. *J. Clin. Endocrinol. Metab. 40:* 450–457, 1975.

25. Glick, S. M. Normal and abnormal secretion of growth hormone. *Ann. N.Y. Acad. Sci. 148:* 471–487, 1968.

26. Goldstein, A. Opioid peptides (endorphins) in pituitary and brain. *Science 193:* 1081–1086, 1976.

27. Graf, L., Ronai, A. Z., Bajusz, S., Cseh, G., and Szekely, J. I. Opioid agonist activity of β-lipotropin fragments: A possible biological source of morphine-like substances in the pituitary. *FEBS Lett. 64:* 181–185, 1976.

28. Graf, L., Szekely, J. I., Ronai, A. Z., Dunai-Kovacs, Z., and Bajusz, S. Comparative study on analgesic effect of Met[5]-enkephalin and related lipotropin fragments. *Nature (Lond.) 263:* 240–242, 1976.

29. Guillemin, R., Bloom, F. E., Rossier, J., Minick, S., Henriksen, S., Burgus, R., and Ling, N. Current physiological studies with the endorphins. In McIntyre, I., and Szelke, M. (eds.), *Molecular Endocrinology*. Amsterdam: Elsevier, North Holland, 1977, pp. 251–267.

30. Guillemin, R., Ling, N., and Burgus, R. Endorphins, peptides, d'origine hypothalamique et neurophypohysaire a activite morphinomimetique. Isolement et structure moleculaire de l'α-endorphine. *C. R. Acad. Sci. Paris Ser. D. 283:* 783β-785, 1976.

31. Guillemin, R., Ling, N., and Vargo, T. M. Radioimmunoassays for α-β-endorphin. *Biochem. Biophys. Res. Commun. 77:* 361–366, 1977.

32. Guillemin, R., Vargo, T., Rossier, J., Minick, S., Ling, N., Rivier, C., Vale, W., and Bloom, F. β-Endorphin and adrenocorticotropin are secreted concomitantly by the pituitary gland. *Science 197:* 1368–1369, 1977.

33. Hokfelt, T., Elde, R., Johansson, O., Terenius, L. and Stein, L. The distribution of enkephalin-immunoreactive cell bodies in the rat central nervous system. *Neuroscience Lett. 5:* 25–31, 1977.

34. Hokfelt, T., Ljungdahl, A., Terenius, L., Elde, R., and Nilsson, G. Immunohistochemical analysis of peptide pathways possibly related to pain and analgesia: Enkephalin and Substance P. *Proc. Natl. Acad. Sci. U.S.A. 74:* 3081–3085, 1977.

35. Hong, J. S., Yang, H. Y. T., and Costa, E. On the location of methionine enkephalin neurons in rat striatum. *Neuropharmacol. 16:* 451–453, 1977.

36. Hughes, J., Smith, T. W., Kosterlitz, H. W., Fothergill, L. A., Morgan, B. A., and Morris, H. R. Identification of two related pentapeptides from the brain with potent opiate agonist activity. *Nature 258:* 577–580, 1975.

37. Krieger, D. T., Liotta, A., and Li, C. H. Human plasma immunoreactive β-lipotropin: Correlation with basal and stimulated plasma ACTH concentrations. *Life Sci. 21:* 1771–1778, 1977.

38. Kuhar, M. J., Pert, C. B., and Snyder, S. H. Regional distribution of opiate receptor binding in monkey and human brain. *Nature 245:* 447–450, 1973.

39. Lazarus, L. H., Ling, N., and Guillemin, R. β-Lipotropin as a prohormone for the morphineminetric peptides endorphins and enkephalins. *Proc. Natl. Acad. Sci. U.S.A. 73:* 2156–2159, 1976.

40. Li, C. H. Lipotropin, a new active peptide from pituitary glands. *Nature 201:* 924, 1964.

41. Li, C. H., Barnafi, L., Chretien, M., and Chung, D. Isolation and amino acid sequence of β-LPH from sheep pituitary gland. *Nature 208:* 1093–1094, 1965.

42. Li, C. H., and Chung, D. Isolation and structure of an untriakontapeptide with opiate activity from camel pituitary glands. *Proc. Natl. Acad. Sci. U.S.A. 73:* 1145–1148, 1976.

43. Li, C. H., Lemaire, S., Yamashiro, D., and Doneen, B. A. The synthesis and opiate activity of β-endorphin. *Biochem. Biophys. Res. Commun. 71:* 19–25, 1976.

44. Li, C. H., Yamashiro, D., Tseng, L. F., and Loh, H. H. Synthesis and analgesic activity of human β-endorphin. *J. Med. Chem. 24:* 324–38, 1977.

45. Ling, N. Solid phase synthesis of porcine α-endorphin and γ-endorphins, two hypothalamic-pituitary peptides with opiate activity. *Biochem. Biophys. Res. Commun. 74:* 248–255, 1977.

46. Ling, N., Burgus, R., and Guillemin, R., Isolation primary structures and synthesis of α-endorphin and γ-endorphin, two peptides of hypothalamic-hypophyseal origin with morphinomimetric activity. *Proc. Natl. Acad. Sci. U.S.A. 73:* 3942–3946, 1976.

47. Ling, N., and Guillemin, R. Morphinomimetric activity of synthetic fragments of β-lipotropin and analogs. *Proc. Natl. Acad. Sci. U.S.A. 73:* 3308–3310, 1976.

48. Loh, H. H., Tseng, L. F., Wei, E., and Li, C. H. β-Endorphin is a potent analgesic agent. *Proc. Natl. Acad. Sci. U.S.A. 73:* 2895–2898, 1976.

49. Lord, J. A. H., Waterfield, A. A., Hughes, J., and Kosterlitz, H. W. Endogeneous opioid peptides: Multiple agonists and receptors. *Nature (Lond.) 267:* 495–499, 1977.

50. Madden, J., IV, Akil, H., Patrick, R. L., and Barchas, J. D. Stress-induced parallel changes in central opioid levels and pain responsiveness in the rat. *Nature (Lond.) 265:* 358–360, 1977.

51. Mains, R., Eipper, E., and Ling, N. Common precursor to corticotropin and endorphins. *Proc. Natl. Acad. Sci. U.S.A. 74:* 3014–3018, 1977.

52. Moon, H. D., Li, C. H., and Jennings, B. M. Immunohistochemical and histochemical studies of β-lipotrophs. *Anat. Rec. 175:* 529–538, 1973.

53. Moriatry, G. C. Adenohypophysis: Ultrastructural cytochemistry. A review. *J. Histochem. Cytochem. 21:* 855–894, 1973.

54. Pelletier, G., Leclerc, R., Labrie, F., Cote, J., Chretien, M., and Lis, M. Immunohistochemical localization of β-lipotropic hormone in the pituitary gland. *Endocrinology 100:* 770–776, 1977.

55. Pert, C. B., and Snyder, S. H. Properties of opiate-receptor binding in rat brain. *Proc. Natl. Acad. Sci. 70:* 2243–2247, 1973.

56. Pert, C. B., and Snyder, S. H. Opiate receptor binding of agonists and antagonists affected differentially by sodium. *Mol. Pharmacol. 10:* 868–874, 1974.

57. Phifer, R. F., Orth, D. N., and Spicer, S. S. Specific demonstration of the human hypophyseal adrenocortico-melanotropic (ACTH/MSH) cell. *J. Clin. Endocrinol. Metab. 39:* 684–692, 1974.

58. Roberts, J. L., and Herbert, E. Characterization of a common precursor to corticotropin and β-lipotropin: Identification of β-lipotropin peptides and their arrangement relative to corticotropin in the precursor synthesized in a cell-free system. *Proc. Natl. Acad. Sci. U.S.A. 74:* 5300–5304, 1977.

59. Ross, M., Dingledine, R., Cox, B. M., and Goldstein, A. Distribution of endorphins

(peptides with morphine-like pharmacological activity) in pituitary. *Brain Res. 124:* 523-532, 1977.

60. Rossier, J., Bayon, A., Vargo, T., Ling, N., Guillemin, R., and Bloom, F. Radioimmunoassay of brain peptides: Evaluation of a methodology for the assay of β-endorphin and enkephalins. *Life Sci. 21:* 847-852, 1977.

61. Rossier, J., French, E., Rivier, C., Ling, N., Guillemin, R., and Bloom, F. Foot-shock induced stress increases β-endorphin in rat blood but not brain. *Nature (Lond.) 270:* 618-620, 1977.

62. Rissier, J., Guillemin, R., and Bloom, F. Foot shock induced stress decreases Leu[5]-enkephalin immunoreactivity in rat hypothalamus. *Europ. J. Pharmacol., 48:* 465-466, 1978.

63. Rossier, J., Vargo, T., Minick, S., Ling, N., Bloom, F., and Guillemin, R. Regional dissociation of β-endorphin and enkephalin contents in rat brain and pituitary. *Proc. Natl. Acad. Sci. U.S.A. 74:* 5162-5165, 1977.

64. Selye, H. *Stress.* Montreal: Acta, 1950.

65. Simantov, R., Kuhar, M. J., Uhl, G. R., and Snyder, S. H. Opioid peptide enkephalin: Immunohistochemical mapping in rat central nervous system. *Proc. Natl. Acad. Sci. U.S.A. 74:* 2167-2171, 1977.

66. Simantov, R., and Snyder, S. H. Morphine-like peptides in mammalian brain: Isolation, structure elucidation and interactions with opiate receptor. *Proc. Natl. Acad. Sci. U.S.A. 73:* 2515-2519, 1976.

67. Simantov, R., and Snyder, S. H. Brain pituitary opiate mechanisms: Pituitary opiate receptor binding, radioimmunoassays for methionine enkephalin and leucine enkephalin, and H-enkephalin interactions with the opiate receptor. In Kosterlitz, H. W. (ed.), *Opiates and Endogeneous opioid peptides.* Amsterdam: Elsevier/North Holland Biomedical Press, 1976, pp. 41-48.

68. Smyth, D. G., and Snell, C. R. Metabolism of the analgesic peptide lipotropin C-fragment in rat striatal slices. *FEBS Lett. 78:* 225-228, 1977.

69. Simon, E. J., Hiller, J. M., and Edelman, I. Stereospecific binding of the potent narcotic analgesic ^{3}H etorphine to rat-brain homogenate. *Proc. Natl. Acad. Sci. 70:* 1947-1949, 1973.

70. Simon, E. J., Hiller, J. M., Groth, J., and Edelman, I. Further properties of stereospecific opiate binding sites in rat brain: On the nature of the sodium effect. *J. Pharmacol. Exp. Ther. 192:* 531-537, 1975.

71. Terenius, L. Characteristics of the "receptor" for narcotic analgesics in synaptic plasma membrane fraction from rat brain. *Acta Pharmacol. Toxicol. 33:* 377-384, 1973.

72. Teschemacher, H., Opheim, K. E., Cox, B. M., and Goldstein, A. A peptide-like substance from pituitary that acts like morphine. I. Isolation. *Life Sci. 16:* 1771-1775, 1975.

73. Tseng, L.-F., Loh, H. H., and Li, C. H. β-Endorphin as a potent analgesic by intravenous injection. *Nature 263:* 239-240, 1976.

74. Watson, S. J., Akil, H., Sullivan, S., and Barchas, J. D. Immunocytochemical localization of methionine enkephalin: Preliminary observations. *Life Sci. 21:* 733-738, 1977.

75. Yang, H. Y., Hong, J. S., and Costa, E. Regional distribution of Leu and Met enkephalin in rat brain. *Neuropharmacol. 16:* 303-307, 1977.

10
Psychophysiologic Mechanisms Regulating the Hypothalamic-Pituitary-Adrenal Response To Stress

Joan Vernikos-Danellis and John P. Heybach
Department of Pharmacology, Wright State University Medical School, Dayton, Ohio 45431 and Biomedical Research Division, NASA-Ames Research Center, Moffett Field, California

INTRODUCTION

Of all the changes that occur in the body in response to stress, the secretions of the pituitary-adrenal cortical and sympathoadrenal systems have been used most extensively as indexes of the presence of a stress. The reliance on these parameters has been based essentially on numerous observations that their response appears to be stimulus-nonspecific. The choice of parameters, however, was based to a great extent on technological developments. The introduction in the early 1950s of a practical technique to measure catecholamines in the urine encouraged a great surge of work measuring catecholamine excretion in the urine of individuals exposed to various stressful situations. The subsequent introduction of considerably simpler techniques for the measurement of plasma corticosteroid concentrations encouraged the almost exclusive use of this parameter in stress studies, both in laboratory and clinical research and in human operational situations. In addition, the discovery by Sayers and Sayers (1948) that corticosteroids inhibited the stress response and that the response of the pituitary-adrenal system was regulated primarily by target-organ negative feedback, encouraged even further reliance on plasma corticosteroid measurements.

It has been generally accepted that the secretion of the adrenal cortex in stressful situations is governed by the adrenocorticotropic activity of the pituitary gland, but the exact mechanisms by which the secretion of corticotropic hormone (ACTH) is controlled are still not adequately understood. Opinions covering the control of ACTH secretion have varied considerably. Furthermore, in more recent years it has become increasingly apparent that not only hypotheses regarding the regulation of ACTH secretion, but also those involving the adrenal cortical changes long believed to be exclusively under pituitary control, have been questioned.

Evidence has been accumulating which provides exceptions to the generally accepted concept of a tightly controlled negative feedback circuit that responds to stress. These exceptions are important not only because they suggest alternative ways in which the pituitary-adrenal system is regulated, but in particular because they emphasize that measurement of changes in plasma corticosteroids or adrenal weight, which have been the most common measures of the stress response, cannot be assumed to reflect in a quantitative manner pituitary ACTH activity.

In view of these recent developments it is appropriate to reevaluate the extensive reliance in physiological and behavioral research on these stress indexes. It is important to point out here that few clinical endocrinologists would rely exclusively on a single plasma corticosteroid value to infer the status of the pituitary-adrenal function of their patients, as the most vocal basic researchers have been so willing to do. In this review various existing hypotheses of pituitary-adrenal regulation will be reconsidered in view of these more recent experimental findings.

I. HYPOTHALAMIC-PITUITARY-ADRENAL INDEXES OF STRESS

(1) Adrenal Size

Increased pituitary ACTH secretion caused by stress results in changes in adrenocortical size, morphology, histology, and chemistry that appear to be associated with increased synthesis and release of corticosteroids (Sayers, et al., 1944; Sayers and Sayers, 1949). These aspects of pituitary-adrenal physiology were reviewed extensively by Sayers (1950). In addition to the adrenal hypertrophy and hyperplasia that follows stress or the administration of ACTH to both normal or hypophysectomized animals, it was observed that removal of one adrenal resulted in compensatory growth of the remaining gland. The requirement for ACTH in this adrenal size phenomenon came from early evidence that it was primarily the fasciculate and reticularis zones that were affected (Mackay and Mackay, 1926; Smith, 1930). Unilateral adrenalectomy in the hypophysectomized rat did not result in the massive increase in weight of the remaining adrenal that is observed in the rat with an intact pituitary (Collip, Anderson, and Thomson, 1933; Shumecker and Firor, 1934). Treatment of intact rats with adrenal cortical extract or glucocorticoids resulted in adrenal atrophy that was prevented by concomitant treatment with ACTH (Ingle, 1950). Such data provided evidence for a profound physiologic effect of ACTH on adrenal weight, primarily through alterations in the inner two zones of the cortex. It was postulated that removal of one adrenal would decrease total corticosteroid secretion. Low circulating corticosteroid levels would then allow increased ACTH secretion by virtue of decreased feedback inhibition. In response to the elevated ACTH levels, the remaining adrenal gland would then grow until total output of corticosteroids was normal again, and the normal feedback relationship between steroids and ACTH was reestablished (Ingle, 1950).

Although several lines of investigation over the years indicated that increased secretion of ACTH was not solely responsible for compensatory adrenal growth, this assumption survived approximately 50 years. Only recently through the elegant work of Dallman and her associates has convincing evidence been provided against ACTH as the sole mediator of compensatory adrenal growth and suggested that this response may be neurally mediated (Dallman, Engeland, and McBride, 1977). As early as 1959, Halasz and Szentágothai obtained data regarding the possibility that adrenal compensatory growth may be in part neurally mediated. They showed that nuclei of cell bodies in the hypothalamic ventromedial nucleus contralateral to the side of unilateral adrenalectomy enlarge and take up greater amounts of [^{3}H]-leucine than those ipsilateral to the adrenalectomy (Halasz and Szentágothai, 1959; Gerendai et al., 1974). Conditions that caused an enlarged adrenal in rats resulted in bilateral decreases in nuclear size of these neurons, whereas adrenalectomy, celiac ganglionectomy, or treatment with corticosteroids increased nuclear size in these cell bodies (Ifft, 1964; Palkovits and Stark, 1972). They proposed that stretch receptors in the adrenal capsule (Kiss, 1951) conveyed, via afferent nerves, information to the hypothalamus, where adrenal size was regulated (Szentágothai et al., 1962). This concept was supported by the studies of Engeland and Dallman (1976), who found that lidocaine, but not saline, pretreatment of the adrenal to be removed prevented the compensatory growth of the other adrenal measured 12 hours later. They also reported (Sato et al., 1975) that hypothalamic corticotropin releasing factor (CRF) activity was decreased within seconds after completion of bilateral adrenalectomy compared to surgical sham operations, where CRF levels were high. Briefly clamping the pedicles of the adrenal glands resulted in changes in CRF and ACTH similar to bilateral adrenalectomy. This response appeared to be specific to pinching the neural and vascular supply of the adrenal either by manipulation or removal.

In addition to the evidence for the presence of afferents mediating the compensatory adrenal growth, there are data supporting the presence of efferent nerves from the hypothalamus to the adrenal. Unilateral hypothalamic lesions lead to a decrease in nuclear volume of cells in the zone fasciculata of the adrenal contralateral to the lesion (Smollich and Docke, 1969). Unilateral hypothalamic lesions or deafferentation, or spinal cord hemisection inhibit compensatory adrenal growth if they are ipsilateral but not contralateral to subsequent adrenalectomy (Engeland and Dallman, 1975, 1976). Further evidence for the involvement of a neural reflex in compensatory adrenal hypertrophy came from the observation (Dallman, Engeland, and Shinsako, 1976) that manipulation of one adrenal results in growth of the contralateral but not the manipulated gland within 12 hours. Dallman et al. (1976) reasoned that since both adrenals would be expected to grow after unilateral manipulation if the signals were humoral, the results suggest that a neural reflex is involved. Evidence against the involvement of ACTH has also been accumulating. Compensatory adrenal hypertrophy appears to involve cell proliferation as evidenced by an increase in the mitotic index and [^{3}H]-thymidine uptake (Carr, 1959; Reiter and Pizzarello, 1966), whereas ACTH-induced adrenal enlargement is not accompanied by an increase in the mitotic index (Cater and Stack-Dunne, 1955). The primary effect of ACTH treatment in vivo is to increase adrenal RNA synthesis (cell hypertrophy) followed by a slower increase in DNA synthesis (Fiala, Spraul, and Fiala, 1956; Bransome and Reddy, 1961; Imrie et al., 1965), whereas unilateral adrenalectomy results in a rapid increase in RNA and DNA content (cell proliferation). Treatment of unilaterally adrenalectomized rats with ACTH during the first 24 hours in fact inhibits the normal increase in DNA content of the remaining gland. Similarly, treatment of cultured adrenal cells with ACTH inhibits [^{3}H]-thymidine uptake (Masui and Garren, 1971; Ramachandran and Suyama, 1975; Hornsby and Gill, 1977).

Finally, there is no evidence that circulating corticosterone levels are reduced after unilateral adrenalectomy or that circulating ACTH increases as the original humoral theory of compensatory growth presumed. In fact, circulating ACTH and corticosterone levels do not differ between unilaterally adrenalectomized and sham-adrenalectomized control rats after the first two hours, although the remaining adrenal is increased in weight (Mialhe et al., 1973; Engeland and Dallman, 1975). Thus it appears that change in adrenal size, particularly that which occurs after unilateral adrenalectomy, is not a reliable index of ACTH activity.

(2) Plasma and Adrenal Corticosteroid Levels

There is no doubt that circulating corticosteroid levels, corticosterone in the rat and cortisol in dog, cat, and human, have replaced adrenal ascorbic acid depletion and adrenal weight as the most frequently used measure to identify the presence of a stress response. It is also well established that stressful conditions stimulate the secretion of adrenocortical steroids, an effect which can also be produced by the administration of ACTH. The reliance on this measure as an accurate reflection of stress-induced ACTH secretion at any time and of hypothalamic-pituitary-adrenal function as a whole has been almost total. Yet the circulating concentration of corticosteroids is affected not only by ACTH secretion but also by a variety of other factors. These include the intrinsic circadian rhythmicity of the adrenal, adrenal secretory mechanisms, and the distribution, binding, and metabolism of corticosterone and factors that alter the responsiveness of the adrenal to ACTH.

More than 25 years ago it was shown that the plasma concentration of cortisol rises in the morning and declines subsequently in the afternoon and evening (Bliss et al., 1953; Migeon et al., 1956). Such an adrenocortical rhythm has been described in many species and is reported to be associated with the 24-hour variations in the secretion rates of ACTH and CRF. Since the plasma level of ACTH and hypothalamic CRF content have been shown to exhibit similar circadian rhythms (Demura et al., 1966; Vernikos-Danellis, Winget, and Hetherington, 1969; Berson and Yalow, 1968; David-Nelson and Brodish, 1969; Hiroshige et al., 1969), this periodicity of the adrenal cortex could arise not only from periodic inputs at the hypothalamic median eminence, but also by the action of autonomous endogenous oscillators in any one of the components of the system (median eminence, adenohypophysis, adrenal cortex, or metabolic processes for ACTH or corticosteroids). For instance, cultured adrenal glands show a circadian rhythm in the conversion of acetate to corticosterone that persists for two days and is obviously independent of ACTH (Andrews and Folk, 1964). On the other hand, Nugent et al., showed many years ago (1959) that if people are given a constant infusion of ACTH that raises and sustains plasma corticosteroids at their maximal circadian level for four days, the plasma glucocorticoid level remains relatively constant, suggesting that distribution binding or metabolism variations do not affect the rhythm in these levels greatly.

Evidence has been accumulating in recent years to indicate that the pituitary-adrenal response to acute stress is functionally independent of the circadian variation in pituitary-adrenal activity. The mechanisms controlling the circadian rhythm of the pituitary-adrenal system as well as the stress response are associated with the hypothalamus, but appear to be independent of each other, just as the stimuli that elicit a stress response are different from those which synchronize pituitary-adrenal circadian rhythms.

For instance, photoperiod is considered a strong synchronizer of pituitary-adrenal rhythmicity. Rats kept for long periods of time in constant light (56 to 90 days) do not show a circadian peak in plasma corticosterone (Cheifetz, Gaffud, and Dingman, 1968; Dunn, Dyer, and Bennett, 1972), but the rhythm is restored after the light-dark cycle is again imposed. There is no evidence that constant light is stressful, since the average plasma corticosterone level in constant light-exposed rats was in fact lower than the controls in these studies.

Feeding and watering have been shown to be potent synchronizers in rats, overriding the effects of a well-regulated photoperiod (Johnson and Levine, 1973; Krieger, 1974). It was first demonstrated by Johnson and Levine (1973) that the plasma corticosterone rhythm was shifted in phase as a result of restricting water consumption to a limited time in the early afternoon. This new rhythm required more than seven days to develop and did not appear immediately as would have been expected of a stress response. Perhaps the most interesting evidence of a dissociation between adrenal cortical rhythmicity and adrenal cortical stress response comes from maturation studies. The response to ether stress appears in both male and female rats as early as five days before weaning, while the circadian rhythm in pituitary-adrenal activity occurs later, 10 to 12 days after weaning (Allen and Kendall, 1967). The late onset of the diurnal rhythm of plasma corticosterone concentration suggests that although the capacity to respond to acute stress is present, certain CNS structural requirements are not sufficiently developed to support circadian periodicity. Furthermore, treatment of the neonatal rat with dexamethasone (Krieger, 1972) or constant light or constant darkness (Vernikos-Danellis, Winget, and Hetherington, 1970) delays the onset of the plasma corticosterone rhythm, although the effect on the stress response under these conditions is not known.

The ontogenetic time lag between the onset of the stress response and the diurnal rhythm suggests that separate neural mechanisms regulate these two responses, and that each develops morphologically at a different rate. This may provide a useful means for identifying and mapping these components. However, the work that provides evidence for neuroanatomical dissociation of the regulation of rhythm and stress response has relied on CNS lesions in adult animals. Lesions of the anterior periventricular nucleus abolish the diurnal rhythm in plasma corticosterone at an intermediate level two or three weeks following surgery (Slusher, 1964) without altering the response to the stress of sound, ether, or electric stimulation of the posterior diencephalon. These were the earliest data indicating that there is an anatomical dissociation between circuits mediating the stress response and those mediating the diurnal variation in corticosteroids.

The participation of the hippocampo-fornix system in the mediation of the pituitary-adrenal rhythm has been studied. Although severing the fornix abolished the diurnal rhythm (Moberg et al., 1971), the normal rhythm returned with time (Lingvari and Halasz, 1973). Rats with septal ablation with concomitant interruption of fornix fibers or with hippocampal lesions showed normal plasma corticosterone rhythms at 3 to 12 weeks after surgery (Wilson and Critchlow, 1973, 1974; Lanier et al., 1975), and normal stress and negative feedback responses. In contrast, complete de-afferentation of the medial basal hypothalamus abolished the diurnal rhythm in plasma corticosterone and reduced but did not abolish the response to stress at four weeks following surgery (Halasz, Slusher, and Gorski, 1967; Palka, Coyer, and Critchlow, 1969). These data suggest that some structure other than the hippocampo-fornix system must be destroyed in order to disrupt the diurnal rhythm permanently. Swanson and Cowan (1975) have described fibers that pass from the suprachiasmatic nuclei to the periventricular nuclei and the median eminence. The suprachiasmatic nucleus (SCN) in turn receives serotonergic projections arising in the median raphe nuclei via the medial forebrain bundle (MFB). Transection of the MFB at the level of the ventromedial nucleus (Moore and Qavi, 1971) or cuts just caudal to the optic chiasm or lesions of the SCN (Moore and Eichler, 1972) abolish the plasma corticosterone rhythm in the rat at three weeks after surgery, suggesting that the connections from the raphe to the SCN play an important role in the maintenance of a normal rhythm. In contrast, we have recently observed that although premammillary MFB lesions do abolish the plasma corticosterone rhythm three days after surgery, the normal rhythm is reinstated by seven days. Evidence from high-affinity synaptosomal uptake studies using hypothalami from such lesioned animals showed that only serotonin uptake was reduced three days after the lesion when the rhythm was disrupted, but both serotonin and norepinephrine uptake were reduced and dopamine uptake was significantly increased seven days after the lesion when the rhythm was reinstated (Heybach et al., unpublished observations). It would appear that the MFB serotonergic pathways are not solely responsible for the regulation of the plasma corticosterone rhythm, and that dopaminergic mechanisms, possibly originating in the arcuate nucleus, may also contribute to this regulation. It is of interest in this regard to mention the recent work of Krieger, who showed that the rhythm in plasma corticosterone which was abolished in rats by lesions in the SCN could be reinstated by alterations in the feeding schedules (Krieger, 1977a). These data suggest that although the SCN may mediate light-regulated rhythmicity, this does not constitute a final common pathway, and other neural or neurohumoral or behavioral mechanisms must also be involved. It is also of interest that lesions of the ventromedial and dorsomedial hypothalamic nuclei (VMH and DMH) in weanling rats disrupt both the feeding and the plasma corticosterone rhythms (Bernardis, 1973; Bellinger, Bernardis, and Mendel, 1976) for up to nine weeks. The authors suggest the possibility that fiber tracts from the SCN could innervate the medial area of the VMH, and that discrete VMH lesions may thus result in disruption in normal diurnal corticosterone studies. They also point out that although the arcuate nucleus was not lesioned, it showed some degeneration after VMH lesions and may also be participating in the disturbance of plasma corticosterone rhythmicity (Bernardis, 1972).

Whatever the central mechanisms that regulate basal plasma corticosterone rhythmicity, they appear to be distinct from those regulating the stress response. However, the adrenocortical response to stress is affected by this diurnal rhythmicity, since not only does ACTH secretion exhibit different characteristics as a function of the pituitary-adrenal circadian rhythm (Engeland et al. 1977), but, in addition, the sensitivity of the adrenal cortex to ACTH also varies in a circadian fashion (Dallman et al., 1976).

The information that the peak plasma corticosterone levels after stress in the rat occur at 15 minutes after application of the stimulus (Guillemin, Dean, and Liebelt, 1959) has been relied on widely in stress research. Use of corticosterone at a single time point after stress as an index of ACTH secretion assumes that the response of the adrenal cortex to ACTH does not change as a function of the time of day, and that this response is not affected if the circadian rhythm in basal plasma corticosterone secretion is disturbed. It is difficult to compare quantitatively plasma corticosterone responses that start from different initial values, whether these are due to diurnal fluctuations or prior experimental treatments. Both increases or maximal level attained at 15 minutes have been used, resulting in dubious interpretations. Assumptions are made that the secretion rate, metabolic clearance rate, and distribution volume of corticosterone are constant throughout the day, that the maximal concentration always occurs at 15 minutes, and that the concentration attained at this time after stress is below ceiling level. As a matter of fact, these assumptions are not valid. Irrespective of the intensity of the stress stimulus, maximal values attained at 15 minutes do not usually exceed 90 $\mu g/100$ ml in females and 60 $\mu g/100$ ml in males. Increasing the intensity of the stimulus merely results in a more sustained response. For example, although plasma corticosterone levels in male rats 15 minutes after 1 minute of ether only, or ether plus laparotomy, are approximately 35 $\mu g/100$ ml, the response to ether has returned to prestress levels by 60 minutes, whereas the response to ether and laparotomy persists for two hours (Vernikos-Danellis, unpublished). This, if one is to use the 15-minute value to determine the effect of a stress-modifying factor, selection of the type of stress stimulus becomes very critical. A stressor producing a submaximal plasma corticosterone response is necessary to detect enhancement of the stress response, and the response to supramaximal stimulation cannot be reliably used to detect inhibition, since considerable reduction in plasma ACTH secretion can occur without any significant evidence of a reduction of the plasma corticosterone response. Although a dose-dependent increase in plasma glucocorticoids secretion that starts within two minutes can be shown in hypophysectomized animals, there is a maximum rate of secretion which is reached with relatively low doses of ACTH; larger ACTH doses or stress of greater intensity only prolong the time of maximum output.

Similarly, the peak plasma corticosterone response does not always occur at 15 minutes. There are genetic differences in the time course of the plasma corticosterone response (Treiman and Levine, 1969). Chronic stress exposure or pretreatments such as the various learning paradigms often used in behavioral research can increase the corticosterone secretion rate in response to a superimposed acute stress (Sakellaris and Vernikos-Danellis, 1974, 1975).

Lastly, not only does the maximal plasma corticosterone level attained after stress in the rat vary with the time of day, but the maximum level is attained earlier in the evening hours than between 0600 and 1200 (Engeland et al., 1977). It is also probable that the nutritional state of the animal will affect the responsiveness of the adrenal, either by interfering with protein synthesis (Ferguson, 1963) or by disturbing the optimal concentrations of cations (Lefkowitz, Roth, and Pastan, 1970), or by other means. For instance, it has been proposed that the postprandial secretion of insulin inhibits adrenal responsiveness to ACTH (Wilkinson, Shinsako, and Dallman, 1977), whereas it increases in alloxan-diabetic rats (L'Age et al., 1974). Pretreatment with ACTH can also alter the sensitivity of the adrenal to the subsequent administration of ACTH, and the time interval between the ACTH stimuli determines the nature of the effect. It has long been known that a prior stimulation by ACTH renders the adrenal more responsive to subsequent ACTH (Nugent et al., 1959). However, a step input of ACTH sustained for about 1 hour, removed, and followed 5 minutes later by a second similar step input of ACTH, will result in a second response that will be less than the first. If 40 minutes is allowed for recovery between the two stimuli, the second response will be like the first (Urquhart and Li, 1968, 1969).

Prior stress may also affect the subsequent responsiveness of the adrenal. Dallman and Jones (1973) reported that the plasma corticosterone response to a second stress was as great as or greater than the first response, whereas an infusion of plasma corticosterone to mimic the first response inhibited the response to the second stress. They concluded that the response to a first stress leaves the adrenal cortex in a hyperexcitable state so that it would be hyperresponsive to a subsequent stress were it not for the inhibitory effects of the increased corticosteroid levels resulting from the first-stress response. In fact, exposure to chronic stress does indeed result in a hyperexcitable pituitary-adrenal system (Daniels-Severs et al., 1973). Thus, careful selection of the intensity of the stress stimulus, knowledge of the prior condition of the animal, and the determination of the time course of the plasma corticosterone response (instead of a single time point) would be a more reliable approach when this parameter is to be used.

(3) Pituitary and Plasma ACTH

Although many of the same considerations apply to quantifying the stress response by measuring circulating ACTH levels rather than corticosteroid levels, ACTH is at least one step closer to the site of the neural initiation of stress responses. It is also likely that there are less dramatic non-linearities in the ACTH distribution, binding, and metabolism systems than those observed in the corticosteroid system (Urquhart, 1974), although this has never been substantiated experimentally.

Subjection of an intact or adrenalectomized animal to an acute stress stimulus has been shown to result in a very rapid increase in the blood level of ACTH, which reaches a maximum within 2 to 2.5 minutes (Sydnor and Sayers, 1954; Hodges and Vernikos, 1959; Vernikos-Danellis, 1963; Jones, Brush, and Neame, 1972). Plasma ACTH has usually returned to prestress levels by 20 minutes, but this varies, depending on the intensity of the stimulus. A similar time course of ACTH secretion has been documented in man (Vernikos-Danellis and Marks, 1962; Gwynup et al., 1967). A diurnal rhythm in the rate of the stress-induced plasma ACTH response has been reported (Vernikos-Danellis, 1968). The peak response occurs later in the evening hours as the plasma corticosterone basal level is rising, and response is faster and generally greater in the morning, although differences have been reported between high and low intensity stimuli (Engeland et al., 1977). Hence, measurement of plasma ACTH at a single time point after a stress stimulus should also be regarded with caution.

One of the factors that used to be considered critical to the ability of the pituitary to release ACTH was its content of the hormone. Pituitary ACTH content decreases following a variety of stressful stimuli (Vernikos-Danellis, 1965a,b), but this does not coincide with the time of maximum blood levels of the hormone; rather it occurs at a time when the stress-induced increased circulating ACTH concentrations have practically disappeared. Maximal reductions occur at one to five hours after the application of the stress and do not recover for 24 hours (Fortier, 1959a,b). This delayed fall in pituitary ACTH content, which becomes apparent one hour after stress in the intact animal, is not due to an inhibitory effect of the increasing titer of circulating corticosteroids or ACTH synthesis, since the stress of adrenalectomy will also result in this delayed, prolonged fall (Fortier, 1959b). Whatever the reason for the decreased pituitary ACTH content after stress, it is considerably greater than could be accounted for by the amount of hormone released. Furthermore, at the time of maximal release, pituitary ACTH is either unchanged or increased (Vernikos-Danellis, 1963). Considerable evidence has accummulated to suggest that the initial response to stress is one of increased synthesis of ACTH, and that the stress-induced release of ACTH is dependent not on preexisting stores of the hormone in the gland, but rather on the ability of the adenohypophysis to synthesize ACTH. In support of this thesis are the results of experiments in which it was shown that the adenohypophysis of intact or adrenalectomized rats takes up a labeled amino acid and incorporates it into what was believed to be rat ACTH (Jacobowitz, Marks, and Vernikos-Danellis, 1963). Acute stress increased the rate of incorporation within 2.5 minutes, at which time pituitary glycogen was greatly reduced (Jacobowitz and Marks, 1964). Both ethionine and actinomycin blocked the stress-induced increases in both circulating and pituitary ACTH (Marks and Vernikos-Danellis, 1963; Vernikos-Danellis, 1965a,b). Furthermore, a stress applied at the time of maximum pituitary TH depletion resulted in blood and pituitary CTH responses that were as great as those occurring in a normal animal (Vernikos-Danellis, 1963), indicating that pituitary ACTH content is no indication of the responsiveness of the gland.

The secretion of ACTH by the pituitary gland is regulated by the hypothalamic neurohumor CRF, whose exact identity is not yet known. Factors that would affect ACTH secretion in response to stress would include those that would alter the responsiveness of adenohypophyseal cells to CRF. Knowledge of the mechanisms by which CRF produces its effect, and the twofold possibility that ACTH may be secreted from sources other than adenohypophyseal cells and that stimulation of ACTH release by means other than CRF can occur, would be important considerations.

Some evidence for direct sympathetic innervation of the pituitary that might under certain circumstances modulate and enhance the release of

ACTH has been reported (Gann and Cryer, 1973). In addition, the possibility that epinephrine may enhance the response of the pituitary to CRF and stress has been suggested by both in vivo (Vernikos-Danellis, 1968) and in vitro studies (Saffran and Schally, 1955). The release of ACTH induced either by exogenous or endogenous hypothalamic extracts can be inhibited locally at the pituitary by corticosteroids under some experimental conditions (De Wied, 1964; Chowers, Conforti, and Feldman, 1967; Russell et al., 1969). Although most of this evidence for a direct steroid action on the pituitary has been obtained using relatively low doses of dexamethasone, relatively large doses of cortisol (Vernikos-Danellis, 1964; Pollock and LaBella, 1966) and corticosterone (Kraicer and Milligan, 1970) are required. Because of this apparent lack of specificity of the site of action of dexamethasone, its use should be considered with reservations.

The ionic environment of the anterior pituitary fundamentally affects the secretion of ACTH and other adenohypophyseal hormones and their response to their respective hypophyseotropic hormones. The critical observations of Kraicer et al. (1969a,b) that increasing external potassium ion concentrations of pituitaries in vitro are associated with enhanced release of ACTH, and that this response is calcium-dependent, and the more recent discovery that anterior cells both neoplastic (Kidokoro, 1975) and normal (Douglas and Taraskevich, 1977) can generate action potentials in response to a hypophyseotropic hormone, have led Douglas and Taraskevich (1977) to propose that the brain, through its hypophysiotropic hormones, regulates the secretory activity of the adenohypophysis by initiating or modulating electrical activity in the form of action potentials. Since calcium ions are seemingly involved as charge carriers in this process, they further proposed that this electrical excitability and impulse generation may be a general property of the many endocrine cells that have embryological origins in the primitive neuroectoderm (such as chromaffin cells), and that the functional significance of impulses in these endocrine cells may be "to provide a mechanism for promoting entry of calcium ions affecting stimulus-secretion coupling and activating exocytosis." Calcium dependence has been shown for pituitary secretions induced by appropriate hypophysiotropic hormones (or crude or purified hormone preparations), and fluxes of Ca^{45} have been stimulated by excess potassium and also, although with less consistency, with hypophysiotropic hormones (Kraicer et al., 1969a,b; MacLeod and Fontham, 1970; Vale, Rivier, and Brown, 1977; Douglas, 1977). There is also evidence that the calcium in the anterior pituitary, as in other secretory cells, is capable of initiating secretion in conditions under which it can penetrate the cells, as suggested from the secretory responses of adenohypophyseal cells to the calcium ionophore A 23187 (Cochrane and Douglas, 1975; Vale et al., 1977). As is true with most peptides (Catt and Dufau, 1977), it would seem likely that hypophyseotrophic peptide hormones would act on the cell surface, and experimental evidence from the anterior pituitary shows that the pure hypophysiotropic hormones tested do indeed bind to surface receptors (Vale et al., 1977).

Substances other than hypophyseotropic peptides of hypothalamic origin have been reported to stimulate ACTH release directly, and although their physiological significance at this time is not known, they should be taken into account in the design and interpretation of experiments. Thus, Hiroshige (1973) has found that a small but not a large dose of histamine, spermidine, angiotensin II, and vasopressin injected into the pituitary region of pentobarbital- and dexamethasone-pretreated rats caused release of ACTH. The doses of these substances required are relatively high. In contrast to tbeir effect in releasing or inhibiting other pituitary hormones, prostaglandins (Hedge, 1972), epinephrine, noreprinephrine, L-dopa, dopamine, serotonin, acetylcholine, carbachol, oxytocin, putrescine, and bradykinin were found to be ineffective in releasing ACTH directly (Hiroshige, 1973). In contrast, it appears that the ACTH localized in the neurointermediate lobe is releasable by substances ineffective on the adenophypophysis (Fischer and Moriarty, 1977). In the rat, both cholinergic and adrenergic synapses have been found on, or in close proximity to, the polyglandular cells in the pars intermedia (Whitaker and LaBella, 1972, 1973; Dahlstrom and Fuxe, 1966). Peptidergic nerve terminals, on the other hand, appear to be few in number and have not been found in synaptic contact with the pars intermedia cells (Kobayashi, 1969). Thus acetylcholine and serotonin, as well as median eminence extracts and antidiuretic hormone, released ACTH from in vitro neurointermediate lobe preparations, dopamine inhibited, and norepinephrine and dexamethasone were ineffective (Moriarty and Moriarty, 1975; Fischer and Moriarty, 1977). Kraicer and Morris (1976) also reported that serotonin stimulated ACTH release over a range of doses that had no effect on the pars distalis, whereas they found carbachol and histamine to be ineffective. These investigators, as had done Van Loon and Kragt (1970) earlier for the pars distalis, raised the very important experimental consideration that the catecholamines dopamine, norepinephrine, and epinephrine appear to inactivate ACTH released during the incubation of tissue in vitro, a fact that could lead to misinterpretation of results unless rigorous controls are conducted.

4. Hypothalamic CRF

The term corticotropin releasing factor (CRF) was first suggested by Saffran, Schally, and Benfey (1955) to describe the hypothalamic neurohumor with the specific function of *releasing* ACTH from the adenohypophysis. By definition (Schally and Guillemin, 1960) CRF acts directly on the cells of the anterior pituitary and therefore is considered as the final common pathway for the neurohumoral control of ACTH secretion (Harris, 1955). The demonstration of the presence of CRF activity in the medial basal hypothalamus (Vernikos-Danellis, 1964) and the variation of the CRF content of this tissue in response to stress would then suggest this measure as the most direct way of quantitating a stress response. It was first observed that exposure of intact, hypophysectomized, or adrenalectomized rats to the stress of ether causes a rapid increase in the CRF activity of the median eminence (Vernikos-Danellis, 1965a). Subsequent studies of hypothalamic CRF content before and after stress have confirmed that large increases occur within two minutes after applying a wide variety of stressful stimuli (Hiroshige et al., 1968, 1969, 1971; Hiroshige and Sato, 1970, 1971; Hiroshige, 1973; Sato and George, 1973). The response, however, is biphasic, returning to prestress levels between 20 and 40 minutes and showing a second rise at 80 minutes. The time course and magnitude of these later changes appear to be dependent on the nature and intensity of the stress (Sato et al., 1975). The system here too appears to show redundancy. Just as considerably more ACTH is secreted during stress than is required to stimulate the adrenal cortex maximally, so also is the CRF increase in relation to pituitary ACTH stimulation. While the very rapid increases in hypothalamic CRF content immediately after stress when ACTH secretion is also at its peak, strongly suggest increased synthesis of CRF, the mechanisms that result in changes in CRF minutes to hours after an acute stress, are uncertain. Problems with measuring the tissue content of this or any hormone are that increased content could reflect either increased synthesis or decreased secretion; and, conversely, that decreased content could reflect decreased synthesis or increased secretion or even increased metabolism. The thesis of increased synthetic activity of the median eminence following stress is consistent with the findings of Jacobowitz and Marks (1964), who found a marked and rapid fall in the glycogen content of the median eminence after stress and a decrease in hypothalamic nucleic acids in response to stress accompanied by a rapid turnover of ATP.

Although CRF content in the blood has occasionally been measured, its short half-life, the relatively low concentrations in peripheral blood of intact animals, and the relative insensitivity of assay systems have been problems discouraging its routine use in stress research. The relative attributes of methods to measure CRF activity in tissue or blood have been critically reviewed (Vernikos-Danellis, 1965a; Vernikos-Danellis and Marks, 1970). Since the exact identity of CRF is not known, and the pituitary apparently responds to substances other than hypothalamic peptides that might be available under physiological conditions, the specificity of the various assay systems for CRF should be considered (Hiroshige, 1973; Seelig and Sayers, 1977). Furthermore, CRF appears to be an inherently unstable molecule (Vernikos-Danellis, 1964), which means that multistage extractions and purifications are liable to result in large losses of biological activity, making quantitative determinations tedious and difficult.

CENTRAL PATHWAYS REGULATING HYPOTHALAMIC PITUITARY-ADRENAL RESPONSE TO STRESS

(1) Central Neurotransmitters

Recent reviews have summarized the available data regarding the central neural mechanisms that regulate hypothalamic CRF activity and hence pituitary-adrenocortical secretion in response to stress (Hodges, 1976; Jones, Hillhouse, and Burden, 1976a; Krieger, 1977b; Sayers, 1977). Since considerable disagreement exists as to the nature of the involvement of various CNS transmitters, this section will focus on the major points of agreement and discrepancy in our current understanding of the neural and neurohumoral interactions within the hypothalamus believed to regulate CRF neurons or within the pituitary to stimulate ACTH secretion directly.

(a) Catecholamines The majority of both in vivo and in vitro studies have been interpreted to indicate that norepinephrine (NE) is involved primarily in the inhibition of CRF release. However, sufficient evidence exists to indicate that catecholamines, in fact, exert multiple effects at several sites within the hypothalamic-pituitary adrenal axis, involving both α- and β-adrenergic receptors.

In phenobarbital-anesthetized dogs, injection into the third ventricle of NE or L-dopa or the central α-adrenergic agonist, clonidine, inhibits the secretion of adrenocortical steroids in response to surgical stress (Van Loon et al., 1971; Ganong et al., 1976). In addition, intraventricular injection of the α-adrenergic antagonist, phenoxybenzamine, prevents this inhibition of corticosteroid secretion seen following L-dopa or clonidine administration. In this preparation systemic administration of NE had no effect on corticosteroid secretion, and these data have therefore been interpreted as indicating a specific intrahypothalamic noradrenergic receptor "within the blood brain barrier." Recently, it has been shown in the anesthetized dog that electrical stimulation of ascending NE fibers to the hypothalamus, located in the ventral NE bundle (VNB), can block the stress-induced secretion of corticosteroids (Rose, Goldsmith, and Ganong, 1976). However, lesions of the VNB produced by intracranial injections of 6-hydroxydopamine (6-OHDA) in the rat do not alter basal corticosterone levels and result in only a transient enhancement of the stress response at one day following surgery (Fuxe et al., 1973).

There is also some question as to whether dopamine (DA) may exert an inhibitory action. In an in vitro preparation of rat hypothalamus, NE had no effect on basal CRF secretion but led to a dose-dependent inhibition of the release of CRF in response to stimulation by serotonin (5HT) and acetylcholine (Ach), whereas DA has no such effect (Hillhouse, Burden, and Jones, 1975). Others have reported that DA, but not NE, profoundly inhibited the release of CRF from hypothalamic synaptosomal preparations (Edwardson and Bennett, 1974). Similarly, some in vivo work suggests a role for DA in the regulation of CRF secretion. Haloperidol, a DA receptor blocker, has been reported to reduce the plasma corticosterone response to injection of ketamine in the rat (Fahringer, Foley, and Redgate, 1974), and intraventricular DA administration in the phenobarbital-anesthetized rat inhibited the plasma corticosterone response to surgical stress (Vermes et al., 1972).

Additional evidence for the interaction between hypothalamic catecholamines and pituitary-adrenal hormones derives from measurement of catecholamines and their biosynthetic enzymes following endocrine manipulations of application of various stressors. Median eminence and arcuate nucleus tyrosine hydroxylase activity was reduced nine days following adrenalectomy in the rat and increased by treatment with dexamethasone (Kizer et al, 1974). In the arcuate nucleus both DA and NE levels were reduced following stress, whereas tyrosine hydroxylase activity was increased only following immobilization stress (Palkovits, et al., 1975). Tyrosine hydroxylase is present in both NE- and DA-containing neurons, whereas dopamine-β-hydroxylase (DBH) is present only in NE neurons. Hypothalamic DBH is decreased two days following adrenalectomy in the rat, and, similarly to the effect of stress on tyrosine hydroxylase, only immobilization decreased anterior hypothalamic DBH (Shen and Ganong, 1976). The relationship between neurotransmitter levels, enzyme activity, and functional changes in the relevant neurons and at the relevant receptors are, however, poorly understood with regard to the significance of such changes in the activity of CRF neurons.

However, other studies have suggested that catecholamines can indeed stimulate ACTH secretion or enhance its secretion in response to other stimuli. In unanesthetized rats or cats intraventricular administration or implantation of NE into the median eminence produced an acute rise in plasma corticosteroids (Hall and Marks, 1968; Krieger and Krieger, 1970a). Using a different approach to manipulate central catecholamines, Van Loon et al. (1971) showed that treatment of rats with a-methyl-p-tyrosine (a-MT), which inhibits tyrosine hydroxylase activity and blocks the biosynthesis of catecholamines, elevated basal levels of plasma corticosterone. However, a-MT treatment had little effect on basal plasma ACTH levels and significantly reduced both ACTH and corticosterone secretion in response to ether stress. In addition, this inhibition of the stress response was more complete and could be shown to be dose-dependent 24 hours following adrenalectomy (Vernikos-Danellis, 1968). Peripherally administered catecholamines stimulate the secretion of ACTH, an effect that has been presumed to be nonspecific and secondary to the changes in blood pressure. In unanesthetized rats, intraperitoneal injection of E or NE or intravenous infusion of E for 1 minute led to dose-dependent increases in plasma ACTH levels, which could be prevented by treatment with phentolamine.

Treatment with E, but not NE or DA, potentiated the increase in plasma ACTH levels seen 2.5 minutes following ether stress, and this potentiation was prevented by pretreatment with a β-adrenergic blocker (Vernikos-Danellis, 1968). This blockage of β-adrenergic receptors reduced the corticotropin-releasing activity of injected crude median eminence extract, suggesting an extrahypothalamic direct action at the pituitary level. This β-adrenergic effect of E argues against vasoconstriction and increased blood pressure as the source of stress-induced activation of this system. A catecholamine-enhancing action of ACTH secretion has also been reported by Hsu, Hsu, and Gann (1976), who found that L-dopa pretreatment enhanced the response to metyrapone in the monkey but did not itself stimulate ACTH secretion. Although there are data to suggest that this potentiating action of catecholamines on ACTH secretion occurs at the pituitary, an additional action on hypothalamic CRF secretion is not ruled out.

Thus far it has been implicit in this and most other discussions that neurally or humorally released CRF and other humoral factors that may effect the relese of ACTH directly at the pituitary act via adenohypophyseal ACTH-containing cells. This, however, may not be entirely the case. The neurointermediate lobe of the pituitary contains biologically active ACTH (Moriarty and Moriarty, 1975). Although median eminence extract, presumably containing CRF, can elicit ACTH secretion from in vitro neurointermediate lobe (Fischer and Moriarty, 1977), this area receives a dense innervation via infundibular fibers (Howe, 1973) which can modify ACTH release. In in vitro preparations of neurointermediate lobe, DA, but not NE, inhibited ACTH release (Fischer and Moriarty, 1977). The physiological significance of this neurointermediate lobe ACTH is unknown, with respect to both corticosteroid secretion from the adrenal cortex and "short-loop" feedback control of adenohypophyseal ACTH or hypothalamic CRF in response to stressful stimuli. Several factors must be considered in any attempt to resolve these apparent discrepancies in the action of catecholamines on the hypothalamic-pituitary-adrenal function. Obviously the possibilities of species differences, presence or absence of anesthesia, type of anesthesia, properties of different in vitro systems, and sites of action of pharmacological tools used, are critical variables. However, it appears that the various catecholamines can exert both stimulatory and inhibitory actions and at several sites. At sites within the pituitary, E and NE appear to enhance ACTH release via β-adrenergic receptors, and DA may inhibit stimulated release of ACTH from the neurointermediate lobe. At sites within the hypothalamus, the majority of the data suggest that NE can inhibit the release of CRF, perhaps via a postsynaptic α-adrenergic receptor system. Norepinephrine does inhibit the release of CRF when applied in vivo in anesthetized dogs and in stimulated in vitro rat hypothalamus. However, intrahypothalamic application of NE stimulates corticosteroid secretion in unanesthetized cats, perhaps a more physiologically relevant preparation.

With the exception of the in vitro hypothalamus test system of Hillhouse et al. (1975), most of the data demonstrating an inhibitory action of catecholamines have been obtained in animals with high circulating corticosteroid levels as a result of the experimental situation, whether it was surgery, α-MT, reserpine, or prior steroid application (Ganong et al., 1976; Rose et al., 1976; Hall and Marks, 1968; Steiner, Pieri, and Kauffman, 1968; Van Loon et al., 1971). In contrast, in intact or chronically adrenalectomized unanesthetized animals, intrahypothalamic or intraventricular NE administration was stimulatory (Hall and Marks, 1968; Daniels-Severs and Vernikos-Danellis, unpublished observations; Krieger and Krieger, 1970b). It is conceivable that the nature of the noradrenergic regulation of the hypothalamic-pituitary response may be modulated by the level of corticosteroids.

(b) Serotonin Extensive evidence indicates a role for hypothalamic serotonin (5HT) with respect to circadian and stress-induced variations in the activity of the hypothalamic-pituitary-adrenal system, but the exact nature of its involvement is the subject of considerable debate (Krieger, 1977b); Vernikos-Danellis et al., 1977). Lateral ventricular injection and medial, but not anterior or posterior, hypothalamic implants of 5HT prevent the rise in corticosterone levels in response to ether and surgical stress in hexobarbital-anesthetized rats (Vermes and Telegdy, 1972). Inhibition of corticosterone release, induced by intraventricular administration of DA or NE in phenobarbital-anesthetized rats, is accompanied by increased hypothalamic 5HT content, and this inhibition is abolished by lowering hypothalamic 5HT levels through pretreatment with p-chlorophenylalanine (PCPA) (Vermes et al., 1972). Similarly, the reduction in plasma cortisol levels and increase in hypothalamic 5HT levels induced by injections of arginine vasotocin in urethane-anesthetized cats is prevented by PCPA treatment (Pavel et al., 1977). However, in unanesthetized cats 5HT microinjection into the ventromedial hypothalamus–median eminence region stimulates corticosteroid secretion (Krieger and Krieger, 1970a). Similarly, in in vitro rat hypothalamus, 5HT results in a dose-dependent increase in CRF release which can be prevented by application of the 5HT receptor blocker methysergide. In this preparation, application of the indolealkylamine metabolite of 5HT, melatonin, also inhibits 5HT-induced CRF release (Jones, Hillhouse, and Burden, 1976a,b).

These in vitro data agree most closely with the stimulatory effect of

5HT seen in unanesthetized cats. Relevant to this point, it has been demonstrated that lateral ventricular injections of 5HT into unanesthetized rats bearing chronic cannulae stimulates CRF release and raises plasma corticosteroid levels, but this effect is abolished by pentobarbitone anesthesia (Abe and Hiroshige, 1974). It appears, then, that anesthesia can alter the hypothalamic-pituitary-adrenal response to intracranial 5HT administration. The effect of application of anesthetics on 5HT-stimulated CRF release in in vitro systems would be of interest regarding this phenomenon. It should be noted, also, that 5HT appears to inhibit hypothalamic-pituitary-adrenal activity following stress, but in non-stress paradigms itself leads to increased activity of this system.

The hypothalamus is densely innervated by 5HT-containing fibers ascending in the medial forebrain bundle (MFB) from the midbrain raphe complex. Destruction of this raphe system reduces brain 5HT levels and tryptophan hydroxylase activity as well as reducing the high-affinity uptake of 5HT in hypothalamic synaptosomes (Kuhar, Roth, and Aghajanian, 1971; Kellar et al., 1977). Electrolytic lesions of the raphe nuclei augmented the plasma corticosterone response to stress as indicated by both supranormal elevation and prolonged secretion, in conjunction with reduced levels of hypothalamic 5HT, following ether plus footshock in rats (Vermes, Telegdy, and Lissak, 1974). Following application of various stressors in intact rats, hypothalamic 5HT levels decrease, with the maximum effect occuring 20-30 minutes following stress initiation, when circulating corticosterone is at peak levels (Vermes, Telegdy, and Lissak, 1973). In agreement with these studies, electrical stimulation of the midbrain raphe reduced the plasma corticosterone response to either stress in conscious, chronically implanted rats, and this inhibition was blocked by methysergide (Kovács et al., 1976). Treatment of rats with PCPA lowered brain 5HT and enhanced the secretion of ACTH in response to ether stress (Berger, Barchas, and Vernikos-Danellis, 1974), while loading with tryptophan, the amino acid 5HT precursor, inhibited the plasma corticosterone response to ether stress in a dose-dependent manner (Vernikos-Danellis et al., 1977).

Alterations in central 5HT system activity following endocrine manipulations have been less well studied. Adrenalectomy does not alter tryptophan hydroxylase activity (Kizer et al., 1976), but has been reported to lower brain 5HT (Pfeifer et al., 1963). Conversely, peripheral corticosterone injections in intact rats increased hypothalamic 5HT levels and returned elevated 5HT levels and 5-hydroxy-indoleacetic acid levels to normal in adrenalectomized rats (Telegdy and Vermes, 1975). Further, ACTH injections raise 5HT levels in the hypothalamus of intact, but not adrenalectomized rats (Vermes et al., 1973), indicating glucocorticoid mediation.

In the in vitro rat pituitary neurointermediate lobe preparation, 5HT stimulated ACTH secretion (Fischer and Moriarty, 1977). In in vitro preparations of dispersed pars intermedia cells, 5HT stimulated ACTH release in a dose-dependent fashion, but 5HT had no effect on pars distalis. The conclusion was drawn that 5HT fibers directly innervate pars intermedia and regulate local ACTH secretion (Kraicer and Morris, 1976).

The nature of hypothalamic 5HT regulation of CRF release, as is evident from this brief review, is not understood. However, several possibilities present themselves which may provide some degree of resolution of discrepant data. It is clear that procedural variables such as the presence or absence of anesthesia as well as the type of anesthesia employed are critical and must be taken into account. Second, the site of action of exogenously administered 5HT and 5HT-active pharmacological agents should also be critically evaluated. Depending upon the site of injection, 5HT can either stimulate or inhibit the hypothalamic-pituitary-adrenal system. Interpretation of these studies is further confounded by whether or not the effects of 5HT are assessed in relation to basal activity of this system or in situations of stress. There is no a priori reason to assume a similar effect should obtain in different endocrine states.

Manipulation of endogenous 5HT systems, in particular treatment with agents or lesions that lower hypothalamic 5HT, augment the response of the pituitary-adrenal system to stress and rather consistently indicate that at least the afferents to the hypothalamus from the midbrain raphe nuclei can function to inhibit stress-induced activity of this system. On the other hand, 5HT may stimulate the release of ACTH directly at the pituitary. Intraperitoneal injections of fenfluramine, a halogenated amphetamine derivative that presumably causes rapid release of central endogenous 5HT stores (Trulson and Jacobs, 1976), induce hypersecretion of corticosterone in the rat for up to four hours after injection. Pretreatment with the glucocorticoid prednisolone does not alter this response, but it is abolished by hypophysectomy. However, at three days following treatment with fenfluramine, when 5HT levels in brain are reduced, reportedly because of selective cytotoxic effects to the β-9 5HT cells in the midbrain (Harvey, McMaster, and Fuller, 1977), the plasma corticosterone response to ether stress is augmented. These data indicate an immediate activation of the hypothalamic-pituitary-adrenal system to released 5HT, perhaps directly at the level of the pituitary, and a later loss of stress-inhibitory mechanisms due to damage to ascending 5HT fibers (Heybach and Vernikos-Danellis, 1978a).

(c) Acetylcholine   With few exceptions, administration of acetylcholine (Ach) and cholinomimetics leads to stimulation of the hypothalamic-pituitary-adrenal system. In cats implantation of carbachol into the median eminence region stimulated corticosteroid secretion, and this effect was blocked by pretreatment with atropine (Krieger and Krieger, 1970a,b). Implants of atrophine in the hypothalamus of rats rostral to the periventricular nuclei inhibited the rise in plasma corticosterone induced by ether stress or intraventricular injection of arginine vasopressin (Hedge and Smelik, 1968). In cats carbachol reduced corticosteroid secretion when injected into the preoptic area but stimulated corticosteroid secretion when applied to the posterior hypothalamic region (Endroczi and Lissak, 1963). Intraventricular carbachol stimulates ACTH secretion, and this effect is enhanced by reserpine pretreatment in rats (Hall and Marks, 1968).

In in vitro preparations ACh stimulated CRF release from rat hypothalamus in a dose-related manner, and this effect was blocked by hexamethonium and only slightly reduced by atropine (Hillhouse et al., 1975; Jones and Hillhouse, 1977). However, ACh fails to effect the release of CRF from in vitro median eminence (Jones et al., 1976a). In addition, ACh stimulates ACTH release from in vitro neurointermediate lobe (Fischer and Moriarty, 1977), but has no effect on dispersed pars intermedia cells (Kraicer and Morris, 1976).

The available evidence suggests a stimulatory role for cholinergic neurons in CRF release from the hypothalamus and ACTH release from the pituitary. The nature of the receptors that mediate these excitatory effects remains to be established, since both atropine and hexamethonium can inhibit the effect of ACh in different preparations. It would appear that multiple cholinergic synapses mediate the hypothalamic secretion of CRF, and that both muscarinic and nicotinic receptors are involved.

(d) GABA   Other central transmitter substances have received much less attention with respect to regulation of CRF release. Gamma-aminobutyrate (GABA) has been reported to elevate corticosteroid levels in unanesthetized cats (Krieger and Krieger, 1970a). However, intraventricular injections of GABA inhibit ACTH release in rats with hypothalamic islands (Makara and Stark, 1974). In the in vitro hypothalamic preparation, Jones and Hillhouse (1977) found that GABA inhibited the CRF release in response to serotonin. The data support the general concept that GABA exerts a tonic inhibitory influence on hypothalamic-pituitary-adrenal activity, both under basal conditions and in response to stressful stimuli.

Models of the anatomy and neurochemistry of the neural systems thought to be involved in the regulation of CRF release have been proposed (Jones et al., 1976a,b), but they fail to resolve completely the discrepancies that exist in the literature. The discovery regarding central monoaminergic regulation of the stress response and concurrent models of the nature of monoaminergic influence developed generally on the basis of the technical and analytical advances in this field. It is more than likely that the well-studied neurotransmitter systems are not the only systems involved in the regulation of the CRF neuron. The recent explosion of evidence of central peptide neurotransmitter systems (particularly endogenous opiate systems) and their close association with the pituitary and ACTH is but one example of possible additional neuroregulatory mechanisms. Furthermore, our current lack of understanding of the complex anatomy of the hypothalamus and the nature of the receptors on the CRF neurons as well as other neurons in the hypothalamus that are involved in this control, presents the possibility of a rather staggering degree of complexity in the hypothalamic mechanisms alone. The further possibility of direct neural innervation and transmitter receptor systems in the pituitary itself certainly precludes firm conclusions as to the nature of the regulatory effect exerted by any one suspected transmitter substance.

(2) Corticosteroids: Role, Site, and Mechanism of Action

Most of the evidence that the secretion of ACTH is controlled by changes in the blood level of corticosteroids has been provided by studies showing that large doses of corticoids depress the secretion of ACTH (Sayers and Sayers, 1945), and that animals with adrenocortical insufficiency have high circulating ACTH levels (Hodges and Vernikos, 1959; Fortier, 1959b). The original hypothesis of a negative feedback control of ACTH secretion suggested that stress causes increased utilization of corticosteroids by peripheral tissues, and that the resulting low blood level of the steroids acts as a stimulus to the pituitary gland to increase its output of ACTH (Sayers and Sayers, 1947). Attempts in the 1950s to demonstrate increased peripheral utilization of corticoids during stress were unsuccessful (Ulrich and Long, 1956; Eik-Nes and Samuels, 1958). Although the thesis that increased adrenocortical activity is essential for the animal to withstand stress has survived, the exact mechanism of this process remains obscure. A notable exception is the recent important series of studies reported by Gann and his coworkers (Gann and Cryer, 1973; Pirkle and Gann, 1976), indicating an essential function of the adrenal cortex in the maintenance of plasma volume and the requirement for increased amounts of circulating cortisol for restoration of plasma protein and the associated restitution of blood volume after hemorrhage in the dog.

It has generally been assumed that the degree of inhibition of pituitary ACTH secretion is directly proportional to the blood corticosteroid concentration. Such an assumption is generally incorrect, and numerous examples exist in the literature demonstrating no direct correlation between circulating ACTH and corticosteroids when the two are measured concomitantly. Of what physiological importance then is this negative feedback system? There appear to be at least three aspects of corticosteroid inhibition of the pituitary-adrenal system that can be dissociated experimentally. The evidence is strong for an effect of corticosteroids in the control of the synthesis and basal secretion of ACTH. This response exhibits a time lag that is evident as a delay between the disappearance of plasma corticosteroids and the rise in plasma ACTH after adrenalectomy (Hodges and Vernikos, 1959; Dallman et al., 1972) and a delay between the administration of a large dose of steroid and the long-lasting inhibition of pituitary ACTH secretion, evident well after the plasma corticosteroid concentration has returned to the resting level (Smelik, 1963; Hodges and Jones, 1964). In addition to this slow or delayed feedback, a fast-responding component of the system has been demonstrated, through a carefully designed series of experiments, to operate under circumstances that closely mimic physiologically attainable levels of circulating corticosteroids. By comparing the magnitude of the stress response in rats at various times after the administration of a small dose of corticosterone, fast feedback inhibition, which possesses the characteristics of rate sensitivity and saturation, can be shown to occur within 20 minutes (Jones et al., 1972). Complete inhibition of stress-induced ACTH secretion during an i.p. infusion of corticosterone was found only when the plasma level was rising at a rate exceeding 1.5 $\mu g/100$ ml/min. Inhibition of ACTH secretion was not related to the absolute plasma concentration of corticosterone. Inhibition of the stress response could be terminated either by increasing the concentration of the infusate or the duration of the infusion. Thus Jones et al. (1972, 1974) concluded that fast feedback possesses characteristics of rate sensitivity and saturation. With the development of more sensitive techniques for the assay of plasma ACTH, it has been possible to demonstrate a fast feedback increase in circulating ACTH 10 minutes after adrenalectomy when the plasma corticosterone concentration is rapidly decreasing (Dallman et al., 1972). The physiological significance of this mechanism in the modulation of the stress response, however, is not readily apparent. Although increasing endogenous plasma corticosterone by an injection of ACTH can mimic fast feedback by exogenous corticosterone administration and has been shown to inhibit the response to a subsequent injection stress (Dallman and Jones, 1973), raising the endogenous corticosterone titer by other means has failed to exert fast feedback inhibition. For instance, when plasma corticosterone was increased by exposure of rats to electric shock or laparotomy or more prolonged restraint, the response to a subsequent minor stress such as an i.p. injection was not inhibited (Dallman and Jones, 1973). Raising circulating corticosterone levels during chronic exposure to cold stress also has no inhibitory effect on a superimposed acute ether stress response. In fact, both ACTH secretion and adrenal responsiveness have been found to be increased rather than suppressed, indicating an ineffectiveness of the high circulating corticosterone level to exert negative feedback (Daniels-Severs et al., 1973; Sakellaris and Vernikos-Danellis, 1975). Dallman and Jones (1973) concluded that although corticosterone does inhibit ACTH secretion, stress *per se* may increase the excitability of the pituitary-adrenal system, thus rendering it more responsive to a subsequent stress stimulus and making inhibition of that response more difficult. In support of this concept is the observation that although a blocking dose of exogenous corticosteroid will inhibit the plasma corticosterone response to an injection stress, the response to a second such stress applied 30 minutes later was not suppressed, suggesting that exposure to one stress stimulus increases the responsiveness to a subsequent stimulus whether plasma corticosterone was increased or not (Vernikos-Danellis, 1966). On the other hand, rats bearing MTT-F$_4$ ACTH-secreting tumors that have circulating corticosterone levels in the range of 60–70 $\mu g/100$ ml plasma are still capable of responding to a stress in spite of a markedly reduced pituitary weight and pituitary ACTH content (Vernikos-Danellis, Anderson, and Trigg, 1967); this stress response is abolished by hypophysectomy (Wherry et al., 1962). These results further emphasize that neither increased circulating corticoid concentrations nor decreased pituitary ACTH content is a reliable index of the inability of the adenohypophysis to respond to stress with increased ACTH secretion. Stress-induced hyperexcitability appears to occur only after certain types of stress stimuli. Dallman (1967) noted that prior exposure to scalding enhanced the increase in circulating corticosterone in response to histamine, whereas prior administration of histamine has no effect on the response to scalding. Similarly, histamine had no effect on the subsequent response to ether. However, pretreatment of rats with isoproterenol, epinephrine, caffeine, or a large dose of vasopressin enhanced the subsequent plasma ACTH response to ether (Vernikos-Danellis, 1968). This hyperexcitability of the pituitary to a subsequent stress, induced by such pretreatment, could be blocked by the administration of a β-adrenergic blocker but not by an α-adrenergic blocker. The thesis was proposed that the hyperexcitability of the pituitary-adrenal system induced by certain types of stress stimuli involved a β-adrenergic receptor cyclic AMP-mediated response, and was an action exerted primarily at the pituitary, although CNS sites of action could not be excluded (Vernikos-Danellis and Harris, 1968).

The nature of the hyperexcitability of the pituitary ACTH response to stress produced by prior stressful exposures seems to differ from that observed soon after adrenalectomy. Adrenalectomized rats exhibit a marked rise in circulating ACTH in response to mild stress stimuli that produce only very small responses in intact rats (Hodges and Vernikos, 1959; Hodges and Jones, 1964). This hyperresponsiveness to stress can be prevented by treatment with large doses of corticosteroids. In contrast, the initial fall in pituitary ACTH concentration after adrenalectomy, and the subsequent rise in the plasma and pituitary ACTH basal secretion, can be prevented by physiological doses of corticosterone or hydrocortisone (Hodges and Vernikos-Danellis, 1962; Hodges and Jones, 1964). This differential sensitivity to corticosteroids of basal and stress-induced release of ACTH has been taken to indicate that corticosteroids are involved in the control of both the synthesis and the basal secretion of ACTH, but that they are of questionable physiological significance in regulating the stress-induced release of the hormone (Buckingham and Hodges, 1974, 1975). Hodges (1976) has further proposed that the time lag in this inhibitory action of corticoids "suggests the existence of a corticoid sensitive controller of adrenocorticotrophic function in some tissue not readily accessible to the systemic circulation." It could equally well imply a mechanism of action mediated by some other biochemical process.

The site of action of negative feedback regulation of ACTH secretion by corticosteroids has been the subject of much controversy over the years. Corticosteroid implants in the basomedial hypothalamus, like electrolytic lesions in the same region, or hypothalamic de-afferentation, as well as implants into the midbrain or septum, have been shown repeatedly to inhibit the pituitary-adrenocortical system (Smelik and Sawyer, 1962; Corbin et al., 1965; Bohus, Nyakas, and Lissak, 1968; Smelik, 1969; Yates et al., 1974). Studies with steroid implants are, however, difficult to interpret. Not only have the amounts of steroid to which a particular brain region was exposed been excessive, but the spread of the steroid to other sites including the pituitary makes interpretation of results questionable. It is, however, apparent that corticosteroids can inhibit the pituitary-adrenal system by acting at the pituitary directly (Vale and Rivier, 1977), the hypothalamus to inhibit CRF secretion (Jones, Gillham, and Hillhouse, 1977), and at other possible CNS sites (McHugh and Smith, 1967; Feldman and Conforti, 1976).

Systematic administration has been used to identify the primary site of action of corticosteroids. By testing the ability of a median eminence extract to release ACTH from animals pretreated with different doses of hydrocortisone, it was found that inhibition of the stress response occurred over a range of doses that did not affect the responsiveness of the pituitary to the ACTH-releasing activity of the extract. Increasing the dose of hydrocortisone above 15 mg/100 g body weight resulted in decreased responsiveness of the pituitary to the extract (Vernikos-Danellis, 1964). Similar findings were reported by Yates et al. (1971) using progressively increasing doses of dexamethasone. Thus, it is obvious that naturally occurring corticosteroids act preferentially by inhibiting hypothalamic CRF activity, rather than by inhibiting directly the release of ACTH at the pituitary. Where and how corticosteroids inhibit CRF activity is certainly not known. One approach has been to try to identify central receptor sites for corticosteroids by following the distribution and uptake of labeled material. Labeled corticosteroids administered systemically are taken up by various brain regions including the hypothalamus, hippocampus, and septum, as well as by the pituitary itself (Eik-Nes and Brizzee, 1965; McEwen et al., 1969, 1970, 1972, 1976; Stevens, Grosser, and Reed, 1971). Tritiated corticosterone has been shown to be taken up in the brains of adrenalectomized rats, concentrated by the hippocampus and septum, and bound to cell nuclei (McEwen et al., 1969, 1970, 1976). Neurons appear to be the primary uptake sites. In these adrenalectomized rats the hypothalamus did not show neurons even moderately labeled with H^3-corticosterone by radioautography. Using the adrenalectomized rat model, McEwen and his associates (DeKloet, Wallach, and McEwen, 1975) discovered marked differences in the labeling characteristics of corticosterone and dexamethasone. The latter was at least five to six times more effective in labeling pituitary cell nuclear sites than were comparable amounts of corticosterone, and was considerably less bound by hippocampal nuclear sites. Furthermore, dexamethasone labeled cell nuclear sites uniformly across all brain regions in contrast to the differential binding of corticosterone and the intensity of the labeling of brain neurons, which was of equal intensity whether the rat was adrenalectomized or not (Rhees, Grosser, and Stevens, 1975; Koch et al., 1975). It has been reported recently (Turner, Shielke, and Carroll, 1977) that the regional brain cytosol binding of endogenous corticosterone differs greatly, not only quantitatively but also qualitatively, between stressed intact and adrenalectomized rats. In the stressed intact rat the pituitary and not the hippocampus showed the highest binding, followed by high binding in the preoptic, septal, and hypothalamic regions. In contrast to dexamethasone, total binding sites for corticosterone were higher in adrenalectomized than in intact rats. McEwen (1976, 1977) concludes that the receptors capable of binding dexamethasone are not substantially occupied by endogenous corticosterone and do not change in response to the absence of circulating corticosterone, and proposes the presence of multiple populations of soluble glucocorticoid receptors. These apparently respond differentially to stress or adrenalectomy and even to immediate or delayed effects of adrenalectomy (McEwen, Wallach, and Magnus, 1974; Olpe and McEwen, 1976), further emphasizing the dissociation in mechanism as well as possible sites of action of these various responses of the pituitary-adrenal system.

It should be pointed out here that the central actions of corticosteroids are by no means limited to inhibition of the pituitary-adrenal system. Hence, the relative distribution of glucocorticoid receptors and their changes after pituitary-adrenal experimental manipulations may be only of secondary or partial relevance in the regulation of the function of this system.

(3) Interaction with Behavior

The effects of pituitary-adrenal hormones on the central nervous system and behavior have been extensively reviewed (Vernikos-Danellis, 1972; Brush and Froehlich, 1975; Rheith et al., 1977; De Wied, 1977). Although for many years it was considered that the behavioral effects of these hormones were exclusively due to the potent adrenocortical steroids, which, after all, gain easy access into the CNS, it is becoming increasingly apparent that ACTH and other ACTH-like peptides of pituitary origin exert extra-adrenal behavioral effects, and that their function in the brain is that of neuroregulators or modulators of neural activity (Rheith et al., 1977; Vernikos-Danellis, 1977). Furthermore, there is evidence (Heybach and Vernikos-Danellis, 1977, 1978c) that the long-established effect of adrenocortical steroid hormones on the sensitivity to sensory stimuli (Henkin and Bartter, 1966; Henkin et al., 1967; Sakellaris, 1972) may be indirect and mediated via the pituitary. Although steroids surely exert direct, extra-pituitary effects on the brain and on behavior, it will be important, in view of these recent findings, to reconsider the existing evidence and unravel the relative importance of pituitary and adrenal hormones to various behaviors. Such a review has already been attempted by Brush and Froehlich (1975), who have astutely pointed out the sources of error in behavioral experiments based on oversimplified interpretation of the workings of the pituitary-adrenal system. They have further pointed out that investigators should refrain from postulating integrating hypotheses governing such hormonal modulation of behavior based merely on correlative studies which ignore the complexities of the system.

All behavioral manipulations are potential modulators of the activity of the pituitary-adrenal system in the experimental setting, with exposure to a novel environment or mere handling of the animal being the simplest and the earliest to be observed (Mason, Harwood, and Rosenthal, 1957; Guillemin et al., 1958). In spite of all the available information, breeding, housing, lighting, shipping, and laboratory environment are still frequently ignored as factors in stress research that may affect the outcome of experimental results. Similarly, in behavioral research the return to a "basal" plasma corticosterone concentration after a training or conditioning period is religiously accepted as tantamount to normalcy, and therefore the response of the pituitary-adrenal system is expected to be similar to that of a naive animal. The information discussed earlier in this review certainly casts serious doubts on this assumption. In fact, not only is the pituitary-adrenal system affected by such manipulations, but as well the entire physiology of the experimental animal is far from normal, with changes in plasma volume, distribution of fluids and electrolytes, and circadian rhythms being some of the most obvious factors.

In addition, it has become apparent in recent years that an animal does not predictably respond to all apparently stressful stimuli. Allowing the animal to express certain types of behavior may either reduce or completely suppress the pituitary-adrenal response resulting from exposure to a stressful stimulus. In 1971 we reported that the plasma ACTH response of rats exposed to the stress of electric shock was greatly reduced if the animals had the opportunity to fight (Conner, Vernikos-Danellis, and Levine, 1971). What was particularly interesting about these findings was that this effect was not a function of learning or expectancy (Levine, Goldman, and Coover, 1972), since it was evident within the first session. Similar observations on the behavioral modulation of the pituitary-adrenal response have been reported using appetitive extinction or reinforcement procedures (Coover, Goldman, and Levine, 1971; Davis et al., 1976) and during the feeding or watering of hungry or thirsty animals on food or water deprivation schedules (Levine and Coover, 1976; Coover, Sutton, and Heybach, 1977). The types of behavior that appear most effective in inhibiting the pituitary-adrenal system are eating, drinking, fighting, escape, and avoidance (Coover, Ursin, and Levine, 1973), which can be classified under the broad category of adaptive behavioral mechanisms. Humans exposed to otherwise highly stressful occupational tasks also show a reduction in cortisol excretion as long as uncontrollable problems do not arise (Vernikos-Danellis, Goldenrath, and Dolkas, 1975). The concept that effective coping behavior can alleviate the consequences of the stress response is not new. Although the data which Weiss (1971) originally used to support his general coping model dealt with stomach ulceration, it is clear that the pituitary-adrenal response, as measured by changes in plasma ACTH and corticosteroid levels, can be attenuated by behavioral mechanisms. These mechanisms can serve an adaptive function by dampening the physiological responses which, uncontrolled, may be excessive and have damaging consequences.

The mechanism of such behavioral inhibition of the pituitary-adrenal system is not known. It is clear, however, that it is independent of adrenal corticosteroid negative feedback, since at the time of maximum inhibition plasma corticosterone levels are reduced or falling (Heybach and

Vernikos-Danellis, 1979). Furthermore, it appears that at the time when maximal inhibition of plasma ACTH and corticosterone is evident, the pituitary-adrenal system is unresponsive to other submaximal stressful stimuli such as an i.p. injection of saline (Heybach and Vernikos-Danellis, unpublished observations).

Several central inhibitory pathways have periodically been postulated and reviewed previously (Naumenko, 1967; Van Loon et al., 1971; Ganong, 1977; Palkovits, 1977). That central noradrenergic inhibitory mechanisms mediate behavioral suppression of the pituitary-adrenal response is certainly a possibility. Weiss, Stone, and Harrell (1970) found that whole brain catecholamine concentrations were higher in animals that could escape and/or avoid electric shock than in those that could not. On the other hand, serotonergic inhibitory involvement has been suggested indirectly (Asberg et al., 1976) by the reported inhibitory effectiveness of serotonin precursor loading (Brodie, Sack, and Siever, 1973) and by the findings of decreased cerebrospinal fluid 5-hydroxyindole acetic acid in some depressive patients (Ashcroft and Sharman, 1960). Any conclusions regarding the corticosteroid-independent mechanisms by which behavioral variables modulate the intensity of the pituitary-adrenal response to stress, would be entirely speculative at this time. There is sufficient experimental evidence at this time, however, to substantiate the long-recognized phenomenon (Sachar, 1970) that successful coping behavior represents yet another mechanism that must be considered not only in terms of the overall regulation of the pituitary-adrenal system but also in the experimental design and interpretation of data using pituitary-adrenal indexes of the stress response.

References

Abe, K., and Hiroshige, T. The effects of various putative neirotransmitters on the release of corticotrophin releasing hormone from the hypothalamus of the rat *in vitro*. I. The effect of acetylcholine and noradrenaline. *Neuroendocrinol. 14:* 195–211, 1974.

Allen, C., and Kendall, J. W. Maturation of the circadian rhythm of plasma corticosterone in the rat. *Endocrinol. 80:* 926–930, 1967.

Andrews, R. V., and Folk, G. E., Jr. Circadian metabolic patterns in cultured hamster adrenal glands. *Comp. Biochem. Physiol. 11:* 393–409, 1964.

Asberg, M., Thoren, P., Traskman, L., Bertilsson, L., and Ringberger, V. "Serotonin depression"—A biochemical subgroup within the affective disorders? *Science 191:* 478–480, 1976.

Ashcroft, G. W., and Sharman, D. 5-Hydroxyindoles in human cerebrospinal fluid. *Nature (Lond.) 186:* 1050–1051, 1960.

Bellinger, L. L., Bernardis, L. L., and Mendel, V. E. Effect of ventromedial and dorsomedial hypothalamic lesions on circadian corticosterone rhythms. *Neuroendocrinol. 22:* 216–225, 1976.

Berger, P. A., Barchas, J. D., and Vernikos-Danellis, J. Serotonin and pituitary-adrenal function. *Nature (Lond.) 248:* 424–426, 1974.

Bernardis, L. L. Delayed ventricular changes in the hypothalamus of the weanling rat following electrolytic lesions of the ventromedial nucleus. *J. Neuro.-Viscer. Rel. 32:* 347–354, 1972.

Bernardis, L. L. Disruption of diurnal feeding and weight gain cycles in weanling rats by ventromedial and dorsomedial hypothalamic lesions. *Physiol. Behav. 10:* 855–861, 1973.

Berson, S. A., and Yalow, R. S. Radioimmunoassay of ACTH in plasma. *J. Clin. Invest. 47:* 2725–2751, 1968.

Bliss, E. L., Sandberg, A. A., Nelson, D. H., and Eik-Nes, K. The normal level of 17-hydroxycorticosteroids in the peripheral blood in man. *J. Clin. Invest. 32:* 818–825, 1953.

Bohus, C., Nyakas, C., and Lissak, K. Involvement of suprahypothalamic structures in the hormonal feedback action of corticosteroids. *Acta Physiol. Hung. 34:* 1–8, 1968.

Bransome, E. D., and Reddy, N. J. Studies of adrenal nucleic acids: The influence of ACTH, unilateral adrenalectomy and growth hormone upon adrenal RNA and DNA in the dog. *Endocrinol. 69:* 997–1008, 1961.

Brodie, H. K. H., Sack, R., and Siever, L. Clinical studies of L-5-hydroxytryptophan in depression. In Barchas, J. D., and Usdin, E. (eds.), *Serotonin and Behavior*. New York and London: Academic Press, 1973, pp. 549–560.

Brush, F. R., and Froehlich, J. C. Motivational effects of the pituitary and adrenal hormones. In Eleftheriou, B., and Spralt, R. L. (eds.), *Hormonal Correlates of Behavior. Vol. II. An Organismic View*. New York: Plenum Press, 1975, pp. 777–806.

Buckingham, J. C., and Hodges, J. R. Interrelationships of pituitary and plasma corticotrophin and plasma corticosterone in adrenalectomized and stressed adrenalectomized rats. *J. Endocrin. 63:* 213–222, 1974.

Buckingham, J. C., and Hodges, J. R. Interrelationships of pituitary and plasma corticotrophin and plasma corticosterone during adrenocortical regeneration in the rat. *J. Endocrin. 67:* 411–417, 1975.

Carr, I. The human adrenal cortex at the time of death. *J. Path. Bact. 78:* 533–541, 1959.

Cater, D. B., and Stack-Dunne, M. P. Mitotic activity in the adrenal cortex studied in the rat. *Ciba Found. Colloq. Endocrinol. 8:* 31–41, 1955.

Catt, K. J., and Dufau, M. L. Peptide hormone receptors. *Ann. Rev. Physiol. 39:* 529–557, 1977.

Cheifetz, P., Gaffud, N., and Dingman, J. F. Effects of bilateral adrenalectomy and continuous light on the circadian rhythm of corticotropin in female rats. *Endocrinol. 82:* 1117–1124, 1968.

Chowers, I., Conforti, N., and Feldman, S. Effects of corticosteroids on hypothalamic corticotropin releasing factor and pituitary ACTH content. *Neuroendocrinol. 2:* 193–199, 1967.

Cochrane, D. E., and Douglas, W. W. Depolarizing effects of the ionophores X537A and A23187 and their relevance to secretion. *Brit. J. Pharmacol. 54:* 400–402, 1975.

Collip, J. B., Anderson, E. M., and Thomson, D. L. Adrenotropic hormone of anterior pituitary lobe. *Lancet 2:* 347–348, 1933.

Conner, R. L., Vernikos-Danellis, J., and Levine, S. Stress, fighting and neuroendocrine function. *Nature (Lond.) 234:* 564–566, 1971.

Coover, G. D., Goldman, L., and Levine, S. Plasma corticosterone levels during extinction of a lever-press response in hippocampectomized rats. *Physiol. and Behav. 7:* 727–732, 1971.

Coover, G. D., Sutton, B. R., and Heybach, J. P. Conditioning decreases in plasma corticosterone in rats by pairing stimuli with daily feedings. *J. Comp. Physiol. Psych. 91:* 716–726, 1977.

Coover, G. D., Ursin, H., and Levine, S. Plasma corticosterone levels during active avoidance learning in rats. *J. Comp. Physiol. Psych. 82:* 170–174, 1973.

Corbin, A., Mangili, G., Motta, M., and Martini, L. Effect of hypothalamic and mesencephalic steroid implantations on ACTH feedback mechanisms. *Endocrinol. 76:* 811–818, 1965.

Dahlstrom, A., and Fuxe, K. Monoamines and the pituitary gland. *Acta Endocrinol. (Kbh.) 51:* 301–314, 1966.

Dallman, M. F. Central neural inputs and feedback pathways of the adrenocortical system in the rat. Ph.D. Thesis, Stanford University, 1967.

Dallman, M. F., Engeland, W. C., and McBride, M. H. The neural regulation of compensatory adrenal growth. In Krieger, D. T., and Ganong, W. F. (eds.), *ACTH and Related Peptides: Structure, Regulation and Action. Ann. N.Y. Acad. Sci. 297:* 373–392, 1977.

Dallman, M. F., Engeland, W. C., and Shinsako, J. Nychtohemeral rhythm in adrenal responsiveness to ACTH. *Proc. 58th Ann. Mtg. Endocrin. Soc.,* San Francisco, 1976, p. 58.

Dallman, M. F., Engeland, W. C., and Shinsako, J. Compensatory adrenal growth: a neurally mediated reflex. *Am. J. Physiol. 231:* 408–414, 1976.

Dallman, M. F., and Jones, M. T. Corticosteroid feedback control of ACTH secretion: Effect of stress-induced corticosterone secretion on subsequent stress responses in the rat. *Endocrinol. 92:* 1367–1375, 1973.

Dallman, M. F., Jones, M. T., Vernikos-Danellis, J., and Ganong, W. F. Corticosteroid feedback control of ACTH secretion: Rapid effect of bilateral adrenalectomy on plasma ACTH in the rat. *Endocrinol. 91:* 961–968, 1972.

Daniels-Severs, A. E., Goodwin, A. L., Keil, L. C., and Vernikos-Danellis, J. Effect of chronic crowding and cold on the pituitary-adrenal system. *Pharmacol. 9:* 348–356, 1973.

David-Nelson, M. A., and Brodish, A. Evidence for a diurnal rhythm of CRF in the hypothalamus. *Endocrinol. 85:* 861–866, 1969.

Davis, H., Memmott, J., Macfadden, L., and Levine, S. Pituitary-adrenal activity under different appetitive extinction procedures. *Physiol. and Behav. 17:* 687–690, 1976.

DeKloet, R., Wallach, G., and McEwen, B. S. Differences in corticosterone and dexamethasone binding in rat brain and pituitary. *Endocrinol. 96:* 598–609, 1975.

Demura, H., West, C. D., Nugent, C. A., Nagakawa, K., and Tyler, F. H. A sensitive radiommunoassay for plasma ACTH levels. *J. Clin. Endocrinol. Metab. 26:* 1297–1301, 1966.

De Wied, D. The site of the blocking action of dexamethasone on stress-induced pituitary ACTH release. *J. Endocrinol. 29:* 29–36, 1964.

De Wied, D. Behavioral effects of neuropeptides related to ACTH, MSH nd β-LPH. In Krieger, D. T., and Ganong, W. F. (eds.), *ACTH and Related Peptides: Structure, Regulation and Action. Ann. N.Y. Acad. Sci. 297:* 263–274, 1977.

Douglas, W. W. Mechanisms of stimulus-secretion coupling: Variations on the theme of calcium-activated exocytosis. *Proc. Int. Congr. Physiol.,* Paris, July, 1977.

Douglas, W. W., and Taraskevich, P. S. Action potentials (probably calcium spikes) in normal and cancerous cells of the anterior pituitary and the stimulant effect of thyrotropin releasing hormone, TRH. *J. Phsyiol. (Lond.), 272:* 41–43, 1977.

Dunn, J. D., Dyer, R., and Bennett, M. Diurnal variation in plasma corticosterone following long term exposure to continuous illumination. *Endocrinol. 90:* 1660–1663, 1972.

Edwardson, J. A., and Bennett, G. W. Modulation of corticotrophin releasing factor release from hypothalamic synaptosomes. *Nature (Lond.) 251:* 425–427, 1974.

Eik-Nes, K. B., and Brizzee, K. R. Concentration of tritium in brain tissue of dogs given [2-^{3}H]-cortisol intravenously. *Biochem. Biophys. Acta. 97:* 320–333, 1965.

Eik-Nes, K. B., and Samuels, L. T. Metabolism of cortisol in normal and "stressed" dogs. *Endocrinol. 63:* 82–88, 1958.

Endroczi, E., and Lissak, K. Effect of hypothalamic and brainstem structures on pituitary-adrenocortical function. *Acta Physiol. Hung. 24:* 67–77, 1963.

Engeland, W. C., and Dallman, M. F. Compensatory adrenal growth is neurally mediated. *Neuroendoctrinol. 19:* 352–362, 1975.

Engeland, W. C., and Dallman, M. F. Neural mediation of compensatory adrenal growth. *Endocrinol. 99:* 1659–1662, 1976.

Engeland, W. C., Shinsako, J., Winget, C. M., Vernikos-Danellis, J., and Dallman, M. F. Circadian patterns of stress induced ACTH secretion are modified by corticosterone responses. *Endocrinol. 100:* 138–147, 1977.

Fahringer, E. E., Foley, E. L., and Redgate, E. S. Pituitary adrenal response to ketamine and the inhibition of the response by catecholaminergic blockade. *Neuroendocrinol. 14:* 151–164, 1974.

Feldman, S., and Conforti, N. Inhibition and facilitation of feedback influences of dexamethasone on adrenocrotical responses to ether stress in rats with hypothalamic deafferentations and brain lesions. *Acta Endocrinol. 82:* 785–791, 1976.

Ferguson, J. J. Protein synthesis and adrenocorticotropin responsiveness. *J. Biol. Chem. 238:* 2754–2759, 1963.

Fiala, S., Sproul, E. E., and Fiala, A. Action of corticotrophin (ACTH) on nucleic acids and subcellular elements of adrenal cortex. *J. Biophys. Biochem. Cytol. 2:* 115–126, 1956.

Fischer, J. L., and Moriarty, C. M. Control of bioactive corticotropin release from the neurointermediate lobe of the rat pituitary *in vitro. Endocrinol. 100:* 1047–1054, 1977.

Fortier, C. Adenohypophysis corticotropin, plasma free corticosteroids and adrenal weight following surgical trauma in the rat. *Archiv. Int. Physiol. 67:* 333–340, 1959a.

Fortier, C. Pituitary ACTH and plasma free corticosteroids following bilateral adrenalectomy in the rat. *Proc. Soc. Exp. Biol. Med. 100:* 13–16, 1959b.

Fuxe, K., Hokfelt, T., Jonsson, G., Levine, S., Lidbrink, F., and Lofstrom, A. Studies on central monoamine neurons. In Brodish, A., and Redgate, E. S. (eds.), *Brain Pituitary-Adrenal Interrelationships*. Basel: Karger, 1973, pp. 239-269.

Gann, D. S., and Cryer, G. L. Feedback control of ACTH secretion by cortisol. In Brodish, A., and Redgate, E. S. (eds.), *Brain Pituitary-Adrenal Interrelationships*. Basel: Karger, 1973, pp. 197-223.

Ganong, W. F. Neurotransmitters involved in ACTH secretion: Catecholamines. In Krieger, D. T., and Ganong, W. F. (eds.), *ACTH and Related Peptides: Structure, Regulation and Action. Ann. N.Y. Acad. Sci. 297:* 509-517, 1977.

Ganong, W. F., Kramer, N., Salmon, J., Reid, A., Lovinger, R., Scapagnini, U., Boryczka., A. T., and Shackelford, R. Pharmacological evidence for inhibition of ACTH secretion by a central adrenergic system in the dog. *Neurosci. 1:* 167-174, 1976.

Gerendai, I., Kiss, J., Molnar, J., and Halasz, B. Further data on the existence of a neural pathway from the adrenal gland to the hypothalamus. *Cell Tissue Res. 153:* 559-564, 1974.

Guillemin, R., Clayton, G. W., Smith, J. D., and Lipscomb, H. S. Measurement of free corticosteroids in rat plasma. Physiological validation of a method. *Endocrinol. 63:* 349-352, 1958.

Guillemin, D., Dean, W. E., and Liebelt, R. A. Nychtohemeral variations in plasma free corticosteroid levels of the rat. *Proc. Soc. Exp. Biol. Med. 101:* 394-395, 1959.

Gwinup, G., Steinberg, T., King, C., and Vernikos-Danellis, J. Vasopressin induced ACTH secretion in man. *J. Clin. Endocrinol. Metab. 27:* 927-930, 1967.

Halasz, B., Slusher, M. A., and Gorski, R. A. Adrenocorticotropic hormone secretion in rats after partial or total deafferentation of the medial basal hypothalamus. *Neuroendocrinol. 2:* 43-55, 1967.

Halasz, B., and Szentágothai, J. Histologischer beweis einer neuroesen signaluebernittlung von der nebenneirenrinde zum hypothalamus. *Z. Zellforsch. Mikrosk. Anat. 50:* 297-306, 1959.

Hall, M. M., and Marks, B. H. Neurotransmitter effects of biogenic amines in the regullation of pituitary ACTH secretion. *Pharmacol. 10:* 225, 1968.

Harris, G. W. *Neural Control of the Pituitary Gland.* London: Amold, 1955.

Harvey, J. A., McMaster, S. E., and Fuller, R. W. Comparison between the neurotoxic and serotonin depleting effects of various halogenated derivatives of amphetamine in the rat. *J. Pharmacol. Exp. Therap. 202:* 581-589, 1977.

Hedge, G. A. The effects of prostaglandins on ACTH secretion. *Endocrinol. 91:* 925-933, 1972.

Hedge, G. A., and Smelik, P. G. Corticotrophin release: Inhibition by intrahypothalamic implantation of atropine. *Science 159:* 891-892, 1968.

Henkin, R. I., and Bartter, F. C. Studies on olfactory thresholds in normal man and in patients with adrenal cortical insufficiency: The role of adrenal cortical steroids and of serum sodium concentration. *J. Clin. Invest. 45:* 1631-1639, 1966.

Henkin, R. I., McGlone, R. E., Daly, R., and Bartter, F. C. Studies on auditory thresholds in normal man and in patients with adrenal cortical insufficiency: The role of adrenal cortical steroids. *J. Clin. Invest. 46:* 429-435, 1967.

Heybach, J. P., and Vernikos-Danellis, J. Modulation of pain sensitivity in the rat by adrenocortical hormones. *Neurosci. Abstracts 3:* 346, 1977.

Heybach, J. P., and Vernikos-Danellis, J. The effects of fenfluramine administration on the activity of the pituitary-adrenal system in the rat. *Proc. West. Pharmacol. Soc. 21:* 19–25, 1978a.

Heybach, J. P., and Vernikos-Danellis, J. Inhibition of the pituitary-adrenal response to stress during deprivation-induced feeding. *Indocrinol.,* in press 1979.

Heybach, J. P. and Vernikos-Danellis, J. The effect of pituitary-adrenal function in the modulation of pain sensitivity in the rat. *J. Physiol. (Lond.), 283:* 331–340, 1978c.

Hillhouse, E. W., Burden, J., and Jones, M. T. The effects of various putative neurotransmitters on the release of corticotrophin-releasing hormone from the hypothalamus of the rat *in vitro.* I. The effect of acetylcholine and noradrenaline. *Neuroendocrinol. 17:* 1–11, 1975.

Hiroshige, T. Assay of corticotropin releasing factor. In Brodish, A., and Redgate, E. S. (eds.), *Brain Pituitary-Adrenal Interrelationships.* Basel: Karger, 1973a, pp. 57–78.

Hiroshige, T., Abe, K., Wada, S., and Kaneko, M. Sex differences in the circadian periodicity of CRF activity in the rat hypothalamus. *Neuroendocrinol. 11:* 306–320, 1973.

Hiroshige, T., Kunita, H., Ogura, C., and Itoh, S. Effects on ACTH release of intrapituitary injections of posterior pituitary hormones and several amines in the hypothalamus. *Jap. J. Physiol. 18:* 606–619, 1968.

Hiroshige, T., Sakakura, M., and Itoh, S. Diurnal variation of corticotropin releasing activity in the rat hypothalamus. *Endocrinol. Jap. 16:* 465–469, 1969.

Hiroshige, T., and Sato, T. Circadian rhythm and stress induced changes in hypothalamic content of corticotropin-releasing activity during postnatal development in the rat. *Endocrinol. 86:* 1184–1186, 1970.

Hiroshige, T., and Sato, T. Changes in hypothalamic content of corticotropin-releasing activity following stress during neonatal maturation in the rat. *Neuroendocrinol. 7:* 257–270, 1971.

Hiroshige, T., Sato, T., and Abe, K. Dynamic changes in hypothalamic content of corticotropin-releasing factor following noxious stimuli: Delayed response in early neonates in comparison with biphasic response in adult rats. *Endocrinol. 89:* 1287–1294, 1971.

Hiroshige, T., Sato, T., Ohta, R., and Itoh, S. Increase in corticotropin-releasing activity in the rat hypothalamus following noxious stimuli. *Jap. J. Physiol. 19:* 866–875, 1969.

Hodges, J. R. The hypothalamic-pituitary-adrenocortical system. *J. Pharm. Pharmac. 28:* 379–382, 1976.

Hodges, J. R., and Jones, M. T. Changes in pituitary corticotropic function in adrenalectomized rats. *J. Physiol. 173:* 190–200, 1964.

Hodges, J. R., and Vernikos, J. Circulating corticotrophin in normal and adrenalectomized rats after stress. *Acta Endocrinol. 30:* 188–196, 1959.

Hodges, J. R., and Vernikos-Danellis, J. Pituitary and blood corticotrophin changes in adrenalectomized rats maintained on physiological doses of corticosteroids. *Acta Endocrinol. (Kbh) 39:* 79–86, 1962.

Hornsby, P. J., and Gill, G. N. Changing hormonal responsiveness of normal bovine adrenocortical cells through 50 generations in tissue culture: Dissociation of ACTH control of steroidogenesis and growth. *Endocr. Soc. Abstracts 289:* 201, 1977.

Howe, A. The mammalian pars intermedia: A review of its structure and function. *J. Endocrinol. 59:* 385–409, 1973.

Hsu, T-H., Hsu, C-K., and Gann, D. S. Potentiation of the ACTH response to metyrapone by L-DOPA in the monkey. *Endocrinol. 99:* 9115–1118, 1976.

Ifft, J. D. The effect of endocrine gland extirpations on the size of nucleoli in the rat hypothalamic neurons. *Anat. Rec. 148:* 599–604, 1964.

Imrie, R. C., Ramaiah, J. R., Antoni, F., and Hutchison, W. C. The effect of adrenocorticotrophin on the nucleic acid metabolism of the rat adrenal gland. *J. Endocrinol. 32:* 303–312, 1965.

Ingle, D. J. Control of regeneration of the adrenal cortex in the rat. *Symposium on Pituitary-Adrenal Function.* AAAS. Baltimore: Horn-Shafer, 1950, pp. 49–50.

Jacobowitz, D. M., and Marks, B. H. Effect of stress on glycogen and phosphorylase in the rat anterior pituitary. *Endocrinol. 75:* 86–88, 1964.

Jacobowitz, D. M., Marks, B. H., and Vernikos-Danellis, J. Effects of acute stress on uptake of serine-1-C^{14} by pituitary and hypothalamus of intact rats. *Fed. Proc. 22:* 507, 1963.

Johnson, J. T., and Levine, S. Influence of water deprivation on adrenocortical rhythms. *Neuroendocrinol. 11:* 268–273, 1973.

Jones, M. T., Brush, F. R., and Neame, R. L. B. Characteristics of fast feedback control of corticotrophin release by corticosteroids. *J. Endocrinol. 55:* 489–497, 1972.

Jones, M. T., Gillham, B., and Hillhouse, E. W. The nature of corticotropin releasing factor from rat hypothalamus *in vitro. Fed. Proc. 36:* 2104–2109, 1977.

Jones, M. T., and Hillhouse, E. W. Neurotransmitter regulation of corticotropin releasing factor *in vitro.* In Krieger, D. T., and Ganong, W. F. (eds.), *ACTH and Related Peptides: Structure, Regulation and Action. Ann. N.Y. Acad. Sci. 297:* 536–558, 1977.

Jones, M. T., Hillhouse, E. W., and Burden, J. Effects of various putative neurotransmitters on the secretion of corticotropin-releasing hormone from the rat hypothalamus *in vitro.* A model of the neurotransmitters involved. *J. Endocrinol. 69:* 1–10, 1976a.

Jones, M. T., Hillhouse, E. W., and Burden, J. Secretion of corticotropin-releasing hormone *in vitro.* In Martini, L., and Ganong, W. F. (eds.), *Frontiers in Neuroendocrinology. New York: Raven Press, 4:* 195–226, 1976b.

Jones, M. T., Tiptaft, E. M., Brush, F. R., Fergusson, D. A. N. and Neame, R. L. B. Evidence for dual corticosteroid receptor mechanisms in the feedback control of adrenocorticotrophin secretion. *J. Endocrinol. 60:* 223–233, 1974.

Kellar, K. J., Brown, P. A., Madrid, J., Berstein, M., Vernikos-Danellis, J., and Mehlar, W. R. Origins of serotonin innervation of forebrain structures. *Exp. Neurol. 56:* 52–62, 1977.

Kidokoro, Y. Sodium and calcium components of the action potential in a developing skeletal muscle cell line. *J. Physiol. (Lond.) 244:* 145–159, 1975.

Kiss, V. T. Experimental-morphologische Analyse der Nerbenin. *Acta Anat. (Basel) 13:* 81–89, 1951.

Kizer, J. S., Palkovits, M., Kopin, J. J., Saavedra, J. M., and Brownstein, M. J. Lack of effect of various endocrine manipulations on tryptophan hydroxylase activity of individual nuclei of the hypothalamus, limbic system and midbrain of the rat. *Endocrinol. 98:* 743–747, 1976.

Kizer, J. S., Palkovits, M., Zivin, J., Brownstein, M., Saavedra, J. M., and Kopin, J. J. The effect of endocrinological manipulations on tyrosine hydroxylase and dopamine-β-hydroxylase activities in individual hypothalamic nuclei of the adult male rat. *Endocrinol. 95:* 799–812, 1974.

Kobayashi, Y. Functional morphology of the pars intermedia of the rat hypophysis as revealed with the electron microscope. IV. Effect of corticosterone on the pars intermedia of intact and adrenalectomized rats. *Gunma Symposium on Endocrinology 6:* 107–121, 1969.

Koch, B, Lutz, B., Briaud, B., and Mialhe, C. Glucocorticoid binding to adenohypophysis receptors and its physiological role. *Neuroendocrinol. 18:* 299–310, 1975.

Kovács, G. L., Kishonti, J., Lissák, K., and Telegdy, G. Dose related dual action of corticosterone on hypothalamic serotonin content in rats. *Neurosci. Lett. 8:* 305–310, 1976.

Kraicer, J., and Milligan, J. V. Suppression of ACTH release from adenohypophysis by corticosterone: An *in vitro* study. *Endocrinol. 87:* 371–376, 1970.

Kraicer, J., Milligan, J. V., Gosbee, J. L., Conrad, R. H., and Branson, C. M. *In vitro* release of ACTH: Effects of potassium, calcium and corticosterone. *Endocrinol. 85:* 1144–1153, 1969a.

Kraicer, J., Milligan, J. V., Gosbee, J. L., Conrad, R. H., and Branson, C. M. Potassium, corticosterone and adrenocorticotropic hormone release *in vitro*. *Science 164:* 426–428, 1969b.

Kraicer, J., and Morris, A. R. *In vitro* release of ACTH from dispersed pars intermedia cells. II. Effect of neurotransmitter substances. *Neuroendocrinol. 21:* 175–192, 1976.

Krieger, D. T. Circadian corticosteroid periodicity: Critical period for abolition by neonatal injection of corticosteroid. *Science 178:* 1205–1207, 1972.

Krieger, D. T. Food and water restriction shifts corticosterone, temperature, activity and brain amine periodicity. *Endocrinol. 95:* 1195–1201, 1974.

Krieger, D. T. Serotonin and regulation of ACTH secretion. In Krieger, D. T., and Ganong, W. F. (eds.), *ACTH and Related Peptides: Structure, Regulation and Action. Ann. N.Y. Acad. Sci. 297:* 527–534, 1977a.

Krieger, D. T. Regulation of circadian periodicity of plasma ACTH levels. In Krieger, D. T., and Ganong, W. F. (eds.), *ACTH and Related Peptides: Structure, Regulation and Action. Ann. N.Y. Acad. Sci. 297:* 561–567, 1977b.

Krieger, D. T., and Krieger, H. P. Effects of dexamethasone on pituitary-adrenal activation following intrahypothalamic implantation of "neurotransmitters." *Endocrinol. 87:* 179–182, 1970b.

Krieger, H. P., and Krieger, D. T. Chemical stimulation of the brain: Effect on adrenal corticoid release. *Am. J. Physiol. 218:* 1632–1641, 1970a.

Kuhar, M. F., Roth, R. H., and Aghajanian, G. K. Selective reduction of tryptophan hydroxylase activity in rat forebrain after midbrain raphe lesions. *Brain Res. 35:* 167–176, 1971.

L'Age, M., Langholz, J., Fechner, W., and Salzmann, H. Disturbances of the hypothalamo-hypophyseal-adrenocortical system in the rat. *Endocrinol. 95:* 760–765, 1974.

Lanier, L. P., Hartesveld, C. V., Weiss, B. J., and Isaacson, R. L. Effects of differential hippocampal damage upon rhythmic and stress-induced corticosterone secretion in the rat. *Neuroendocrinol. 18:* 154–160, 1975.

Lefkowitz, R. S., Roth, J., and Pastan, I. Effects of calcium on ACTH stimulation of the adrenal: Separation of hormone binding from adenylcyclase activation. *Nature (Lond.)* *228:* 864–866, 1970.

Levine, S., and Coover, G. D. Environmental control of suppression of the pituitary-adrenal system. *Physiol. Behav. 17:* 35–37, 1976.

Levine, S., Goldman, L., and Coover, G. D. Expectancy and the pituitary-adrenal system. In *Physiology, Emotion and Psychosomatic Illness.* CIBA Foundation Symp. 8. Amsterdam: Elsevier, 1972, pp. 281–296.

Lingvari, I., and Halasz, B. Evidence for a diurnal fluctuation in plasma corticosterone levels after fornix transection in the rat. *Neuroendocrinol. 11:* 191–196, 1973.

McEwen, B. S. Steroid receptors in neuroendocrine tissues: Topography, subcellular distribution and functional implications. In Naftolin, F., Ryan, K. J., and Davis, J. (eds.), *Int. Symp. on Subcellular Mechanisms in Reproductive Neuroendocrinology.* Amsterdam: Elsevier, 1976, pp. 277–304.

McEwen, B. S. Adrenal steroid feedback on neuroendocrine tissues. In Krieger, D. T., and Ganong, W. F. (eds.), *ACTH and Related Peptides: Structure, Regulation and Action. Ann. N.Y. Acad. Sci. 297:* 567–579, 1977.

McEwen, B. S., DeKloet, R., and Wallach, G. Interactions *in vivo* and *in vitro* of corticoids and progesterone with cell nuclei and soluble macromolecules from rat brain regions and pituitary. *Brain Res. 105:* 129–136, 1976.

McEwen, B. S., Wallach, G., and Magnus, C. Corticosterone binding to hippocampus: Immediate and delayed influences of the absence of adrenal secretion. *Brain Res. 70:* 321–334, 1974.

McEwen, B. S., Weiss, J. M., and Schwartz, L. S. Uptake of corticosterone by rat brain and its concentration by certain limbic structures. *Brain Res. 16:* 227–241, 1969.

McEwen, B. S., Weiss, J. M., and Schwartz, L. S. Retention of corticosterone by cell nuclei from brain regions of adrenalectomized rats. *Brain Res. 17:* 471–482, 1970.

McEwein, B. S., Zigmond, R. E., and Gerlach, J. L. Sites of steroid binding and action in the brain. In Bourne, G. H. (ed.), *Structure and Function of Nervous Tissue.* Vol. 5. New York: Academic Press, 1972, pp. 205–291.

McEwen, B. S., Zigmond, R. E., Azmitia, E. C., Jr., and Weiss, J. M. Steroid hormone interaction with specific brain regions. In Bowman, R. E., and Dutta, S. P. (eds.), *Biochemistry of Brain and Behavior.* New York: Plenum Press, 1970, pp. 123–167.

McHugh, P. R., and Smith, G. P. Negative feedback in adreno-cortical response to limbic stimulation in *macacca mulatta. Am. J. Physiol. 213:* 1445–1450, 1967.

Mackay, E. M., and Mackay, L. L. Compensatory hypertrophy of the adrenal cortex. *J. Exp. Med. 43:* 395–402, 1926.

MacLeod, R. M., and Fontham, E. H. Influence of ionic environment on the *in vitro* synthesis and release of pituitary hormones. *Endocrinol. 86:* 863–869, 1970.

Makara, G. B., and Stark, E. Effect of gamma aminobutyric acid (GABA) and GABA antagonist drugs on ACTH release. *Neuroendocrinol. 16:* 178–190, 1974.

Marks, B. H., and Vernikos-Danellis, J. Effects of acute stress on the pituitary gland: Action of ethionine on stress-induced ACTH release. *Endocrinol. 72:* 582–587, 1963.

Mason, J. W., Harwood, C. T., and Rosenthal, N. R. Influence of some environmental factors on plasma and urinary 17-hydroxycorticosteroid levels in the rhesus monkey. *Am. J. Physiol. 190:* 429–433, 1957.

Masui, H., and Garren, L. D. Inhibition of replication in functional mouse adrenal tumor cells by adrenocorticotropic hormone mediated by adenosine $3':5'$-cyclic monophosphate. *Proc. Nat. Acad. Sci. USA 68:* 3206–3210, 1971.

Mialhe, C., Koch, B., Bucher, B., and Briand, B. Etude de la secretion corticotrope au cours de l'hypertrophie compensatrice de la surrenale. *C.R. Acad. Sci. Paris 276:* 589–592, 1973.

Migeon, C. J., Tyler, F. H., Mahoney, J. P., Florentin, A. A., Castle, H., Bliss, E. L., and Samuels, L. T. The diurnal variation of plasma levels and urinary excretion of 17-OHCS in normal subjects, night workers and blind subjects. *J. Clin. Endocrinol. Metab. 17:* 1051–1057, 1956.

Moberg, G. P., Scapagnini, U., DeGroot, J., and Ganong, W. F. Effect of sectioning the fornix on diurnal fluctuations in plasma corticosterone levels in the rat. *Neuroendocrinol. 7:* 11–15, 1971.

Moore, R. Y., and Eichler, V. B. Loss of a circadian adrenal corticosterone rhythm following suprachiasmatic lesions in the rat. *Brain Res. 42:* 201–206, 1972.

Moore, R. Y., and Qavi, H. B. Circadian rhythm in adrenal adenyl cyclase and corticosterone abolished by median forebrain bundle transection in the rat. *Experientia 27:* 249–250, 1971.

Moriarty, C. M., and Moriarty, G. C. Bioactive and immunoactive ACTH in the rat pituitary: Influence of stress and adrenalectomy. *Endocrinol. 96:* 1419–1425, 1975.

Naumenko, E. V. Role of adrenergic and cholinergic structures in the control of the pituitary-adrenal system. *Endocrinol. 80:* 69–76, 1967.

Nugent, C. A., Eik-Nes, K., Samuels, L. T., and Tyler, F. H. Changes in plasma levels of 17-hydroxycorticosteroids during the intravenous administration of ACTH. IV. Response to prolonged infusion of small amounts of ACTH. *J. Clin. Endocrinol. Metab. 19:* 334–343, 1959.

Olpe, H. R., and McEwen, B. S. Glucocorticoid binding to receptor-like proteins in rat brain and pituitary: ontogenetic and experimentally induced changes. *Brain Res. 105:* 121–128, 1976.

Palka, Y., Coyer, D., and Critchlow, V. Effects of isolation of medial basal hypothalamus on pituitary-adrenal and pituitary-ovarian functions. *Neuroendocrinol. 5:* 333–349, 1969.

Palkovits, M., and Stark, E. Quantitative histological changes in the rat hypothalamus Ganong, W. F. (eds.), *ACTH and Related Peptides: Structure, Regulation and Action.* Ann. N.Y. Acad. Sci. 297: 455–476, 1977.

Palkovits, M., Kobayashi, R. M., Kizer, J. S., Jacobowitz, D. M., and Kopin, I. J. Effects of stress on catecholamines and tyrosine hydroxylase activity of individual hypothalamic nuclei. *Neuroendocrinol. 18:* 144–153, 1975.

Pakkovits, M., and Stark, E. Quantitative histological changes in the rat hypothalamus following bilateral adrenalectomy. *Neuroendocrinol. 10:* 23–30, 1972.

Pavel, S., Cristoveanu, A., Goldstein, R., and Calb, M. Inhibition of release of corticotrophin releasing hormone in cats by extremely small amounts of vasotocin injected into the third ventricle of the brain: Evidence for the involvement of 5-hydroxytryptamine-containing neurons. *Endocrinol. 101:* 672–678, 1977.

Pfeiffer, A. K., Vizi, E. S., Satoty, E., and Galambos, E. The effect of adrenalectomy on the norepinephrine and serotonin content of the brain and on reserpine action in rats. *Experientia 9:* 182–183, 1963.

Pirkle, J. C., Jr., and Gann, D. S. Restitution of blood volume after hemorrhage: Role of adrenal cortex. *Am. J. Physiol. 230:* 1683–1687, 1976.

Pollock, J. J., and Labella, F. S. Inhibition by cortisol of ACTH release from anterior pituitary tissue *in vitro. Can. J. Physiol. Pharmacol. 44:* 549–556, 1966.

Ramachandran, J., and Suyama, A. T. Inhibition of replication of normal adrenocortical cells in culture by adrenocorticotropin. *Proc. Nat. Acad. Sci. USA 72:* 113–117, 1975.

Reiter, I. R., and Pizzarello, D. J. Radioautographic study of cellular replacement in the adrenal cortex of male rats. *Texas Rep. Biol. Med. 24:* 189–194, 1966.

Rhees, R. W., Grosser, B. I., and Stevens, W. The autoradiographic localization of [^{3}H]-dexamethasone in the brain and pituitary of the rat. *Brain Res. 100:* 151–156, 1975.

Rheith, M. E. A., Schotman, P., Gispen, W. H., and De Wied, D. Pituitary peptides as modulators of neural functioning. *TIBS 2:* 56–58, 1977.

Rose, J. C., Goldsmith, P. C., and Ganong, W. F. Inhibition of stress induced ACTH secretion by electrical stimulation of the brainstem of dogs. *Fed. Proc. 35:* 459, 1976.

Russell, S. M., Dhariwal, A. P. S., McCann, S. M., and Yates, F. E. Inhibition by dexamethasone of the *in vitro* pituitary response to corticotropin releasing factor (CRF). *Endocrinol. 85:* 512–521, 1969.

Sachar, E. J. Psychological factors relating to activation and inhibition of the adrenocortical stress response in man: A review. *Progr. Brain Res. 32:* 316–324, 1970.

Saffran, M., and Schally, A. V. The release of corticotrophin by anterior pituitary tissue *in vitro. Can. J. Biochem. Physiol. 33:* 408–415, 1955.

Saffran, M., Schally, A. V., and Benfey, B. G. Stimulation of release of corticotropin from the adenohypophysis by a neurohypophysial factor. *Endocrinol. 57:* 439–444, 1955.

Sakellaris, P. C. Olfactory thresholds in normal and adrenalectomized rats. *Physiol. Behav. 9:* 495–500, 1972.

Sakellaris, P. C., and Vernikos-Danellis, J. Alteration of pituitary-adrenal dynamics induced by a water deprivation regimen. *Physiol. Behav. 12:* 1067–1070, 1974.

Sakellaris, P. C., and Vernikos-Danellis, J. Increased rate of response of the pituitary-adrenal system in rats adapted to chronic stress. *Endocrinol. 97:* 597–602, 1975.

Sato, T., and George, J. C. Evidence for the existence of a corticotropin-releasing factor in the pigeon hypothalamus. *Can. J. Physiol. Pharmacol. 51:* 737–742, 1973.

Sato, T., Sato, M., Shinsako, J., and Dallman, M. F. Corticosterone induced changes in hypothalamic corticotropin-releasing factor (CRF) content after stress. *Endocrinol. 97:* 265–274, 1975.

Sayers, G. Adrenal cortex and homeostasis. *Physiol. Rev. 30:* 241–320, 1950.

Sayers, G. Nature of corticotropin releasing factor (symposium). *Fed. Proc. 36:* 2087–2109, 1977.

Sayers, G., and Sayers, M. A. Regulatory effect of adrenal cortical extract on elaboration of pituitary adrenotropic hormone. *Proc. Soc. Exp. Biol. Med. 60:* 162–163, 1945.

Sayers, G., and Sayers, M. A. Regulation of pituitary adrenocorticotrophic activity during the response of the rat to acute stress. *Endocrinol. 40:* 265–273, 1947.

Sayers, G., and Sayers, M. A. Pituitary-adrenal system. *Recent Prog. Horm. Res. 2:* 81–115, 1948.

Sayers, G., and Sayers, M. A. Pituitary-adrenal system. *Ann. N.Y. Acad. Sci. 50:* 522–539, 1949.

Sayers, G., Sayers, M. A., Fry, E. G., White, A., and Long, C. N. H. Effect of adrenotropic hormone of anterior pituitary on cholesterol content of adrenals. *Yale J. Biol. Med. 16:* 361–392, 1944.

Schally, A. V., and Guillemin, R. Studies on corticotropin releasing factor: Ion exchange chromatography of pituitary preparations. *Texas Rep. Biol. Med. 18:* 133–136, 1960.

Seelig, S., and Sayers, G. Bovine hypothalamic corticotropin releasing factor: Chemical and biological characteristics. *Fed. Proc. 36:* 2100–2103, 1977.

Shen, J. T., and Ganong, W. F. Effect of variations in pituitary-adrenal activity on dopamine-β-hydroxylase activity in various regions of rat brain. *Neuroendocrinol. 20:* 311–318, 1976.

Shumacker, H. B., and Firor, W. M. Interrelationship of adrenal cortex and anterior lobe of hypophysis. *Endocrinol. 18:* 676–692, 1934.

Slusher, M. A. Effects of chronic hypothalamic lesions on diurnal and stress corticosteroid levels. *Am. J. Physiol. 206:* 1161–1164, 1964.

Smelik, P. G. Failure to inhibit corticotrophin secretion by experimentally induced increases in corticoid levels. *Acta Endocrinol. 44:* 36–46, 1963.

Smelik, P. G. The regulation of ACTH secretion. *Acta Physiol. Pharmacol. Neerl. 15:* 123–135, 1969.

Smelik, P. G., and Sawyer, C. H. Effects of implantation of cortisol into the brain stem or pituitary gland on the adrenal response to stress in the rabbit. *Acta Endocrinol. (Kbh.) 41:* 561–570, 1962.

Smith, P. E. Hypophysectomy and replacement therapy in the rat. *Am. J. Anat. 45:* 205–273, 1930.

Smollich, A., and Docke, F. Nerale Einflussnahme des Hypothalamus auf die Funktion der Nebennierenrinde. *J. Neurovisc. Rel. 31:* 128–135, 1969.

Steiner, F. A., Pieri, L., and Kaufmann, L. Effects of dopamine and ACTH on steroid sensitive single neurones in basal hypothalamus. *Experientia 24:* 1133–1134, 1968.

Stevens, R., Grosser, B. I., and Reed, D. J. Corticosteroid-binding molecules in rat brain cytosols: Regional distribution. *Brain Res. 35:* 602–607, 1971.

Swanson, L. W., and Cowan, W. M. The efferent connections of the suprachiasmatic nucleus of the hypothalamus. *J. Comp. Neurol. 160:* 1–12, 1975.

Sydnor, K. L., and Sayers, G. Blood and pituitary ACTH in intact and adrenalectomized rats after stress. *Endocrinol. 55:* 621–636, 1954.

Szentágothai, J., Flerko, B., Mess, B., and Halasz, B. *Hypothalamic Control of the Anterior Pituitary.* Budapest: Akademi Kiado, 1962.

Telegdy, G., and Vermes, I. Effect of adrenocortical hormones on activity of the serotonergic system in limbic structures in rats. *Neuroendocrinol. 18:* 16–26, 1975.

Treiman, D. M., and Levine, S. Plasma corticosterone response to stress in four species of wild mice. *Endocrinol. 84:* 676–680, 1969.

Trulson, M. E., and Jacobs, B. L. Behavioral evidence for the rapid release of CNS serotonin by PCA and fenfluramine. *Europ. J. Pharmacol. 36:* 149–154, 1976.

Turner, B., Schielke, J., and Carroll, B. J. Endogenous corticosterone in intact stressed rats: regional brain cytosol binding. *Soc. Neurosciences Abstracts 3:* 463, 1977.

Ulrich, F., and Long, C. N. H. Effects of stress on serum C^{14} levels in rats following administration of hydrocortisone-4-C^{14} and corticosterone-4-C^{14}. *Endocrinol. 59:* 170–180, 1956.

Urquhart, J. Physiological actions of adrenocorticotropic hormone. In Greep, R. O., and Astwood, E. B. (eds.), *Handbook of Physiology,* Section 7, Vol. IV, Part 2. Washington, D.C.: Am. Physiol. Soc., 1974, pp. 133–157.

Urquhart, J. and Li, C. C. The dynamics of adrenocortical secretion. *Am. J. Physiol. 214:* 73–85, 1968.

Urquhart, J. and Li, C. C. Dynamic testing and modeling of adrenocortical secretory function. *Ann. N.Y. Acad. Sci. 156:* 756–758, 1969.

Vale, W., and Rivier, C. Substances modulating the secretion of ACTH by cultured anterior pituitary cells. *Fed. Proc. 36:* 2094–2099, 1977.

Vale, W., Rivier, C., and Brown, M. Regulatory peptides of the hypothalamus. *Ann. Rev. Physiol. 39:* 473–527, 1977.

Van Loon, G. R., and Kragt, C. L. Effect of dopamine on the biological activity and *in vitro* release of ACTH and FSH. *Proc. Soc. Exp. Biol. Med. 133:* 1137–1141, 1970.

Van Loon, G. R., Scapagnini, U., Cohen, R., and Ganong, W. F. Effect of the intraventricular administration of adrenergic drugs on the adrenal venous 17-hydroxycorticosteroid response to surgical stress in the dog. *Neuroendocrinol. 8:* 257–272, 1971. 257–272, 1971.

Van Loon, G. R., Scapagnini, U., Moberg, G. P., and Ganong, W. F. Evidence for central adrenergic neuronal inhibition of ACTH secretion in the rat. *Endocrinol. 89:* 1464–1469, 1971.

Vermes, I., Dull, G., Telegdy, G., and Lissak, K. Possible role of serotonin in the monoamine-induced inhibition of the stress mechanism in the rat. *Acta Physiol. Hung. 42:* 219–233, 1972.

Vermes, I., and Telegdy, G. Effect of intraventricular injection and intrahypothalamic implantation of serotonin on the hypothalamo-hypophysial-adrenal system in the rat. *Acta Physiol. Hung. 42:* 49–59, 1972.

Vermes, I., Telegdy, G., and Lissak, K. Correlation between hypothalamic serotonin content and adrenal function during acute stress. Effect of adrenal corticosteroids on hypothalamic serotonin content. *Acta Physiol. Hung. 43:* 33–42, 1973.

Vermes, I., Telegdy, G., and Lissak, K. Effect of midbrain raphe lesion on diurnal and stress-induced changes in serotonin content of discrete regions of the limbic system and in adrenal function in the rat. *Acta Physiol. Hung. 45:* 217–224, 1974.

Vernikos-Danellis, J. Effect of acute stress on the pituitary gland: Changes in blood and pituitary ACTH concentrations. *Endocrinol. 72:* 574–581, 1963.

Vernikos-Danellis, J. Estimation of corticotropin-releasing activity of rat hypothalamus and neurohypophysis before and after stress. *Endocrinol. 75:* 514–520, 1964.

Vernikos-Danellis, J. Effect of stress, adrenalectomy, hypophysectomy and hydrocortisone on the corticotropin-releasing activity of rat median eminence. *Endocrinol. 76:* 122–126, 1965a.

Vernikos-Danellis, J. The regulation of the synthesis and release of ACTH. In Harris, R. S., Wool, I. G., and Loraine, J. A. (eds.), *Vitamins and Hormones,* New York: Academic Press, *23:* 97–152, 1965b.

Vernikos-Danellis, J. Competitive antagonism of caffeine and hydrocortisone on the hypothalamic-pituitary stress response. *Proc. 48th Endocrin. Soc. Mtg.,* Chicago, 1966, p. 24.

Vernikos-Danellis. J. The pharmacological approach to the study of mechanisms regulating ACTH secretion. In Martini, L. (ed.), *The Pharmacology of Hormonal Polypeptides and Proteins.* New York: Plenum Press, 1968, pp. 175–189.

Vernikos-Danellis, J. Effects of hormones on the central nervous system. In Levine, S. (ed.), *Hormones and Behavior.* New York: Academic Press, 1972, pp. 11–62.

Vernikos-Danellis, J. Peptide substances as neuroregulators. In Usdin, E., Hamburg, D. A., and Barchas, J. D. (eds.), *Neuroregulators and Psychiatric Disorders.* New York: Oxford University Press, 1977, pp. 284–286.

Vernikos-Danellis, J., and Marks, B. H. Epinephrine induced release of ACTH in normal human subjects: A test of pituitary function. *Endocrinol. 70:* 525–531, 1962.

Vernikos-Danellis, J., and Marks, B. H. The assay of CRF. In Meites, J. (ed.), *Hypophysiotropic Hormones of the Hypothalamus: Assay and Chemistry.* Baltimore: Williams & Wilkins, 1970, pp. 60–68.

Vernikos-Danellis, J., Anderson, E., and Trigg, L. Feedback mechanisms regulating ACTH secretion in rats bearing transplantable pituitary tumors. *Endocrinol. 80:* 345–350, 1967.

Vernikos-Danellis, J., and Harris, C. G, III. The effect of *in vitro* and *in vivo* caffeine, theophylline and hydrocortisone on the phosphodiesterase activity of the pituitary, median eminence, heart and cerebral cortex of the rat. *Proc. Soc. Exp. Biol. Med. 128:* 1016–1021, 1968.

Vernikos-Danellis, J., Winget, C. M., and Hetherington, N. W. Diurnal rhythmicity of negative feedback mechanisms regulating ACTH secretion. *Proc. 51st Endocrin. Soc. Mtg.,* New York, 1969, p. 90.

Vernikos-Danellis, J., Winget, C. M., and Hetherington, N. W. Diurnal rhythm of the pituitary adrenocortical response to stress: Effect of constant light and constant dark. *Life Sci. and Space Res. 8:* 240–246, 1970.

Vernikos-Danellis, J., Goldenrath, W. L., and Dolkas, C. B. The physiological cost of flight stress and flight fatigue. *U.S. Navy Med. J. 66:* 12–16, 1975.

Vernikos-Danellis, J., Kellar, K. J., Kent, D., Gonzales, C., Berger, P. A., and Barchas, J. D. Serotonin involvement in pituitary-adrenal function. In Krieger, D. T., and Ganong, W. F. (eds.), *ACTH and Related Peptides: Structure, Regulation and Action. Ann. N.Y. Acad. Sci. 297:* 518–526, 1977.

Weiss, J. M. Effects of coping behavior in different warning signal conditions on stress pathology in rats. *J. Comp. Physiol. Psychol. 77:* 1–13, 1971.

Weiss, J. M., Stone, E. A., and Harrell, N. Coping behavior and brain norepinephrine level in rats. *J. Comp. Physiol. Psychol. 72:* 153–160, 1970.

Wherry, F. E., Trigg, L. N., Grindeland, R. E., and Anderson, E. Identification of the hormones secreted by an autonomous mammotropic pituitary tumor in rats. *Proc. Soc. Exp. Biol. Med. 110:* 362–365, 1962.

Whitaker, S., and LaBella, F. S. Electron microscopic histochemistry of cholinesterase in the posterior, intermediate and anterior lobes of the rat pituitary. *Z. Zellforsch. 130:* 152–170, 1972.

Whitaker, S., and LaBella, F. S. Cholinesterase in the posterior and intermediate lobes of the pituitary. Species differences as determined by light and electron microscopic histochemistry. *Z. Zellforsch. 142:* 69–88, 1973.

Wilkinson, C. W., Shinsako, J., and Dallman, M. F. Insulin, corticosterone and ACTH rhythms in rats fed 2 hr/day. *The Physiologist 20:* 102, 1977.

Wilson, M., and Critchlow, V. Effect of fornix transection or hippocampectomy on rhythmic pituitary-adrenal function in the rat. *Neuroendocrinol. 13:* 29–40, 1973.

Wilson, M., and Critchlow, V. Effect of septal ablation on rhythmic pituitary-adrenal function in the rat. *Neuroendocrinol. 14:* 333–334, 1974.

Yates, F. E., Maran, J. W., Cryer, G. L., and Gann, D. S. The pituitary adrenal cortical system: Stimulation and inhibition of secretion of corticotrophin. In McCann, S. M. (ed.), *Physiology Series One: Endocrine Physiology Vol. 5* Baltimore: University Park Press, 1974, pp. 109–150.

Yates, F. E., Russell, S. M., Dallman, M. F., Hedge, G. A., McCann, S. M., and Dhariwal, A. P. S. Potentiation by vasopressin of corticotropin release induced by corticotropin releasing factor. *Endocrinol. 88:* 3–15, 1971.

11.
Pituitary-Adrenal System Hormones and Behavior

D. de Wied
Rudolf Magnus Institute for Pharmacology
Medical Faculty, University of Utrecht,
Vondellaan 6, Utrecht, The Netherlands

INTRODUCTION

The pituitary-adrenal system plays an essential role in homeostatic functions. Numerous aspects of stress-induced pituitary-adrenal activation in relation to peripheral mechanisms of adaptation have been studied since Selye's first observations on the general adaptation syndrome (for review see Selye, 1950). The nonspecific character of the pituitary-adrenal response to stress was deduced from observations that pituitary-adrenal activity could be induced by a great variety of noxious stimuli such as trauma, hemorrhage, cold, heat, exercise, infections, drugs, and so on. Although Selye commented that ''mere'' emotional stress activates the pituitary-adrenal system, somatic stress has long been regarded as the most important stimulus. However, psychological stimuli which affect emotionality and which result in fear, anxiety or frustration are among the most potent stressors that activate the pituitary-adrenal system (Selye, 1950; Mason, 1968; Levine, Goldman, and Coover, 1972). The response pattern of the pituitary-adrenal system depends on both the quality and the strength of the emotional stimulus. Thus, the increase in plasma corticosterone levels is very rapid and pronounced in rats that are prevented from coping behaviorally with a fear-provoking situation, while the response is slower in the animal that is allowed to cope (Bohus, 1975a). In addition, plasma ACTH levels are related to the intensity of the aversive stimulus in rats (Van Wimersma Greidanus et al., 1977).

In the early days of therapy with ACTH and adrenocortical steroids, psychological changes, including mood alterations and psychotic reactions, were frequently seen (for review see Von Zerssen, 1976). This suggested that hormones of the pituitary-adrenal system influenced brain function. Behavioral effects of ACTH in monkeys and rats were reported by Mirsky, Miller, and Stein in 1953. Although these first studies suggested the implication of pituitary-adrenal system hormones in conditioned behavior, it took many years before the brain was recognized as a target tissue of pituitary-adrenal system hormones. The fact that removal of neither the pituitary nor the adrenal cortex visibly alters the animal's gross behavior probably explains the delayed recognition. Adrenalectomy does not influence either exploratory behavior in an open field or the rate of habituation that normally occurs in this situation (Paul and Havlena, 1962; Davis and Zolovick, 1972; Tamásey et al., 1973), although defecation (emotionality?) can be somewhat increased (Moyer, 1958; Joffe, Mulick, and Rawson, 1972). Hypophysectomy may sometimes lead to an increase in exploratory behavior of rats in a solitary situation, but it does not affect maintenance behavior (grooming, and so forth), play, or fear (Gispen, Van der Poel, and Van Wimersma Greidanus, 1973). Learned behavior, however, appeared to be affected by the absence of pituitary-adrenal system hormones.

EFFECT OF ADRENALECTOMY ON CONDITIONED AND AGGRESSIVE BEHAVIOR

Removal of the adrenals did not substantially affect the acquisition of conditioned avoidance behavior in rats maintained with either sodium chloride in the drinking water or mineralocorticosteroid treatment (Fuller, Chambers, and Fuller, 1958; Moyer and Moshein, 1963; Bohus and Endröczi, 1965; De Wied, 1967; Van Delft, 1970; Weiss et al., 1970). A more or less normal salt balance seems necessary to secure the physical fitness of the rats to execute a conditioned avoidance response. Bohus and Lissák (1968) showed that adrenalectomized rats not receiving maintenance therapy have difficulty in acquiring a one-way active avoidance response. However, adrenalectomized rats with a normal salt balance could perform even better than the controls in either rewarded (Paul and Havlena, 1962) or avoidance situations (Beatty et al., 1970). Paul and Havlena (1962) found that adrenalectomized rats maintained on salt water made fewer errors in a maze-learning situation than did the controls. They suggested that adrenalectomized rats had fewer irrelevant fear-motivated responses which interfered with food-seeking behavior. Beatty et al. (1970) reported that adrenalectomy attenuated the deleterious effect of severe punishment (electric shocks) during shuttle-box avoidance training. This in turn suggested that it was high circulating levels of ACTH rather than the absence of adrenocortical steroids in adrenalectomized rats (Hodges and Vernikos-Danellis, 1962; Dallman, Demanincor, and Shinsako, 1974) which were associated with improved performance. This is consistent with the observation that adrenocortical steroids in doses which suppress ACTH release in adrenalectomized rats only slightly facilitated one-way active avoidance behavior (Van Delft, 1970).

Adrenalectomy interferes with the maintenance of avoidance behavior in the absence of shock punishment. Adrenalectomized rats are resistant to the extinction of active (De Wied, 1967; Bohus, Nyakas, and Endröczi, 1968; Weiss et al., 1970; Silva, 1974) and of passive avoidance behavior (Bohus, 1974). Retention of passive avoidance behavior is facilitated in rats adrenalectomized prior to the learning trial (Weiss et al., 1970; Silva, 1973). Treatment with corticosterone that normalizes the level of ACTH in blood also normalizes the extinction of active avoidance behavior of adrenalectomized rats (Weiss et al., 1970).

Aggressive behavior is also affected by adrenalectomy. In mice, isolation aggression is either attenuated (Brain, Nowell, and Wouters, 1971; Harding and Leshner, 1972; Leshner et al., 1973) or takes longer to develop in the absence of the adrenals (Sigg, Day, and Colombo, 1966). Burge and Edwards (1971), however, found no difference in the aggressiveness of isolated adrenalectomized mice. This may be due to the use of different methods for measuring aggression and of different strains of mice. Differential plasma corticosterone responses to stress have been found in different strains of mice (Levine and Treiman, 1964), and the behavioral response and effectiveness of hormone treatment are also strain-dependent (Levine and Levin, 1970). Thus, an improved performance of learned behavior and an increased resistance to extinction were found in adrenalectomized rats possibly as a result of high circulating levels of ACTH. This suggestion gains support from experiments on learned behavior in hypophysectomized rats.

HYPOPHYSECTOMY AND BEHAVIOR

A serious impairment in the acquisition of conditioned avoidance behavior follows the removal of the pituitary gland. Applezweig and Baudry
(1955) and Applezweig and Moeller (1959) performed experiments in a
few rats and found that hypophysectomy reduced the ability to acquire
shuttle-box avoidance behavior. Bélanger (1958) could not confirm these
observations but had used a longer conditioned-unconditioned stimulus
interval. Subsequent experiments on adenohypophysectomized (De
Wied, 1964) or totally hypophysectomized rats (De Wied, 1969a; Bohus,
Gispin, and De Wied, 1973), however, demonstrated clearly that such
animals were markedly inferior to sham-operated control rats in the acquisition of conditioned avoidance behavior. Hypophysectomy also at-
tenuates passive avoidance behavior (Anderson, Winn, and Tam, 1968;
Weiss et al., 1970). Passive avoidance behavior was impaired in rats that
received weak or moderate electric shocks during the learning trial (Lissák and Bohus, 1972) but not in rats subjected to high shock levels. These
authors suggested that fear-motivation rather than learning was impaired
in the hypophysectomized rat. Observations in other than fear-motivated
situations are scarce and less conclusive. Stone and King (1954) reported
that hypophysectomy at the age of 40 days did not affect learning in a
relatively simple maze, but hypophysectomy at 15, 30, and 35 days
reduced learning in a 13-choice swimming maze during the second part of
the trial series. However, discrimination behavior, which was tested in a
five-unit discrimination problem with food reward, was not affected in
the hypophysectomized rat.

Since hypophysectomy results in multiple metabolic deficiencies and
consequently in physical weakness, the deficiency in learning behavior
may be caused by these factors. Indeed, substitution therapy of the
adenohypophysectomized rats with thyroxine, cortisone, and testosterone
improved avoidance learning in the shuttle-box and normalized the impaired sensory and/or motor function as measured in a straight runway
under continuous shock punishment (De Wied, 1964). It was found subsequently that either testosterone, thyroxine, or growth hormone alone
improved the avoidance acquisition of hypophysectomized rats in the
shuttle-box (De Wied, 1969b, 1971). Testosterone and growth hormone
both reduced the loss of body weight of hypophysectomized rats. Furthermore, when hypophysectomized rats were fed a special diet that ensured their good health, their avoidance performance was improved (Har-

ris, 1973). Deterioration of the physical condition may not be the primary cause of the behavioral deficit of hypophysectomized rats; studies using passive avoidance behavior which requires a reduction in motor behavior instead of the increase required in active avoidance behavior, suggest this possibility. Hypophysectomized rats are superior rather than inferior in passive avoidance behavior (Weiss et al., 1970; Lissák and Bohus, 1972).

It was initially thought that the pituitary-adrenal dysfunction caused the behavioral impairment of hypophysectomized rats. Treatment of adenohypophysectomized rats (De Wied, 1964) and of hypophysectomized animals (De Wied, 1969b, Weiss et al., 1970) with doses of ACTH sufficient to maintain the size of the adrenal cortex restored their avoidance learning in the shuttle-box. The absence of corticosteroids could not, however, account for the behavioral deficit of the hypophysectomized rat. As we have seen, adrenalectomy did not impair avoidance acquisition, and treatment of hypophysectomized rats with the potent synthetic glucocorticosteroid dexamethasone failed to improve their avoidance learning (De Wied, 1971). The behavioral influence of ACTH therefore seemed to be due to an extra-adrenal effect of the hormone. Such an effect was demonstrated in experiments in which peptides structurally related to ACTH but devoid of corticotrophic actions were used. Treatment of hypophysectomized rats with ACTH 1-10 or ACTH 4-10 (Table 11.1) or with α-MSH: was as effective as treatment with the whole ACTH molecule to correct the behavioral impairment of the hypophysectomized rat (De Wied, 1964). These results were not due to metabolic or endocrine effects, since the heptapeptide ACTH 4-10 in amounts that normalized avoidance learning, failed to affect body growth, adrenal and testes weights, glucose, insulin, or free fatty acid levels in the plasma of hypophysectomized rats. The motor and sensory capacities of hypophysectomized rats were also inferior when studied in a straight runway under continuous shock punishment, and were only partially restored by ACTH 4-10 (De Wied, 1969b). On the basis of these observa-

Table 11.1 Amino Acid Sequences of a Number of Peptides Related to ACTH/MSH

	1	2	3	4	5	6	7	8	9	10	11	12	13
α-MSH	Ac-Ser-	Tyr-	Ser-	Met-	Glu-	His-	Phe-	Arg-	Trp-	Gly-	Lys-	Pro-	Val-OH
ACTH 1-10	H-Ser-	Tyr-	Ser-	Met-	Glu-	His-	Phe-	Arg-	Trp-	Gly-OH			
ACTH 4-10				H-Met-	Glu-	His-	Phe-	Arg-	Trp-	Gly-OH			
ACTH 4-7				H-Met-	Glu-	His-	Phe-OH						

tions, it was postulated (De Wied, 1969b) that the pituitary manufactures peptides with neurogenic activities (neuropeptides) which may be involved in the formation and maintenance of learned and other adaptive behavioral responses. These neuropeptides may be derived from pituitary hormones which may act as their prohormones (Greven and De Wied, 1973).

EFFECTS OF ACTH AND RELATED PEPTIDES ON BEHAVIOR IN INTACT RATS

Behavioral effects of ACTH and related peptides have also been observed in intact rats in a variety of behavioral situations. ACTH and related peptides delay the extinction of shuttle-box avoidance behavior (De Wied, 1969b), pole-jumping avoidance behavior (Greven and De Wied, 1973), passive avoidance behavior (Levine and Jones, 1965; Lissák and Bohus, 1972; De Wied, 1974; Kastin et al., 1973), food-motivated behavior (Sandman, Kastin, and Schally, 1969; Leonard, 1969; Guth, Levine, and Seward, 1971; Gray, 1971; Garrud, Gray, and De Wied, 1974), and sexually motivated approach behavior (Bohus et al., 1975). On the basis of these observations we suggested that ACTH and related peptides are involved in motivational processes (De Wied, 1974).

There is evidence that ACTH and related peptides affect memory processes as well. These peptides alleviate the amnesia for passive avoidance behavior produced in rats by CO_2 inhalation or electroconvulsive shock, or that produced in mice by intracerebral administration of the protein synthesis inhibitor puromycin (Flexner and Flexner, 1971; Rigter, Van Riezen, and De Wied, 1974; Keyes, 1974; Rigter and Van Riezen, 1975). Rigter, Elbertse, and Van Riezen (1975) demonstrated that CO_2 inhalation–induced retrograde amnesia could be reversed by ACTH 4–10 given one hour prior to the retention test. These authors interpreted the effect of ACTH 4–10 as an influence on retrieval processes, i.e., the reproduction of stored information. These findings are not in conflict with a motivational hypothesis, since motivational effects operate in most of the paradigms used. Observations made in the human suggest that ACTH 4–10 facilitates selective visual attention (Kastin et al., 1975), but there is also evidence for a motivational hypothesis (Gaillard and Sanders, 1975).

In our opinion, ACTH and related peptides temporarily increase the motivational significance of environmental cues. There would then be a greater probability that stimulus-specific behavioral responses will occur. Thus the mechanism by which these neuropeptides exert their behavioral effects is by facilitation of a selective arousal state. Bradycardia accompanies passive avoidance behavior. The rate of bradycardia depends on the intensity and duration of the aversive stimulus during the learning trial. The stronger the punishment, the more bradycardia occurs and the longer the passive avoidance latencies remain. ACTH 4–10 facilitates passive avoidance behavior, but the effect of the peptide is accompanied by tachycardia. This suggests that ACTH 4–10 increases the state of arousal (Bohus, 1975b). Electrophysiological experiments support the suggestion. ACTH 4–10 induces a frequency shift in the theta activity which is evoked in the hippocampus and thalamus by stimulation of the reticular formation in freely moving rats (Urban and De Wied, 1976). Similar shifts can be obtained by increasing the stimulus intensity, indicating that ACTH 4–10 facilitates transmission in midbrain limbic structures.

STRUCTURE-ACTIVITY STUDIES WITH ACTH AND RELATED PEPTIDES

Structure-activity studies were performed to determine the essential elements required for the behavioral effect of ACTH; the pole-jumping avoidance test was used as a measure of the behavioral activity of ACTH fragments (Greven and De Wied, 1977; De Wied, Witter, and Greven, 1975). Not more than four amino acid residues (ACTH 4–7) were found to be needed for the behavioral effect, i.e., delay of extinction of the avoidance response (Table 11.1). Replacement of the amino acid residue phenylalanine in ACTH 1–10 by its D-enantiomer (Bohus and De Wied, 1966) caused an effect opposite to that found with ACTH 1–10. This peptide facilitates extinction of shuttle-box avoidance behavior (De Wied, 1974). The same was found for ACTH 4–10 and ACTH 4–7 in which Phe[7] was replaced by the D-enantiomer (Greven and De Wied, 1973). Replacement of other amino acids in the D-configuration failed to facilitate extinction. Thus, successive substitution of each of the amino acids in [Lys[8]] ACTH 4–9 by their D-enantiomers delayed extinction of the avoidance response in the same way as did treatment with the original molecule. Such peptides are even more potent than the parent molecule. The amino acid residue phenylalanine in position 7 therefore seems to play a key role in the behavioral effect of ACTH. These observations further indicated a dissociation between the requirements for steroidogenic, MSH, and behavioral activity. Substitution of His[6] or Arg[8] by D-enantiomers decreases MSH activity, and substitution of Arg[8] by Lys[8] is accompanied by loss of steroidogenic activity in ACTH 1-24 (Tesser et al., 1973) and of MSH activity in ACTH 1-17 (Chung and Li, 1967). When Trp[9] is replaced by Phe, a marked decrease in steroidogenic potency is found (Hofmann et al., 1970), but in the presence of D-Lys[8] the behavioral potency rises a hundredfold. Oxidation of Met[4] to the sulfoxide level (Dedman, Farmer, and Morris, 1955; Lo, Dixon, and Li, 1961) decreases the steroidogenic and MSH activity but potentiates the behavioral action. Combination of the various substitutions in the same molecule, i.e., methionine sulfoxide for Met[4], D-Lys for Arg[8], and Phe for Trp[8] yielded the peptide H-Met (O)-Glu-His-Phe-D-Lys-Phe-OH (Org 2766). This peptide is behaviorally a thousand times more potent than ACTH 4-10 (Table 11.2), but contains a thousand times less MSH activity and has a markedly reduced steroidogenic effect (Greven and De Wied, 1973). A partial explanation for the potentiating effect on behavior is that the peptide is protected against enzymatic degradation. The in vitro half-life of the various substituted analogues of [Lys[8]] ACTH 4-9 correlates with the behavioral potency (Witter, Greven, and De Wied, 1975).

The sequence ACTH 7-10 still exhibits behavioral activity, although much less than do ACTH 4-7 or ACTH 4-10. This suggests that the features essential for behavioral activity are not restricted to the locus ACTH 4-7 but are present in ACTH 7-10 as well. This latter sequence may contain information for behavioral activity in a dormant form that needs potentiating modifications, e.g., chain elongation, to become ex-

Table 11.2 Amino Acid Sequence of Various Modified ACTH Analogues

		POTENCY RATIO*
	4 5 6 7 8 9 10	
ACTH 4–10	H-Met-Glu-His-Phe-Arg-Trp-Gly-OH	1
Org 2766	(O) H-Met-Glu-His-Phe-(D)Lys-Phe-OH	1000
ACTH 7–10	H-Phe-Arg-Trp-Gly-OH	0.1
ACTH 7–16	H-Phe-Arg-Trp-Gly-Lys-Pro-Val-Gly-Lys-Lys-NH$_2$	1
WB 1438	(O) (D) (D) H-Met-Glu-His-Phe-Lys-Phe-Gly-Lys-Pro-Val-Gly-Lys-Lys-NH$_2$	300,000

*Potency ratio determined in the pole-jumping test. For details see Greven and De Wied (1973, 1977).

posed. Indeed, the sequence ACTH 7–16 is as active as ACTH 4–10 in delaying extinction of pole-jumping avoidance behavior (De Wied et al., 1975). In addition, the tripeptide Phe-D-Lys-Phe, which is the major breakdown product of the highly potent modified hexapeptide Org 2766 (Witter et al., 1975), has only minor behavioral effects. However, chain elongation with ACTH 10–16 again induces a thousandfold potentiation (Greven and De Wied, 1977). Substitution of Lys^{11} by the D-enantiomer augments the behavioral effect a hundredfold. Extension of the NH_2 terminal with Org 2766 appeared to increase the potency further by a factor of 30. In this way a peptide was obtained that was three hundred thousand times stronger than the original ACTH 4–10 molecule. The potency of this peptide depends on the presence of the Gly^{10} and Lys^{16} residues. Removal of either of these amino acids markedly reduced the behavioral potency. A doublet of basic residues apparently is needed at exactly the same distance from the region ACTH 7–9 as in ACTH. Thus the requirements for activity on extinction of pole-jumping avoidance behavior are related more to the structure of ACTH than to that of α-, β-MSH or β-LPH.

BEHAVIORAL EFFECTS OF HORMONES RELATED TO β-LPH

ACTH is part of a much larger precursor glycoprotein (Mains, Eipper, and Ling, 1977). ACTH 1–39 and β-lipotropin (β-LPH 1–91) and peptides related to β-LPH are all present in the same cells in the pituitary gland (Bloom et al., 1977). Guillemin et al. (1977) recently showed that the plasma and pituitary concentration of ACTH and β-LPH 61–91 (β-endorphin) varied concomitantly and in a remarkably parallel fashion, with both ACTH and β-endorphin increasing in response to stress and decreasing after dexamethasone. ACTH 4–10 is not only present in ACTH but also in α- and β-MSH and in β-LPH as the sequence β-LPH 47–53. Which of these peptides is the precursor of ACTH 4–10 is not known. The C-terminal peptides of β-LPH have an opiate-like activity (Hughes et al., 1975; Guillemin, Ling, and Burgus, 1976; Li and Chung, 1976; Bradbury et al., 1976; Wei and Loh, 1976; Van Ree et al., 1976). The endorphins exhibit behavioral effects similar to those of ACTH fragments (De Wied et al., 1978). Interestingly, the behavioral effect of the endorphins is obtained with amounts much lower than those needed to induce the opiate-like activity. For example, the analgesic effects of β-endorphin are obtained following intraventricular administration of microgram quantities, while nanogram amounts of the same peptide given via the same route are sufficient to delay extinction of pole-jumping avoidance behavior (De Wied et al., 1978). In contrast to the opiate-like activity of the endorphins, the behavioral effects cannot be blocked by the specific opiate antagonist naltrexone. This suggests that the influence on avoidance behavior involves other receptor sites in the brain.

ACTH and related peptides also have an appreciable affinity for brain opiate binding sites in rat brain synaptosomal membrane fraction (Terenius, 1975). Structure-activity studies pointed to an active site in ACTH 4–10 (Terenius, Gispen, and De Wied, 1975). Analysis of the binding characteristics of ACTH 1–24 revealed a relatively low selectivity of the peptide for an agonist or antagonist (Terenius, 1976). The affinity constants of ACTH appeared to be of the order of 10^{-5} to 10^{-6} M. While the physiological significance of these relationships can be questioned, these data are nevertheless consistent with findings by Zimmermann and Krivoy (1973) and Gispen et al. (1976) that ACTH-like peptides interfere with morphine at the CNS level. Thus, the various peptides related to ACTH and β-LPH overlap considerably with respect to brain receptor sites. This suggests a redundancy of information in peptides derived from the same pituitary glycoprotein. The behavioral activity of ACTH can in any event be separated from the steroidogenic, MSH, fat mobilizing, and opiate-like activity, since the potent ACTH 4–9 analog Org 2766 is practically devoid of any of the latter effects.

These results indicate that a family of pituitary peptides shares a multitude of effects as indicated by their overlapping activities. The one thousand- or one millionfold increase in behavioral potency that was obtained by modifying ACTH 4–9 (Org 2766) or ACTH 4–16 respectively (Greven and De Wied, 1977) may be explained not only by a reduction in metabolic degradation but also by a greater affinity and/or intrinsic activity for receptor sites in the brain. Such considerations tempt one to speculate about the existence in the pituitary and/or brain of more potent neuropeptides involved in motivational, learning, and memory processes.

LOCUS OF ACTION OF PEPTIDES RELATED TO ACTH AND RECEPTOR SITES IN THE BRAIN

The brain sites for the behavioral action of the peptides related to ACTH have been explored either by attempting to block the peptide effects on extinction of avoidance behavior by destroying various brain regions or by implanting the peptides directly in the brain. The thalamic parafascicular region appeared to mediate the behavioral effects of ACTH-like peptides in experiments with rats having bilateral lesions in this area (Bohus and De Wied, 1967a). It was found that α-MSH (Bohus and De Wied, 1967b) or ACTH 4–10 (Van Wimersma Greidanus, Bohus, and De Wied, 1975) failed to affect extinction of pole-jumping avoidance behavior. Conversely, implanting ACTH 1–10 or [D-Phe⁷] ACTH 1–10 into the nucleus parafascicularis respectively delayed or facilitated the extinction of pole-jumping avoidance behavior (Van Wimersma Greidanus and De Wied, 1971). These studies failed to demonstrate effective sites in the brain other than the parafascicular area, but more recent experiments indicated that the limbic forebrain may be involved as well (Van Wimersma Griedanus and De Wied, 1976). These studies showed that bilateral destruction of the antero-dorsal hippocampus prevented the effect of ACTH 4–10 on extinction of pole-jumping avoidance behavior. In addition, systemic administration of ACTH was found to normalize the deficient shuttle-box acquisition of rats bearing lesions in the amygdaloid nuclei (Bush, Lovely, and Pagano, 1973). Accordingly, the primary locus of action of peptides related to ACTH may be in the posterior thalamic area, but the behavioral effects seem to require intact midbrain limbic structures.

Receptor sites for ACTH in the brain have not yet been demonstrated. However, the tritium-labeled ACTH 4–9 analog (Org 2766) was taken up preferentially in the septal region following intraventricular administration. Hypophysectomy enhanced the uptake of radioactivity in the septum. This increased uptake could be prevented by chronic treatment of hypophysectomized rats with ACTH 1–24 or ACTH 4–10 given as a long-acting zinc phosphate preparation (Verhoef, Witter, and De Wied, 1977). Treatment with [D-Phe⁷] ACTH 4–10, ACTH 11–24, desglycinamide⁹-Lys⁸ vasopressin, or α-endorphin failed to compete with the facilitated uptake of the radiolabeled compound in hypophysectomized rats. These results are evidence for a specific uptake or binding of the ACTH 4–9 analog in the septal region because competitive displacement occurred only with peptides that were structurally closely related to N-terminal ACTH fragments. Studies such as these indicated the presence in the brain of putative receptor sites for these neuropeptides. The inability of [D-Phe⁷] ACTH 4–10 and of α-endorphin to compete with the ACTH 4–9 analog suggests the existence of different receptors for

ACTH and related peptides and for C-terminal β-LPH fragments for the same behavioral effect.

THE PITUITARY OR THE BRAIN AS SOURCE OF NEUROPEPTIDES

ACTH has been detected in the CSF (Kleerekoper, Donald, and Posen, 1972; Allen et al., 1974). Because of the relative impermeability of the blood-brain barrier for ACTH, pituitary peptides may be transported from the pituitary to the brain. This appeared to be an efficient route to the brain for ACTH (Mezey et al., 1978). Intrasellar and intrapituitary administration of the ^{3}H-ACTH 4–9 analog (Org 2766) resulted in a significantly higher radioactivity in the brain than did the intravenous injection of equimolar amounts of labeled peptide. Intrapituitary injection resulted in an uptake with clear regional differences. The highest uptake was found in the hypothalamus. Twenty-four hours after pituitary stalk section, the uptake of radioactivity was markedly depressed in the hypothalamus but not in other brain regions. Hypothalamic uptake was, however, restored at eight days after stalk section. A significant backflow of peptide from the pituitary to the brain and particularly to the hypothalamus was thus demonstrated. Transport to the hypothalamus is presumably partly vascular via the stalk. Transport to other brain areas may occur via the CSF, but a neural route cannot be excluded.

Neuropeptides related to ACTH may, however, be produced by the brain itself. The presence of biologically- and immunoactive ACTH and MSH-like material in the brain has been reported (Guillemin et al., 1962; Schally et al., 1962; Rudman et al., 1973; Swaab, 1976; Oliver, Mical, and Porter, 1977; Kreiger, Liotta, and Brownstein, 1977a,b). Immunoactive MSH-like material and both immuno- and bioactive ACTH-like material appeared to be present in the brain even long after hypophysectomy (Swaab, 1976; Krieger et al., 1977a,b). These observations suggest that the brain is not dependent on the pituitary for its supply of these neuropeptides. As mentioned before, removal of the pituitary results in an impairment in avoidance behavior which can be corrected by the peripheral administration of ACTH and related peptides (De Wied, 1969a; Bohus et al., 1973; Gold et al., 1977). It is thus possible that the generation of behaviorally active neuropeptides in the brain is impaired in the absence of the pituitary. Gel filtration patterns of hypothalamic, preoptic, and amygdala extracts containing ACTH-like immunoactive material are not identical to the pattern obtained from whole pituitaries (Krieger et al.,

1977a,b). On the other hand, the dominant trichloroacetic acid–precipitable MSH-like peptide from intact rat brain co-migrates with α-MSH on gel electrophoresis (Loh and Gainer, 1977). A very potent, but as yet unidentified MSH-like factor was detected by these authors in rat brain. This peptide may be derived from α-MSH: by enzy;matic cleavage. Similarly, enkephalins with regional variations in receptor binding closely parallelling those of opiate receptor binding have been found in brain fractions containing nerve terminals (Hughes, 1975; Pasternak, Goodman, and Snyder, 1975; Simantov et al., 1976a,b, 1977). β-Endorphin has been isolated from the brain, but the levels found were much lower than those of enkephalin (Bradbury et al., 1976). Conversely, the pituitary contains negligible amounts of enkephalins but considerable amounts of opiate-like peptides (for review see Snyder and Simantov, 1977). Whether the behavioral effects of peptides related to ACTH, α-, β-MSH, and β-LPH are mediated by pituitary backflow of neuropeptides originating from these pituitary hormones, or whether they are the result of local production and release of related materials in the brain, remains to be elucidated.

EFFECTS OF ADRENOCORTICAL STEROIDS ON BEHAVIOR

Early experiments involving the whole ACTH molecule suggested that the behavioral effect was mediated by the adrenal cortex. Murphy and Miller (1955) were the first to demonstrate that ACTH delayed the extinction of shuttle-box avoidance behavior in rats. In view of this, Miller and I (unpublished observations, 1958) studied the effect of the synthetic corticosteroid prednisolone on extinction of shuttle-box avoidance behavior in rats. We found that this steroid facilitated the extinction of avoidance behavior and thus acted in a manner opposite to that of ACTH. This was an indication that the influence of ACTH might be of an extra target nature. That this was the case was later demonstrated by Miller and Ogawa (1962), who found that ACTH delayed extinction of shuttle-box avoidance behavior in adrenalectomized rats as well. The preliminary observations on the effects of adrenocortical steroids were subsequently expanded. The administration of corticosterone or cortisone rapidly extinguished active avoidance or approach behavior (De Wied, 1967; Bohus and Lissák, 1968; Garrud et al., 1974; Kovács, Telegdy, and Lissák, 1976), attenuated passive avoidance behavior (Bohus, 1971; Kovács,

Telegdy, and Lissák, 1977; Van Wimersma Greidanus, 1977), and facilitated the extinction of nonrewarded approach behavior after reversal of a discriminative conditioned response (Bohus, 1973). However, steroids other than glucocorticosteroids appeared to have similar behavioral effects. Thus, dexamethasone, progesterone, and pregnenolone facilitated extinction of pole-jumping avoidance behavior in an equipotent manner (Van Wimersma Greidanus, 1970). Testosterone and estradiol were without effect. Common features of the steroids effective on extinction are the double bond in ring A or B and a ketone or hydroxy group at C_3. A ketone group at C_{20} is important but not essential for the effect. Thus, the influence of adrenal steroids on behavior is associated with neither glucocorticosteroid nor mineralocorticosteroid nor gestagenic properties. The effect is not associated with anesthetic properties either, since the steroid anesthetic hydroxydione (Viadril[R]) in equivalent amounts failed to affect the extinction of pole-jumping avoidance behavior. The behavioral effects of corticosteroids are independent of the property of these steroids to suppress ACTH release, since corticosterone also facilitates extinction of avoidance behavior in hypophysectomized rats (De Wied, 1967). In addition, local implantation of corticosteroids in the brain mimics the behavioral effect of systemically administered steroids without producing marked changes in circulating ACTH levels (Bohus, 1970, 1973).

CORTICOSTEROID RECEPTORS AND BEHAVIOR

The site of the behavioral effect of corticosteroids is localized in the same brain areas as the site for the effect of ACTH fragments. Corticosteroid-sensitive areas are present in the septal area, in the hippocampus, amygdala, anterior hypothalamus, medial thalamus, and in the mesencephalic reticular formation (Bohus, 1970, 1973; Endröczi, 1972). Putative receptor sites for corticosteroids are found in particular in the hippocampus (McEwen, Weiss, and Schwartz, 1969). In this structure uptake by the cell nucleus is highly selective for corticosterone, the steroid naturally occurring in the rat. The hippocampal binding system is already saturated within the range of physiological plasma levels of corticosterone (McEwen et al., 1975). These receptor sites may provide a molecular basis for the behavioral effect of corticosteroids. However, as we have seen, various steroids, related as well as unrelated to corticosterone, affect avoidance behavior in the same way as does corticosterone. It should, however, be borne in mind that hippocampal dexamethasone uptake is low while progesterone, although it is bound to hippocampal cytoplasmic receptor proteins, does not enter the cell nucleus. Furthermore, these steroids inhibit the binding of corticosterone to cytosol receptors in the hippocampus (De Kloet, Wallach, and McEwen, 1975; McEwen, de Kloet, and Wallach, 1976). It is conceivable that the effect of corticosterone on adaptive behavior is of a more physiological nature than is that of related steroids. Evidence for this has been obtained recently in a series of elegant experiments performed by Bohus and De Kloet (1977a). These authors found that adrenalectomy one hour prior to forced extinction does not abolish one-trial passive avoidance behavior as is normally observed after forced extinction in intact rats. The administration of physiological amounts of corticosterone immediately after adrenalectomy corrects for the behavioral deficiency of the adrenalectomized rat and facilitates the elimination of passive avoidance behavior as a result of forced extinction. Similar low doses of dexamethasone or progesterone are ineffective in this respect. These steroids if given prior to corticosterone, even block the effect of corticosterone treatment of adrenalectomized rats (Bohus and De Kloet, 1977a). This block could be explained by assuming that dexamethasone and progesterone prevent the binding of corticosterone to hippocampal cytosol receptors (De Kloet and McEwen, 1976). Biochemical observations showed that one hour after adrenalectomy when the behavioral deficit was already present, only 35% of the binding sites were occupied by corticosterone in hippocampal cytosol receptors, while the cell nuclear concentration of corticosterone was still unchanged. Administration of a low dose of corticosterone restored the occupation of hippocampal cytosol receptor sites up to the level of that of intact control rats (Bohus and De Kloet, 1977b). Thus, the behavioral and biochemical observations relate putative receptor sites in the hippocampus with extinction of passive avoidance behavior. That the uptake by the cell nucleus is not affected by adrenalectomy while behavior is impaired indicates that the adaptive process which is under the control of corticosterone is independent of an action at the genomic level. The effect elicited by higher amounts of other steroids on extinction of avoidance behavior may be due to influences on brain structures other than the hippocampus. Various limbic midbrain regions may be the loci of action for the behavioral effect of pharmacological amounts of steroids (Bohus, 1970, 1973; Stumpf and Sar, 1975; Rees, Stumpf, and Sar, 1975; McEwen et al., 1975; De Kloet and McEwen, 1976).

RELATION BETWEEN ADAPTIVE BEHAVIOR AND ONGOING PITUITARY ADRENAL ACTIVITY

Pituitary and adrenal activity are increased during the acquisition and extinction of conditioned emotional responses. Experimentally produced behavioral arousal is accompanied by increased circulating levels of adrenocortical hormones (Mason, 1959; Mason, Brady, and Sidman, 1957). There was a quantitative relation between glucocorticosteroid levels and avoidance rate (Sidman et al., 1962) and a perfect rank-order correlation between these levels and the percent shock avoidances (Wertheim, Conner, and Levine, 1969). Johnston, Miya, and Paolino (1974) reported a positive correlation between the pituitary-adrenal response to ether stress and the conditioned avoidance performance of rats as a function of age. Furthermore, high corticosterone levels have been associated with superior passive avoidance learning (Endröczi, 1972; Lissák, Endröczi, and Medgyesi, 1957; Endröczi, Telegdy, and Lissák, 1957). In contrast, several authors found a poor relationship between operant avoidance behavior and steroid levels (Levine et al., 1970; Mason, Brady, and Tolliver, 1968), while others found an inverse relation between the avoidance performance of an animal and its circulating corticosteroid levels (Dupont, Endröczi, and Fortier, 1971; Van Delft, 1970; Endröczi, 1972). Coover, Ursin, and Levine (1973) suggested that the level of plasma corticosterone was a function of the strength of the classically conditioned components of avoidance behavior because pituitary-adrenal activity is high in the beginning of training and declines when the instrumental response improves. This is consistent with the findings of Ursin et al. (1975), who demonstrated a progressive decline in plasma corticosterone levels in the rat in the course of shuttle-box avoidance training. According to these authors this decline occurs in three stages. In the beginning the rats receive a high number of aversive stimuli which then become predictable owing to classical conditioning. When the performance is finally high and the rat is efficiently coping with the situation, the steroid level in the blood is lowest. Auerbach and Carlton (1971) reported that electroshock-induced amnesia for a passive avoidance response also reduced the rise in plasma corticosterone that normally occurs during retention of passive avoidance behavior. The results obtained by Rigter (1975) using CO_2 as the amnesic agent were similar in principle. The rise in plasma corticosterone reappeared if the amnesia was counteracted by previous administration of ACTH 4–10. Natelson, Krasnegor, and Holaday (1976) argued that corticosteroid levels were of little use, since these authors frequently found a dissociation between cortisol levels and behavioral arousal in monkeys. Indeed, pituitary-adrenal activity depends on many nonspecific factors associated with conditioned behavior rather than on a specific stimulus such as the conditioned stimulus which ultimately elicits the behavioral response. Although physiological variations in pituitary-adrenal activity do not seem to determine subsequent behavior, one may assume that variations in the level of these hormones in some way modulate ongoing behavior.

CONCLUDING REMARKS

The behavioral effect of ACTH, MSH, and their fragments which were detected more than 15 years ago led to the understanding that pituitary hormones apart from their effects on target organs possess central nervous system activity. It subsequently appeared that these central effects are dissociated from the endocrine activities of these hormones and could be localized in a part of the molecule. The term neuropeptides was coined for hormone fragments with central effects.

The Nature of Pituitary Hormones Related to ACTH and β-LPH

The polypeptides ACTH 1–39 and β-LPH are found in the same cells in the pituitary gland. These hormones probably are generated from a large glycoprotein precursor molecule (Mains et al., 1977). ACTH 1–39 in turn may be the precursor for α-MSH (Scott et al., 1973), while β-LPH is the precursor for β-endorphin and γ-LPH. The latter again may be the precursor for β-MSH (Crine et al., 1977). Further degradation of these polypeptides may generate neuropeptides of short-sequence amino acids such as ACTH 4–10, γ- and α-endorphin, and so on. Precursor molecules thus serve as a form of storage from which various neuropeptides are released by enzymatic cleavage. The nature of this process is not clear, and the relation between enzyme activity and pituitary function needs to be studied in detail.

The Origin of Neuropeptides

One has to visualize that neuropeptides are generated in the pituitary and released to the brain. Evidence for this has been obtained by Oliver et al.

(1977), who showed that pituitary hormones are transported retrograde in certain vascular channels of the pituitary stalk toward the hypothalamus. Our findings that a radioactive ACTH 4–9 analog following intrapituitary infusion is readily transported to the brain are in accord with this suggestion (Mezey et al., 1978). However the pituitary is not the only source of neuropeptides. Highly sophisticated immunochemical techniques made it possible to detect small quantitities of peptides in nerve tissue. Such developments led to the discovery that the brain contains a multitude of neuropeptides which may be identical or closely related to several of the pituitary hormones. The concentration of these hormones does not materially fall following hypophysectomy, suggesting that these entities are produced in the brain and may function as neurotransmitters or neuromodulators. The contribution of these "brain-born" neuropeptides and those of pituitary origin in behavioral adaptation remains to be established.

Role of Pituitary Adrenal System Hormones in Behavioral Adaptation

A number of behavioral effects have been observed with ACTH, β-endorphin, and their degradation products. These concern learned behavior such as active and passive avoidance behavior, maze learning, approach behavior motivated by food or water, or sexually motivated behavior. In addition, these peptides alleviate amnesia, and reduce aggressive behavior. Neuropeptides related to ACTH and β-endorphin may therefore be involved in the formation and maintenance of these behaviors.

Several hypotheses have been put forward to explain the effect of ACTH and related peptides such as influences on motivational processes, on learning and memory processes, and on attention and concentration. Interestingly, in man, effects on concentration, (visual) attention, and motivation have been observed following treatment with ACTH 4–10 (Kastin et al., 1975; Van Riezen, Rigter, and De Wied, 1977).

Corticosteroids in general act in a manner opposite to that of neuropeptides and facilitate extinction of active avoidance behavior and approach behavior, and attenuate passive avoidance behavior. These effects may be best explained by assuming that these steroids increase the discriminative capacity of the organism (Bohus, 1973). This may be achieved by a decreased arousal state or normalization of an increased arousal in limbic midbrain structures (see for review Bohus and De Wied, 1978).

Just as the behavioral action of ACTH, MSH, and β-LPH is dissociated from their endocrine and opiate-like effects, so is the action of corticosteroids on behavior not restricted to the glucocorticosteroids. Other steroids, like progesterone and even pregnenolone, have effects on avoidance behavior similar to those of natural and synthetic glucocorticosteroids. However, under certain conditions evidence has been obtained that corticosterone, the glucocorticosteroid naturally occurring in the rat, may be physiologically involved in the modulation of adaptive behavior.

In conclusion, behavioral responses to changes in the environment may be classified as adaptive behavior. Not only motivation, learning, and memory, but also extinction or repression, are expressions of the highest form of behavioral adaptation. Stimuli that elicit fear or anxiety, hope or disappointment, frustration or aggression play an important part in the formation of adaptive behavior. The influence of pituitary and brain neuropeptides and of glucocorticosteroids should therefore be considered in the framework of adaptation. This could be achieved through a modulating influence of these principles on limbic midbrain structures which would allow the organism to select the most adequate behavior in a given situation.

ACKNOWLEDGMENT

Dr. Marie-Louise Desbarats-Schönbaum is gratefully acknowledged for her linguistic assistance.

References

Allen, J. P., Kendall, J. W., McGilvra, R., and Vancura, C. Immunoreactive ACTH in cerebrospinal fluid. *J. Clin. Endocr. 38:* 586–593, 1974.

Anderson, D. C., Winn, W., and Tam, T. Adrenocorticotrophic hormone and acquisition of a passive avoidance response. *J. Comp. Physiol. Psychol. 66:* 497–499, 1968.

Applezweig, M. H., and Baudry, F. D. The pituitary-adrenocortical system in avoidance learning. *Psychol. Rep. 1:* 417–420, 1955.

Applezweig, M. H., and Moeller, G. The pituitary-adrenocortical system and anxiety in avoidance learning. *Acta Psychol. 15:* 602–603, 1959.

Auerbach, P., and Carlton, P. L. Retention deficits correlated with a deficit in the corticoid response to stress. *Science 173:* 1148–1149, 1971.

Beatty, D. A., Beatty, W. A., Bowman, R. E., and Gilchrist, J. C. The effects of ACTH, adrenalectomy and dexamethasone on the acquisition of an avoidance response in rats. *Physiol. Behav. 5:* 939–944, 1970.

Bélanger, D. Effets de l'hypophysectomie sur l'apprentissage d'un réaction échappement-évitement. *Canad. J. Psychol. 12:* 171–178, 1958.

Bloom, F., Battenberg, E., Rossier, J., Ling, N., Leppaluoto, J., Vargo, T. M., and Guillemin, R. Endorphins are located in the intermediate and anterior lobes of the pituitary gland, not in the neurohypophysis. *Life Sci. 20:* 43–47, 1977.

Bohus, B. Central nervous structures and the effect of ACTH and corticosteroids on avoidance behavior: A study with intracerebral implantation of corticosteroids in the rat. In de Wied, D., and Weijnen, J. A. W. M. (eds.), *Progress in Brain Research 32:* 171–184. Amsterdam: Elsevier, 1970.

Bohus, B. Adrenocortical hormones and central nervous function. The site and mode of their behavioural action in the rat. In James, V. H. T., and Martini, L. (eds.), *Hormonal Steroids*. Proceedings Third Int. Congress on Hormonal Steroids. Excerpta Medica International Congress Series No. 219. Amsterdam: Excerpta Medica, 1971, pp. 752–758.

Bohus, B. Pituitary-adrenal influences on avoidance and approach behavior of the rat. In Zimmermann, E., Gispen, W. H., Marks, B. H., and de Wied, D. (eds.), *Drug Effects on Neuroendocrine Regulation. Progress in Brain Research 39:* 407–420. Amsterdam: Elsevier, 1973.

Bohus, B. Pituitary-adrenal hormones and the forced extinction of a passive avoidance response in the rat. *Brain Res. 66:* 366–367, 1974.

Bohus, B. Environmental influences on pituitary-adrenal system function. In Klotz, H.-P (ed.), *Les Endocrines et le Milieu*. Problèmes Actuels d'Endocrinologie et de Nutrition, série no. 19. Paris: Expansion Scientifique Française, 1975a, pp. 55–62.

Bohus, B. Pituitary peptides and adaptive autonomic responses. In Gispen, W. H., van Wimersma Greidanus, Tj. B., Bohus, B., and de Wied, D. (eds.), *Hormones, Homeostasis and the Brain. Progress in Brain Research 42:* 275–283. Amsterdam: Elsevier, 1975b.

Bohus, B., and Endröczi, E. The influence of pituitary-adrenocortical function on the avoiding conditioned reflex activity in rats. *Acta physiol. Acad. Sci. hung. 26:* 183–189, 1965.

Bohus, B., and de Kloet, E. R. Behavioral effect of corticosterone related to putative glucocorticoid receptor properties in the rat brain. *J. Endocrin. 72:* 64P–65P, 1977a.

Bohus, B., and de Kloet, E. R. Hippocampal glucocorticoid receptors and the behavioral effects of corticosterone in the rat. Abstract. 18th Dutch Federative Meeting, Leiden, April, 1977b, p. 153.

Bohus, B., and Kissák, K. Adrenocrotical hormones and avoidance behaviour in rats. *Int. J. Neuropharmacol. 7:* 301–306, 1968.

Bohus, B., and de Wied, D. Inhibitory and facilitatory effect of two related peptides on extinction of avoidance behavior. *Science 153:* 318–320, 1966.

Bohus, B., and de Wied, D. Failure of α-MSH to delay extinction of conditioned avoidance behavior in rats with lesions in the parafascicular nuclei of the thalamus. *Physiol. Behav. 2:* 221–223, 1967a.

Bohus, B., and de Wied, D. Avoidance and escape behavior following medial thalamic lesions in rats. *J. Comp. Physiol. Psychol. 64:* 26–29, 1967b.

Bohus, B., and de Wied, D. Pituitary-adrenal system hormones and adaptive behavior. In Chester Jones, I., and Henderson, I. W., (eds.), *General, Comparative and Clinical Endocrinology of the Adrenal Cortex,* Vol. 3. London: Academic Press, 1978.

Bohus, B., Gispen, W. H., and de Wied, D. Effect of lysine vasopressin and ACTH 4–10 on conditioned avoidance behavior of hypophysectomized rats. *Neuroendocrinology* *11:* 137–143, 1973.

Bohus, B., Hendrickx, H. H. L., van Kolfschoten, A. A., and Krediet, T. G. Effect of ACTH 4–10 on copulatory and sexually motivated approach behavior in the male rat. In Sandler, M., and Gessa, G. L. (eds.), *Sexual Behavior: Pharmacology and Biochemistry.* New York: Raven Press, 1975, pp. 269–275.

Bohus, B., Nyakas, Cs., and Endröczi, E. Effects of adrenocorticotropic hormone on avoidance behaviour of intact and adrenalectomized rats. *Int. J. Neuropharmacol. 7:* 307–314, 1968.

Bradbury, A. F., Smyth, D. G., Snell, C. R., Birdsall, N. J. M., and Hulme, E. C. C-fragment of lipotropin has a high affinity for brain opiate receptors. *Nature 260:* 793–795, 1976.

Brain, P. F., Nowell, N. W., and Wouters, A. Some relationships between adrenal function and the effectiveness of a period of isolation in inducing intermale aggression in albino mice. *Physiol. Behav. 6:* 27–29, 1971.

Burge, K. G., and Edwards, D. A. The adrenal gland and the pre and post castrational aggressive behavior of male mice. *Physiol. Behav. 7:* 885–888, 1971.

Bush, D. F., Lovely, R. H., and Pagano, R. R. Injection of ACTH induces recovery from shuttle-box avoidance deficits in rats with amygdaloid lesions. *J. Comp. Physiol. Psychol. 83:* 168–172, 1973.

Chung, D., and Li, C. H. Adrenocorticotropins, XXXVII. The synthesis of 8-lysine-ACTH 1–7 NH_2 and its biological properties. *J. Am. Chem. Soc. 89:* 4208–4213, 1967.

Coover, G. D., Ursin, H., and Levine, S. Plasma-corticosterone levels during active-avoidance learning in rats. *J. Comp. Physiol. Psychol. 82:* 170–174, 1973.

Crine, P., Benjannet, S., Seidah, N. G., Lis, M., and Chrétien, M. *In vitro* biosynthesis of β-endorphin, γ-lipotropin, and β-lipotropin by the pars intermedia of beef pituitary glands. *Proc. Nat. Acad. Sci., Wash. 74:* 4276–4280, 1977.

Dallman, M. F., Demanincor, D., and Shinsako, J. Diminishing corticotrope capacity to release ACTH during sustained stimulation: The twenty-four hours after bilateral adrenalectomy in the rat. *Endocrinology 95:* 65–73, 1974.

Davis, M., and Zolovick, A. J. Habituation of the startle response in adrenalectomized rats. *Physiol. Behav. 8:* 579–584, 1972.

Dedman, M. L., Farmer, T. H., and Morris, C. J. O. R. Oxidation-reduction properties of adrenocorticotrophic hormone. *Biochem. J. 59:* xii, 1955.

van Delft, A. M. L. Voorwaardelijk vluchtgedrag en het hypofyse-bijniersysteem bij de rat. Thesis, University of Utrecht, 1970.

Dupont, A., Endröczi, E., and Fortier, C. Relationship of pituitary-thyroid and pituitary-adrenocortical activities to conditioned behaviour in the rat. In Ford, D. H., (ed.), *Influence of Hormones on the Nervous System.* Basel: Karger, 1971, pp. 451–462.

Endröczi, E. *Limbic System Learning and Pituitary-Adrenal Function.* Budapest: Akadémiai Kiadó, 1972.

Endröczi, E., Telegdy, G., and Lissák, K. Analysis of the individual variations of adaptation in the rat, on the basis of conditioned reflex and endocrine studies. *Acta physiol. Acad. Sci hung. 11:* 393–398, 1957.

Flexner, J. B., and Flexner, L. B. Pituitary peptides and the suppression of memory by puromycin. *Proc. Nat. Acad. Sci., Wash. 68:* 2519–2521, 1971.

Fuller, J. L., Chambers, R. M., and Fuller, R. P. Effects of cortisone and of adrenalectomy on activity and emotional behavior of mice. *Psychosom. Med. 29:* 323–328, 1956.

Gaillard, A. W. K., and Sanders, A. F. Some effects of ACTH 4–10 on performance during a serial reaction task. *Psychopharmacologia, Berl. 42:* 201–208, 1975.

Garrud, P., Gray, J. A., and de Wied, D. Pituitary-adrenal hormones and extinction of rewarded behaviour in the rat. *Physiol. Behav. 12:* 109–119, 1974.

Gispen, W. H., Buitelaar, J., Wiegant, V. M., Terenius, L., and de Wied, D. Interaction between ACTH fragments, brain opiate receptors and morphine-induced analgesia. *Europ. J. Pharmacol. 39:* 393–397, 1976.

Gispen, W. H., van der Poel, A., and van Wimersma Greidanus, Tj.B. Pituitary-adrenal influences on behavior. Responses to test situations with or without electric footshock. *Physiol. Behav. 10:* 345–350, 1973.

Gold, P. E., Rose, R. P., Spanis, C. W., and Hankins, L. L. Retention deficit for avoidance training in hypophysectomized rats: Time-dependent enhancement of retention performance with ACTH injections. *Horm. Behav. 8:* 363–371, 1977.

Gray, J. A. Effect of ACTH on extinction of rewarded behaviour is blocked by previous administration of ACTH. *Nature, Lond. 229:* 52–54, 1971.

Greven, H. M., and de Wied, D. The influence of peptides derived from corticotropin (ACTH) on performance. Structure activity studies. In Zimmermann, F., Gispen, W. H., Marks, B. H., and de Wied, D. (eds.), *Drug Effects on Neuroendocrine Regulation. Progress in Brain Research 39:* 429–442. Amsterdam: Elsevier, 1973.

Greven, H. M., and de Wied, D. Influence of peptides structurally related to ACTH and MSH on active avoidance behavior in rats. A structure-activity relationship study. In Tilers, F. J. H., Swaab, D. F., and van Wimersma Greidanus, Tj. B. (eds.), *Melanocyte Stimulating Hormone: Control, Chemistry and Effects. Frontiers of Hormone Research,* Vol. 4. Basel: S. Karger, 1977, pp. 140–152.

Guillemin, R., Ling, N., and Burgus, R. Endorphines, peptides d'origine phypothalamique et neurohypophysaire a activité morphinomimetique. Isolement et structure moleculaire d' α-endorphine. *C.R. Acad. Sci., Ser. D. 282:* 783–785, 1976.

Guillemin, R., Schally, A. V., Lipscomb, H. S., Andersen, R. N., and Long, J. M. On the presence in hog hypothalamus of β-corticotropin releasing factor, α- and β-melanocyte stimulating hormones, adrenocorticotropin, lysine-vasopressin and oxytocin. *Endocrinology 70:* 471–477, 1962.

Guillemin, R., Vargo, T., Rossier, J., Minick, S., Long, N., Rivier, C., Vale, W., and Bloom, F. β-Endorphin and adrenocorticotropin are secreted concomitantly by the pituitary gland. *Science 197:* 1367–1369, 1977.

Guth, S., Levine, S., and Seward, J. P. Appetitive acquisition and extinction effects with exogenous ACTH. *Physiol. Behav. 7:* 195–200, 1971.

Harding, C. F., and Leshner, A. I. The effects of adrenalectomy on the aggressiveness of differentially housed mice. *Physiol. Behav. 8:* 437–440, 1972.

Harris, R. K. Acquisition of conditioned avoidance responses by hypophysectomized rats. *J. Comp. Physiol. Psychol. 82:* 254–260, 1973.

Hodges, J. R., and Vernikos-Danellis, J. Pituitary and blood corticotrophin changes in adrenalectomized rats maintained on physiological doses of corticosteroids. *Acta Endocrin., Kbh. 39:* 79–86, 1962.

Hofmann, K., Andreatta, R., Bohn, H., and Moroder, L. Studies on polypeptides. XLV. Structure-function studies in the β-corticotropin series. *J:. Med. Chem. 13:* 339–345, 1970.

Hughes, J. Isolation of an endogenous compound from the brain with pharmacological properties similar to morphine. *Brain Res. 88:* 295–308, 1975.

Hughes, J., Smith, T. W., Kosterlitz, H. W., Fothergill, L. A., Morgan, B. A., and Morris, H. R. Identification of two related pentapeptides from the brain with potent opiate agonist activity. *Nature, Lond. 258:* 577–579, 1975.

Joffe, J. M., Mulick, J. A., and Rawson, R. A. Effects of adrenalectomy on open-field behavior in rats. *Horm. Behav. 3:* 87–96, 1972.

Johnston, R. E., Miya, T. S., and Paolino, R. M. Facilitated avoidance learning and stress-induced corticosterone levels as a function of age in rats. *Physiol. Behav. 12:* 305–308, 1974.

Kastin, A. J., Miller, L. H., Nockton, R., Sandman, C. A., Schally, A. V., and Stratton, L. O. Behavioral aspects of melanocyte stimulating hormone (MSH). In Zimmermann, E., Gispen, W. H., Marks, B. H., and de Wied, D. (eds.), *Drug Effects on Neuroendocrine Regulation. Progress in Brain Research 39:* 461–470. Amsterdam: Elsevier, 1973.

Kastin, A. J., Sandman, C. A., Stratton, L. O., Schally, A. V., and Miller, L. H. Behavioral and electrographic changes in rat and man after MSH. In Gispen, W. H., van Wimersma Greidanus, Tj. B., Bohus, B., and de Wied, D. (eds.), *Hormones, Homeostasis and the Brain. Progress in Brain Research 42:* 143–150. Amsterdam: Elsevier, 1975.

Keyes, J. B. Effect of ACTH on ECG-produced amnesia of a passive avoidance task. *Physiol. Psychol. 2:* 307–309, 1974.

Kleerekoper, M., Donald, R. A., and Posen, S. Corticotrophin in cerebrospinal fluid of patients with Nelson's syndrome. *Lancet 1:* 74–76, 1972.

de Kloet, E. R. and McEwen, B. S. Glucocorticoid interactions with brain and pituitary. In Gispen, W. H. (ed.), *Molecular and Functional Neurobiology.* Amsterdam: Elsevier, 1976, pp. 258–306.

de Kloet, E. R., Wallach, G., and McEwen, B. S. Differences in corticosterone and dexamethasone binding to rat brain and pituitary. *Endocrinology 96:* 598–609, 1975.

Kovács, G. L., Telegdy, G., and Lissák, K. 5-Hydroxytryptamine and the mediation of pituitary-adrenocortical hormones in the extinction of active avoidance behaviour. *Psychoneuroendocrinology 1:* 219–230, 1976.

Kovács, G. L., Telegdy, G., and Lissák, K. Dose-dependent action of corticosteroids on brain serotonin content and passive avoidance behavior. *Horm. Behav. 8:* 155–165, 1977.

Krieger, D. R., Liotta, A., and Brownstein, M. J. Presence of corticotropin in brain of normal and hypophysectomized rats. *Proc. Nat. Acad. Sci., Wash. 74:* 648–652, 1977a.

Krieger, D. T., Liotta, A., and Brownstein, M. J. Presence of corticotropin in limbic system of normal and hypophysectomized rats. *Brain Res. 128:* 575–579, 1977b.

Leonard, B. E. The effect of sodium-barbitone alone and together with ACTH and amphetamine on the behavior of the rat in the multiple "T" maze. *Int. J. Neuropharmacol. 8:* 427–435, 1969.

Leshner, A. I., Walker, W. A., Johnson, A. E., Kelling, J. S., Kreisler, S. J., and Svare, B. B. Pituitary adrenocortical activity and intermale aggressiveness in isolated mice. *Physiol. Behav. 11:* 705–711, 1973.

Levine, M. D., Gordon, T. P., Peterson, R. H., and Rose, R. M. Urinary 17-OHCS response of high- and low-aggressive rhesus monkeys to shock avoidance. *Physiol. Behav. 5:* 919–924, 1970.

Levine, S., and Jones, L. E. Adrenocorticotropic hormone (ACTH) and passive avoidance learning. *J. Comp. Physiol. Psychol. 59:* 357–360, 1965.

Levine, S., and Levin, R. Pituitary-adrenal influences on passive avoidance in two inbred strains of mice. *Horm. Behav. 1:* 105–110, 1970.

Levine, S., and Treiman, D. M. Differential plasma corticosterone response to stress in four inbred strains of mice. *Endocrinology 75:* 142–144, 1964.

Levine, S., Goldman, L., and Coover, G. D. Expectancy and the pituitary-adrenal system. In *Physiology, Emotion and Psychosomatic Illness.* CIBA Foundation Symposium 8 (new series). Amsterdam: Elsevier/Excerpta Medica/North Holland, 1972, pp. 281–291.

Li, C. H., and Chung, D. Isolation and structure of an untriakontapeptide with opiate activity from camel pituitary glands. *Proc. Nat. Acad. Sci., Wash. 73:* 1145–1148, 1976.

Lissák, K., and Bohus, B. Pituitary hormones and avoidance behavior of the rat. *Int. J. Psychobiol. 2:* 103–115, 1972.

Lissák, K., Endröczi, E., and Medgyesi, P. Somatisches Verhalten und Nebennierenrindentätigkeit. *Pflügers Arch. ges. Physiol. 265:* 117–124, 1957.

Lo, T. B., Dixon, J. S., and Li, C. H. Isolation of methionine sulfoxide analogue of α-melanocyte stimulating hormone from bovine pituitary glands. *Biochim. Biophys. Acta 53:* 584–586, 1961.

Loh, Y. P., and Gainer, H. Heterogeneity of melanotropic peptides in the pars intermedia and brain. *Brain Res. 130:* 169–175, 1977.

Mains, R., Eipper, B. A., and Ling, N. Common precursor to corticotropins and endorphins. *Proc. Nat. Acad. Sci., Wash. 74:* 3014–3018, 1977.

Mason, J. W. Psychological influences on the pituitary-adrenal cortical system. *Recent Progr. Hormone Res. 15:* 345–389, 1959.

Mason, J. W. A review of psychoendogene release of the pituitary-adrenal cortical system. *Psychosom. Med. 30:* 576–608, 1968.

Mason, J. W., Brady, J. V., and Sidman, M. Plasma 17-hydroxycorticosteroid levels and conditioned behavior in the rhesus monkey. *Endocrinology 60:* 741–752, 1957.

Mason, J. W., Brady, J. V., and Tolliver, G. A. Plasma and urinary 17-hydroxycorticosteroid response to 72 hr avoidance session in the monkey. *Psychosom. Med. 30:* 608–630, 1968.

McEwen, B. S., de Kloet, E. R., and Wallach, G. Interactions in vivo and in vitro of corticoids and progesterone with cell nuclei and soluble macromolecules from rat brain regions and pituitary. *Brain Res. 105:* 129–136, 1976.

McEwen, B. S., Luine, V. N., Plapinger, L., and de Kloet, E. R. Putative estrogen and glucocorticoid receptors in the limbic brain. *J. Ster. Biochem. 6:* 971–979, 1975.

McEwen, B. S., Weiss, J. M., and Schwartz, L. S. Uptake of corticosterone by rat brain and its concentration by certain limbic structures. *Brain Res. 16:* 227–241, 1969.

Mezey, E., Palkovits, M., de Kloet, E. R., Verhoef, J., and de Wied, D. Evidence for pituitary-brain transport of a behaviorally potent ACTH analog. *Life Sci., 22:* 831–838, 1978.

Miller, R. E., and Ogawa, N. The effect of adrenocorticotropic hormone (ACTH) on avoidance conditioning in the adrenalectomized rat. *J. Comp. Physiol. Psychol. 55:* 211–213, 1962.

Mirsky, I. A., Miller, R., and Stein, M. Relation of adrenocortical activity and adaptive behavior. *Psychosom. Med. 15:* 574–588, 1953.

Murphy, J. V., and Miller, R. E. The effect of adrenocorticotropic hormone (ACTH) on avoidance conditioning in the rat. *J. Comp. Physiol. Psychol. 48:* 47–49, 1955.

Moyer, K. E. The effect of adrenalectomy on anxiety-motivated behavior. *J. Genet. Psychol. 92:* 11–16, 1958.

Moyer, K. E., and Moshein, P. Effect of adrenalectomy on the attenuation of a conditioned avoidance response by ECS in the rat. *J. Comp. Physiol. Psychol. 56:* 163–166, 1963.

Natelson, B. H., Krasnegor, N., and Holaday, J. W. Relations between behavioral arousal and plasma cortisol levels in monkeys performing repeated free-operant avoidance sessions. *J. Comp. Physiol. Psychol. 90:* 958–969, 1976.

Oliver, C., Mical, R. S., and Porter, J. C. Hypothalamic-pituitary vasculature: evidence for retrograde blood flow in the pituitary stalk. *Endocrinology 101:* 598–604, 1977.

Pasternak, G. W., Goodman, R., and Snyder, S. H. An endogenous morphine-like factor in mammalian brain. *Life Sci. 16:* 1765–1769, 1975.

Paul, C., and Havlena, J. Maze learning and open field behavior of adrenalectomized rats. *J. Psychosom. Res. 6:* 153–156, 1962.

van Ress, J. M., de Wied, D., Bradbury, A. F., Hulme, E. C., Smyth, D. G., and Snell, C. R. Induction of tolerance to the analgesic action of lipotropin C-fragment. *Nature 264:* 792–794, 1976.

Rees, H. D., Stumpf, W. E., and Sar, M. Autoradiographic studies with ^{3}H-dexamethasone in the rat brain and pituitary. In Stumpf, W. E., and Grant, L. D. *Anatomical Neuroendocrinology.* Basel: S. Karger, 1975, pp. 262–269.

van Riezen, H., Rigter, H., and de Wied, D. Possible significance of ACTH fragments for human mental performance. *Behav. Biol. 20* (3): 311–324, 1977.

Rigter, H. Plasma corticosterone levels as an index of ACTH 4–10-induced attenuation of amnesia. *Behav. Biol. 15:* 207–211, 1975.

Rigter, H., and van Riezen, H. Anti-amnesic effect of ACTH 4–10. Its dependence of the nature of the amnesic agent and the behavioral test. *Physiol. Behav. 14:* 563–566, 1975.

Rigter, H., Elbertse, R., and van Riezen, H. Time-dependent anti-amnesic effect of ACTH 4–10 and desglycinamide-lysine vasopressin. In Gispen, W. H., van Wimersma Greidanus, Tj. B., Bohus, B., and de Wied, D. (eds.), *Hormones, Homeostasis and the Brain. Progress in Brain Research 42:* 163–171. Amsterdam: Elsevier, 1975.

Rigter, H., van Riezen, H., and de Wied, D. The effects of ACTH and vasopressin analogues on CO_2-induced retrograde amnesia in rats. *Physiol. Behav. 13:* 381–388, 1974.

Rudman, D., Del Rio, A. E., Hollins, B. M., Houser, D. H., Keeling, M. E., Sutin, J., Scott, J. W., Sears, R. A., and Rosenberg, M. Z. Melanotropic-lypolytic peptides in various regions of bovine, simian and human brains and in simian and human cerebrspinal fluids. *Endocrinology 92:* 372–379, 1973.

Sandman, C. A., Kastin, A. J., and Schally, A. V. Melanocyte-stimulating hormone and learned appetitive behavior. *Experientia 25:* 1001–1002, 1969.

Schally, A. V., Lipscomp, H. S., Long, J. M., Dear, W. E., and Guillemin, R. Chromatography and hormonal activities of dog hypothalamus. *Endocrinology 70:* 478–480, 1962.

Scott, A. P., Ratcliffe, J. G., Rees, L. H., Landon, J., Bennett, H. P. J., Lowry, P. J., and McMartin, C. Pituitary peptide. *Nature, New Biology 244:* 65–67, 1973.

Selye, H. *Stress. The Physiology and Pathology of Exposure to Stress.* Montreal: Acta Inc., 1950.

Sidman, M., Mason, J. W., Brady, J. V., and Thach, J. Quantitative relations between avoidance behavior and pituitary-adrenal cortical activity. *J. Exp. Anal. Behav. 5:* 353–362, 1962.

Sigg, E. B., Day, C., and Colombo, C. Endocrine factors in isolation-induced aggressiveness in rodents. *Endocrinology 78:* 679–684, 1966.

Silva, M. T. A. Extinction of a passive avoidance response in adrenalectomized and demedullated rats. *Behav. Biol. 9:* 553–562, 1973.

Silva, M. T. A. Effects of adrenal demedullation and adrenalectomy on an active avoidance response of rats. *Physiol. Psychol. 2:* 171–174, 1974.

Simantov, R., Kuhar, M. J., Pasternak, G. W., and Snyder, S. H. The regional distribution of a morphine-like factor enkephalin in monkey brain. *Brain Res. 106:* 189–197, 1976a.

Simantov, R., Kuhar, M. J., Uhl, G. R., and Snyder, S. H. Opioid peptide enkephalin: Immunohistochemical mapping in rat central nervous system. *Proc. Nat. Acad. Sci., Wash. 74:* 2167–2171, 1977.

Simantov, R., Snowman, A. M., and Snyder, S. H. A morphine-like factor "enkephalin" in rat brain: Subcellular localization. *Brain Res. 107:* 650–657, 1976b.

Snyder, S. H., and Simantov, R. The opiate receptor and opioid peptides. *J. Neurochem. 28:* 13–20, 1977.

Stone, C. P., and King, F. A. Effects of hypophysectomy on behavior in rats: I. Preliminary survey. *J. Comp. Physiol. Psychol. 47:* 213–219, 1954.

Stumpf, W. E., and Sar, M. Anatomical distribution of corticosterone-concentrating neurons in rat brain. In Stumpf, W. E., and Grant, L. D. (eds.), *Anatomical Neuroendocrinology.* Basel: S. Karger, 1975, pp. 254–261.

Swaab, D. F. Localization of an α-MSH-like compound in the nervous system by immunofluorescence. (Abstr. no. 285.) *Vth Int. Congress of Endocrinology,* Hamburg, July 18–24, 1976.

Tamásy, V., Korányi, L., Lissák, K., and Jandala, M. Open-field behavior, habituation and passive avoidance learning: Effect of ACTH and hydrocortisone on normal and adrenalectomized rats. *Physiol. Behav. 10:* 995–1000, 1973.

Terenius, L. Effect of peptides and aminoacids on dihydromorphine binding to the opiate receptor. *J. Pharm. Pharmacol. 27:* 450–452, 1975.

Terenius, L. Somatostatin and ACTH are peptides with partial agonist-like selectivity for opiate receptors. *Europ. J. Pharmacol. 38:* 211–213, 1976.

Terenius, L., Gispen, W. H., and de Wied, D. ACTH-like peptides and opiate receptors in the rat brain: Structure-activity studies. *Europ. J. Pharmacol. 33:* 395–399, 1975.

Tesser, G. I., Maier, R., Schenkel-Hulliger, R., Barthe, P. L., Kamber, B., and Rittel, W. Biological activity of corticotrophin peptides with hono-arginine or ornithine substitutes for arginine in position 8. *Acta Endocrin., Kbh. 74:* 56–66, 1973.

Urban, I., and de Wied, D. Changes in excitability of the theta activity generating substrate by ACTH 4–10 in the rat. *Exp. Brain Res. 24:* 325–344, 1976.

Ursin, H., Coover, G. D., Køhler, C., Deryck, M., Sagvolden, T., and Levine, S. Limbic structures and behavior: Endocrine correlates. In Gispen, W. H., van Wimersma Greidanus, Tj. B., Bohus, B., and de Wied, D. (eds.), *Hormones, Homeostasis and the Brain. Progress in Brain Research 42:* 263–274. Amsterdam: Elsevier, 1975.

Verhoef, J., Witter, A., and de Wied, D. Specific uptake of a behaviorally potent [^{3}H]-ACTH 4–9 analog in the septal area after intraventricular injection in rats. *Brain Res. 131:* 117–128, 1977.

Wei, E., and Loh, H. Physical dependence on opiate-like peptides. *Science 193:* 1262–1263, 1976.

Weiss, J. M., McEwen, B. S., Silva, M., and Kalkut, M. Pituitary-adrenal alterations and fear responding. *Am. J. Physiol. 218:* 864–868, 1970.

Wertheim, G. A., Conner, R. L., and Levine, S. Avoidance conditioning and adrenocortical function in the rat. *Physiol. Behav. 4:* 41–44, 1969.

de Wied, D. Influence of anterior pituitary on avoidance learning and escape behavior. *Am. J. Physiol. 207:* 255–259, 1964.

de Wied, D. Opposite effects of ACTH and glucocorticosteroids on extinction of conditioned avoidance behavior. *Proceedings Second Int. Congress on Hormonal Steroids,* Milan, May, 1966. Excerpta Medica Int. Congress Series No. 132, 1967, p. 945.

de Wied, D. The anterior pituitary and conditioned avoidance behavior. *Proceedings 3rd Int. Congress of Endocrinology,* Mexico D.F., June/July 1968. Excerpta Medica Int. Congress Series no. 184, 1969a, pp. 310–316.

de Wied, D. Effects of peptide hormones on behavior. In Ganong, W. F., and Martini, L. (eds.), *Frontiers in Neuroendocrinology 1969.* London/New York: Oxford University Press, 1969b, pp. 97–140.

de Wied, D. Pituitary-adrenal hormones and behavior. In Stoelinga, G. B. A., and van der Werff ten Bosch, J. J. (eds.), *Normal and Abnormal Development of Brain and Behavior.* Boerhaave Series for Postgraduate Medical Education. Leiden: University Press, 1971, pp. 315–322.

de Wied, D. Pituitary-adrenal system hormones and behavior. In Schmitt, F. O., and Worden, F. G. (eds.), *The Neurosciences, Third Study Program.* Cambridge, Massachusetts: MIT Press, 1974, pp. 653–666.

de Wied, D., Bohus, B., van Ree, J. M., and Urban, I. Behavioral and electrophysiological effects of peptides related to lipotropin (β-LPH). *J. Pharmacol. Exp. Ther., 204:* 570–580, 1978.

de Wied, D., Witter, A., and Greven, H. M. Behaviourally active ACTH analogues. *Biochem. Pharmacol. 24:* 1463–1468, 1975.

van Wimersma Greidanus, Tj. B. Effect of steroids on extinction of an avoidance response in rats. A structure-activity relationship study. In de Wied, D., and Weijnen, J. A. W. M. (eds.), *Pituitary, Adrenal and the Brain. Progress in Brain Research 32:* 185–191. Amsterdam: Elsevier, 1970.

van Wimersma Greidanus, Tj. B. Pregnene-type steroids and impairment of passive avoidance behavior in rats. *Horm. Behav. 9:* 49–56, 1977.

van Wimersma Greidanus, Tj. B., and de Wied, D. Effects of systemic and intracerebral administration of two opposite acting ACTH-related peptides on extinction of conditioned avoidance behavior. *Neuroendocrinology 7:* 291–301, 1971.

van Wimersma Greidanus, Tj. B., and de Wied, D. Dorsal hippocampus: A site of action of neuropeptides on avoidance behavior? *Pharmacol. Biochem. Behav. 5,* Suppl. 1: 29–33, 1976.

van Wimersma Greidanus, Tj. B., Bohus, B., and de Wied, D. CNS sites of action of ACTH, MSH and vasopressin in relation to avoidance behavior. In Stumpf, W. E., and Grant, L. D. (eds.), *Anatomical Neuroendocrinology.* Basel: S. Karger, 1975, pp. 284–289.

van Wimersma Greidanus, Tj. B., Rees, L. H., Scott, A. P., Lowry, P. J., and de Wied, D. ACTH release during passive avoidance behavior. *Brain Research Bulletin 2:* 101–104, 1977.

Witter, A., Greven, H. M., and de Wied, D. Correlation between structure, behavioral activity and rate of biotransformation of some ACTH 4–9 analogs. *J. Pharmacol. Exp. Ther. 193:* 853–860, 1975.

von Zerssen, D. Mood and behavioral changes under corticosteroid therapy. In Itil, T. M., Laudahn, G., and Herrmann, W. M. (eds.), *Psychotropic Action of Hormones.* New York: Spectrum Publications Inc., 1976, pp. 195–222.

Zimmermann, E., and Krivoy, W. A. Antagonism between morphine and the polypeptides ACTH, ACTH 1–24 and β-MSH in the nervous system. In Zimmermann, E., Gispen, W. H., Marks, B. H., and de Wied, D. (eds.), *Drug Effects on Neuroendocrine Regulation. Progress in Brain Research 39:* 383–394. Amsterdam: Elsevier, 1973.

12.

The Endocrine Hypothalamus and the Hormonal Response to Stress

G. B. Makara,[+] M. Palkovits,[++] and J. Szentágothai[++]

[+]*Institute of Experimental Medicine of the Hungarian Academy of Sciences, Budapest and [++]1st Department of Anatomy, Semmelweis University Medical School, Budapest*

1. INTRODUCTION

It was reported by Selye in 1936 that a variety of noxious stimuli elicit a generalized syndrome consisting of the hypertrophy and hyperfunction of the adrenal cortex, the involution of the thymus and the lymph nodes, and ulcerations in the stomach and intestines (Selye, 1936, 1946). This syndrome is a nonspecific response of the body to intense (noxious) demand and has been named the general adaptation syndrome (G.A.S.), or, subsequently, the biological *stress* syndrome, consisting of three more or less distinct phases: the alarm reaction, the phase of resistance, and the phase of exhaustion. The characteristic nonspecific changes during the development of G.A.S. are mediated by two main mechanisms: the release of corticotropin (ACTH) which causes the increased secretion of glucocorticoids; and the activation of the autonomous nervous system to liberate catecholamines by the peripheral sympathetic nerve endings and by the adrenal medulla. Most other components of the G.A.S. are consequences of or corollary to the main mechanism.

It is evident that the hormonal response is a salient feature of the stress syndrome, and an understanding of the hormonal events and their control is necessary to understand how the body organizes its defense against noxious stimulation.

The central position of the hypothalamus in the control of many endocrine mechanisms has become increasingly clear over the last 30 years. With the advent of radioimmunoassays, changes in the blood levels of most anterior pituitary hormones have been demonstrated during the response to stress. The first effect of the various stressors acting upon the body is not as stereotyped as the response (G.A.S.), and it may reach the hypothalamo-hypophyseal complex either over neural pathways or a variety of chemical signals, which may be again chemical substances liberated in various parts of the body, or simply the lack of an important metabolic factor otherwise present. It is assumed that the "first mediator" of the stressful stimulus is likely to be specific to the stimulus, and it is probably in the endocrine hypothalamus that a large variety of inputs are translated into a more limited number, or a more highly organized spectrum, of hormonal responses.

This chapter is an attempt at summarizing what is known today about the hormonal response to stress, with emphasis on the events occurring during the alarm reaction, much less being known of the hormonal changes during the phases of resistance and exhaustion. Subsequently data will be summarized on the location of the cells producing the hypophysiotrophic factors, and the pathways and mechanisms over which information on stress is conveyed and processed. In the last few years, new techniques have revealed important new details about the angio- and neuroarchitectonics of the endocrine hypothalamus which make it necessary to reconsider some of the traditional concepts.

2. THE HORMONAL RESPONSE DURING THE ALARM REACTION

2.1. Corticotropin in Stress

The rapid release of corticotropin (ACTH) following exposure of an animal to any potentially noxious stimulus is the main indicator of the onset of the stress syndrome; in other words, anything that activates (nonspecifically) the chain of the hypothalamus → hypophysis → adrenal cortex ought to be considered, by definition, as a "stressor." Any direct (artificial) influence upon the adrenal control system, such as injection of purified corticotropin-releasing factor (CRF, corticoliberin) or of ACTH itself, or interventions resulting in a depression of blood corticoid hormone levels, cannot, by the same token, be considered as "stress." The response to stress depends on the anatomical integrity and orderly functioning of at least three major entities: hypothalamus, anterior pituitary, and adrenal cortex—and of their circulatory connections.

In the last decade it has been customary to regard the hypothalamus-pituitary-adrenal axis as controlled mainly, or perhaps exclusively, by peptide-producing cells of the medial basal hypothalamus (MBH) that project to the median eminence of the hypothalamus, where the mediator substance would be released into the primary plexus of the hypothalamo-hypophyseal portal circulation and carried to the corticotropin-producing cells of the anterior lobe of the pituitary. This simplistic view is no longer adequate even for summarizing the essential features of the hypothalamo-pituitary complex and a number of recent findings make it necessary to reevaluate our earlier concepts of the functional architecture and of the mechanisms for central control of adrenal cortical secretion.

For the purposes of this paragraph it may suffice to emphasize that according to recent evidence the cells producing (or at least giving rise to the nerve terminals releasing) CRF may be localized outside the mediobasal region of the hypothalamus (MBH). Similarly, the view that CRF is liberated exclusively by nerve terminals in the surface zone of the median eminence (and the proximal part of the pituitary stalk) has now to be questioned. However, the pertinent data will be discussed in paragraph 4.2.1.

Obviously, all stressors have to generate some signal(s) at their site of impact by interacting with the mechanisms of the organism. The possible mechanism was the subject of some specultion for a considerable period (see Selye, 1950; Selye and Heuser, 1955). Considering the variety of stressors capable of activating the endocrine defense system and the variety of mechanisms by which they are put to action, it seems probable that there are a wide number of mechanisms by which corticotropin release can be achieved by various stressors; moreover the same stressful influence may activate various mechanisms.

The site of integration of various signals about any stressful situation and particularly the "decision-making site" for the release of corticotropin may be distributed at some points of convergence of several pathways of information and, from there on, over a sequence of functional links of the central control mechanism.

Much effort was spent to elucidate the pathways that convey information from the site of impact of the stressors to the hypothalamus-pituitary unit. This resulted in various classifications of the stressors according to their pathways or mechanisms. Fortier (1951) distinguished neural and systemic stimuli, according to whether they were mediated by the nervous system or whether they had a direct impact upon the pituitary, supposedly via the systemic circulation. The basic experimental model for this distinction was the difference in the response of the in situ and the heterotopically transplanted pituitary. Other experimental models were based on the consequences for stress reactions of sectioning the pituitary stalk, of removing the neurointermediate lobe (Smelik et al., 1962), and of chronic isolation of the hypothalamo-hypophyseal complex from the rest of the nervous system (Halász, Slusher, and Gorski, 1967; Feldman et al., 1968; Makara et al., 1969). A detailed diagram summarizing one version of this concept by Szentágothai et al. (1962) is reproduced here in Figure 12.1.

Unfortunately, the use by the various workers of the same or very similar terminology for classification based on the study of dissimilar parameters, caused much confusion in the literature and made it difficult to evaluate what was real and what was only apparent in the differences. In virtually all kinds of experimental approach two main mechanisms of stress or stressor action could be distinguished, one associated with the type of response corresponding generally to stimuli that are apparently neural (or neurogenic or neurotropic) and another associated with the type of response to stressors that may generate more pronounced general changes, and that are more likely to act via the general circulation and thus might be called systemic or humoral.

A more sophisticated subdivision of stressors might be based on substantial differences in the pathways activated, or on the site of their action upon the central control mechanism of the pituitary-adrenal system. The following options might be considered: (1) a certain group of stressors activate corticotropin release via both hypothalamic corticoliberin release and another mechanism acting via nonhypothalamic (systemic) mediation, such as the assumed ''tissue-CRF'' (Lymangrover and Brodish, 1973); (2) one might assume the presence of several corticoliberin release mechanisms in the hypothalamus activated by different mechanisms; (3) there might be the mentioned subdivision between humoral and neural mechanisms all reaching the same pool of CRF cells (Makara et al., 1969); or (4) further various combinations of the three mechanisms might

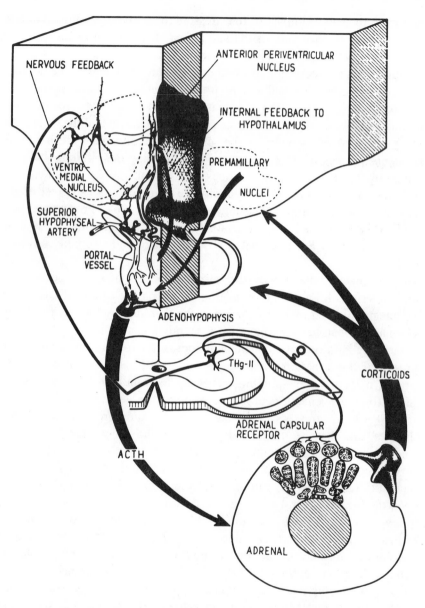

Figure 12.1. Schematic drawing illustrating the former concept about several modes of feedback observed in adrenocorticotropic mechanisms (Szentágothai et al., 1968).

occur. For the time being, none of these explanations would seem to be clearly preferable to any other because most of the original experimental models need careful reevaluation with the modern methods of assays.

Ironically, the most recent data give the best support to the original concept of Fortier (1951). Although Fortier (1966) himself pointed out that his subdivision of the stressors based on the response of heterotopic pituitary did not consider the possible consequences of a rise in systemic plasma levels of hypothalamic CRF, and that the indirect indices of corticotropin release used in those experiments make interpretation difficult, the concept that some stressors might act "directly" on the pituitary has received some experimental foundation later. It appears that many stressors require a normal hypothalamic and CNS function to elicit corticotropin release, but that there are some, such as injection of *E. coli* endotoxin, a large toxic dose of formaldehyde (Makara, Stark, and Mészáros, 1971; Stark et al., 1973/74, and severe surgical trauma (Lymangrover and Brodish, 1973), that are effective in stimulating corticotropin release even after removal or extensive destruction of those areas of the hypothalamus considered necessary for the neural control of the pituitary-adrenal system.

In theory, the subdivision of stressors into two groups, one activating the CRF-producing cells via neural pathways and the other acting via humoral pathways, could also be verified experimentally. Unfortunately, surgical isolation of the MBH or the median eminence was applied throughout, so that if CRF were produced and released by nerve cells located outside the isolated region, this would be no adequate procedure for the detection of CRF release via blood-borne mediation. Another difficulty arises from the possibility that stressors might be mediated initially over neural and subsequently over humoral channels.

In the absence of stress, corticotropin secretion is inversely related to plasma glucocorticoid levels, i.e., a decrease in adrenal hormone concentration leads to a rise in corticotropin secretion and vice versa. This relation is referred to as regulation by negative feedback and is accepted as fully operational under resting conditions. However, the role of negative feedback during the stress response has been subject to protracted debates.

The participation of the feedback regulation in stress-induced release of corticotropin was first suggested by Sayers and Sayers in 1947; they hypothesized that increased peripheral utilization of glucocorticoids might precede the triggering of corticotropin release during stress. Finding no decrease in blood corticoid level after exposure to stressors, Yates et al. (1961) reformulated the hypothesis about the role of feedback, suggesting that stressors reset the feedback controller of the pituitary-adrenal system. A sequence of careful studies has shown, however, that during stress there is no simple relationship between elevated blood corticoid level and inhibition of corticotropin release, and instead of a simple resetting of the threshold of the glucocorticoid-sensitive elements it is better to conceptualize the central control of corticotropin secretion as consisting of several feedback loops as well as having various excitatory (stress) inputs.

The inhibitory effect of glucocorticoid administration has a dual character: it may exert a fast inhibitory effect if the gradient of change in plasma levels is sufficiently steep, but this effect wears off soon after reaching a constant high hormone level. Inhibition becomes effective again after a delay, when the blood level of glucocorticoids is returning to normal (Yates and Maran, 1974). Using simultaneous measurement of immunoreactive corticotropin and corticosterone after exposure to various stressors, Engeland et al. (1977) suggested that if adrenal hormone secretion occurs sufficiently fast, it may feed back within minutes and modify the pattern of corticotropin release produced by mild fast-acting stressors. When the animal is exposed twice within a few hours to the same stressor, the response may seem unchanged; but this is the consequence of two contrary factors acting simultaneously: a "delayed" feedback inhibition produced by the corticoid secreted, and an increased sensitivity to stimuli as a consequence of the first exposure (Dallman and Jones, 1973).

More potent stimuli may be less susceptible to the fast feedback mechanism, and the fact that they elicit a prolonged and sustained rise in blood corticoid levels probably reflects the sustained stimulation of the system which overrides the feedback signal generated when plasma corticoids rise during the response to stress. Large doses of corticoids, administered many hours before the stressor, may decrease or prevent pituitary-adrenal response even to potent stimuli (Hodges and Jones, 1963; Smelik, 1963; Stark and Fachet, 1963).

The feedback signal may be acting upon several sites of the control system. There are reports that glucocorticoid implants at extrahypothalamic sites in a rather diffuse region of the forebrain inhibit compensatory adrenal hypertrophy (Davidson and Feldman, 1967). Both fast and delayed feedback have been demonstrated at the hypothalamic level, using an in vitro system in which CRF release from the isolated hypothalamus was studied (Jones and Hillhouse, 1976). That glucocorticoids may inhibit corticotropin also, by acting directly on the pituitary, has been amply demonstrated in a variety of in vitro systems (see Yates and Maran, 1974).

Extrahypothalamic sites for inhibitory effects of glucocorticoids are also suggested by experiments using rats with acute removal of the whole medial hypothalamus, which ought to prevent hypothalamic CRF from reaching the corticotropin-producing cells. In such animals corticotropin release can be increased by *E. coli* endotoxin injection, and both basal and endotoxin-stimulated ACTH release were strongly inhibited by dexamethasone pretreatment (Stark et al., 1973/74). Similar findings were published by Kendall, Tang, and Cook (1975). These data point to the possibility that in vivo the delayed inhibitory effect of the glucocorticoids might be exerted at the level of the anterior pituitary.

Such intricacies of the pituitary-adrenal response to stress may be important in determining the response of the system when stress is sustained, repeated, or chronic, since under such conditions both persistent drive and feedback signals generated earlier are present.

2.2. Somatotropin Secretion in Stress

The secretion of somatotropin (growth hormone, GH) appears to be under dual hypothalamic control by a factor stimulating its release (somatotropin-releasing factor, somatoliberin, GH-RF) and an inhibitory factor, somatostatin (Martin, 1976). So far, only the latter has been fully characterized, as a polypeptide containing 14 amino acids. It is generally assumed that the changes in somatotropin secretion are due to the changing balance between these two factors.

The early studies of pituitary somatotropin content by bioassay methods have led to numerous and conflicting views. With the introduction of exact, sensitive radioimmunoassays for the measurement of circulating hormone levels, it became evident that somatotropin secretion is most sensitive to various influences, and that certain metabolic adjustments during acute stress may be mediated by this mechanism.

The response to stress of plasma content of immunoreactive somatotropin may be diametrically opposite in various species—decreased in rodents but increased in primates—although it is consistent within a species.

In humans, the application of radioimmunoassay techniques to the study of circulating somatotropin has demonstrated unexpectedly acute and substantial *elevations* after exposure to various stressful stimuli. The somatotropin level has risen in response to hypoglycaemia, intense exercise (Roth et al., 1963; Hunter and Greenwood, 1964), surgery (Roth et al., 1963; Schalch, 1967), electroconvulsive therapy, acute trauma (Schalch, 1967), and pyrogen injection (Kohler et al., 1967; Frohman, Horton, and Lebovitz, 1967). The stress-induced release of growth hormone seems closely to parallel the release of corticotropin under similar conditions. The amount released may be quite substantial. Schalch (1967) calculated that 1.08 mg, i.e., about 21% of the normal daily production, can be released during an acute episode of stress or exercise.

In unanesthetized rhesus monkeys, environmental perturbations, painful stimuli, hemorrhage, as well as injections of histamine, vasopressin, epinephrine, or chlorpromazine lead to an abrupt increase in plasma GH levels (Meyer and Knobil, 1967).

In the rat, various stressful stimuli such as ether, cold, or hypoglycemia exert a strong *inhibitory* influence (Schalch and Reichlin, 1966). Further studies have extended the list of stressors inhibiting the release of this hormone to auditory stimulation (Collu et al., 1973) and immobilization–blood-withdrawal (Rice and Critchlow, 1976).

The application of bioassays led to claims that rat pituitary somatotropin would rapidly decrease during stress (see Müller, 1973), suggesting a rapid, stress-induced release of this hormone. Later studies using specific chemical techniques failed to substantiate these observations (Nagy et al., 1970a). Recent findings suggest that in the rat the decrease is mediated by an acute discharge into the blood of somatostatin. Forced swimming at 37°C for 30 minutes completely suppressed the normal pulsatile secretory pattern of somatotropin; but this is partially restored by injection of somatostatin antiserum (Terry et al., 1976). In rats treated with antiserum and then given electroshock, the plasma GH levels decreased significantly less than in the purely shocked controls (Arimura, Smith, and Schally, 1976).

The role of extrahypothalamic brain structures in the inhibition of growth hormone secretion in the rat was studied by electrical stimulation of various CNS sites, and ablations in and surgical cuts around the medial basal hypothalamus. Electrical stimulation in the hippocampus, basolateral amygdala, and interpeduncular nucleus produced an increase in plasma growth hormone, whereas stimulation in the preoptic region gave opposite results (Martin, 1972). Serial ablation of the septum, striatum, hippocampus, and amygdala failed to prevent the decrease in response to stress by immobilization + blood withdrawal. However, ablation of the preoptic region consistently blocked the somatotropin response and led to its reversal; the same effect was obtained in the complete absence of the telencephalon. These data strongly suggest that the preoptic region contains neural elements that have a major inhibitory influence on somatotropin secretion (Rice and Critchlow, 1976). Some experiments using surgical cuts around the MBH led to findings in apparent conflict with the above interpretation. Collu et al. (1973) observed an ether-induced decrease in plasma somatotropin in rats with complete surgical isolation of the MBH; however, Mitchell et al. (1973) failed to confirm this finding which would suggest a mediation over humoral pathways. In contrast, auditory stimulation failed to decrease plasma somatotropin after complete surgical isolation (Collu et al., 1973) of the MBH, while after a frontal cut only the inhibition occurred, as in the controls. This suggested that auditory stress is probably transmitted only via neural pathways, and that such pathways reach the MBH by a lateral, a dorsal, or a posterior route.

2.3. Prolactin in Stress

Prolactin secretion seems to be under a rather complex hypothalamic control exerted via the release of stimulating and inhibiting factors. There is some evidence from passive immunization experiments for a physiological stimulatory role for thyrotropin-releasing hormone (TRH) in the regulation of both rat prolactin and thyrotropin (Koch et al., 1977); but others (Harris et al., 1978) have obtained data contradicting a dominant role of TRH in prolactin release. There is also evidence for the existence of a separate prolactin-releasing factor (PRF). But, more important, prolactin secretion seems to be under tonic inhibition by the hypothalamus.

Prolactin release–inhibiting factor (PIF) activity has been demonstrated in hypothalamic extracts from a variety of animal species (see Meites et al., 1972). Dopamine, localized in the stalk–median eminence, is a probable candidate for being a PIF. However, the presence of a nondopaminic factor has been also demonstrated (Enjalbert, Priam, and Kordon, 1977).

Early data regarding prolactin secretion during stress remained inconclusive as long as they were based on the determination of pituitary prolactin stores by bioassay, hardly an adequate way to assess its possible pattern of secretion during stress. Chemical measurements of pituitary prolactin content appeared to show no appreciable change within an hour of exposure to a variety of stressors (Nagy et al., 1970b). However, sensitive radioimmunoassays demonstrated that substantial rises of plasma prolactin level occur soon after the exposure to stress in both rats and humans. This is not in contradiction to the unchanged pituitary content because the release of a small fraction of the prolactin content of the pituitary could account for substantial changes in blood plasma levels. Ether inhalation, for example, results in a rapid prolactin release in diestrus female (Neill, 1970; Morishige and Rotchild, 1974), in male (Dunn, Arimura, and Scheving, 1972; Krulich et al., 1974) and in gonadectomized rats (Ajika et al., 1972; Euker, Meites, and Riegle, 1975). Ether-induced prolactin release is manifest within 1.5 minutes after exposure (Wakabayashi, Arimura, and Schally, 1971), a speed comparable to that of corticotropin release. The speed and magnitude of the response appear to vary somewhat with the time of day and the sex of the animals. In males, hormone levels reached their peak 10 minutes later. The higher prolactin levels of females were also rapidly elevated, and returned to resting levels 15 minutes after short exposure to ether. Even the high serum levels measured on the afternoon of proestrus were further elevated (Turpen, Johnson, and Dunn, 1976). Rats "handled" daily before testing for stress-induced effects showed a blunted prolactin rise when compared to nonhandled controls (Turpen et al., 1976). Other stressors, such as restraint, may also elevate blood prolactin levels (Riegle and Meites, 1976a,b). Very little is known about the pathways by which the "message" of stress reaches the hypothalamus and is transmitted to the pituitary. It is not known whether the stress-induced prolactin release is due to PRF release or to the removal of a tonic inhibition. The speed of the response in certain cases, i.e., substantial release within 1.5 minutes, points to the role of a positive drive rather than to a removal of inhibition; however, in many cases the peak of the rise occurs with a delay that might suggest the other mechanism.

The pathways for prolactin release during etherization + bleeding may reach the medial basal hypothalamus either from the lateral or from posterior directions. The elegant study of Krulich, Hefco, and Aschenbrenner (1975) demonstrated that complete surgical isolation of the medial basal hypothalamus does not change significantly the basal prolactin level in the rat, and that a tonic inhibition by the neural tissue within the isolated piece of the hypothalamus may maintain normal basal levels. The response to etherization and serial bleeding is completely prevented by total isolation of the MBH from the rest of the brain even if the connections with the pituitary via the stalk are left intact. Interrupting the anterior neural connections had little if any effect on the stress responses of prolactin.

2.4. Thyrotropin Secretion in Stress

Thyrotropin secretion of the pituitary is thought to be controlled by release into the primary plexus of the portal vessels of hypothalamic TRH. There is good evidence from passive immunization experiments (Koch et al., 1977; Harris et al., 1978) for a tonic secretion of TRH under a variety of conditions.

Early observations of an inverse relationship between the secretion of the adrenal cortex and the thyroid gland led to the conclusion that thyrotropin secretion is inhibited during, and possibly in consequence of, the stimulation by stressors (see Dewhurst et al., 1968).

Recent advances in methods made it possible to reevaluate and to confirm some of the earlier data. In the rat, mild stressors, such as injections or room transfer, were found to depress the thyrotropin level in the blood (Docummun, Sakiz, and Guillemin, 1966). The stress caused by transfer of rats from their home cage to the laboratory or to a jar, produced no change, or a transient elevation for 2 to 5 minutes followed by a decrease in thyrotropin levels 30 minutes later (McCann et al., 1973). A rapid rise of serum thyrotropin and in triiodothyronine levels 60 minutes after disturbing the animals (Döhler et al., 1977) has not been substantiated in male rats after exposure to a novel environment (Fenski and Wuttke, 1977). Exposure to ether depressed blood thyrotropin levels in male (McCann et al., 1973) and in female rats (Mannistö, Saarinen, and Ranta, 1976), again not substantiated in other experiments (Fenske and Wuttke, 1977). In the female rat, ether and other anesthetics inhibited the rise in thyrotropin normally elicited by exposure to cold (Mannistö et al., 1976). Contrary to the usual inverse relationship between corticotropin and thyrotropin, exposure to cold stimulates the release of both hormones in the rat (Dupont et al., 1972; Takeuchi, Kajihara, and Suzuki, 1977); but adding minor stresses, such as anesthesia or painful stimuli, may inhibit or suppress the thyrotropin response to a cold environment while further increasing the plasma corticosterone level (Dupont et al., 1972).

In humans, treadmill exercise, gastroscopy, and other surgery depressed serum thyrotropin levels (Sowers et al., 1977). The post-stress depression may result from the suppressive effect of stress-induced high levels of serum cortisol.

2.5. Gonadotropins in Stress

Despite earlier, very generally held, simplistic views, it is being realized increasingly that these relations are complex. In acute exposure to ether of rats, a rapid rise in blood luteinizing hormone (LH, or lutropin) levels is experienced in male (Dunn et al., 1973/74; Krulich et al., 1974) and in female rats (Neill, 1970; Morishige and Rotchild, 1974; Turpen et al., 1976). Ether anesthesia caused a small rise in serum follicle stimulating hormone (FSH, follitropin) in both male and ovariectomized female rats in some (Krulich et al., 1974; Ajika et al., 1972), but not in other studies (Turpen et al., 1976). The lack of consistency of these data may be due to individual variations, to the transient nature of the responses, and to the possible dependence of the response pattern on previous history (handling, and so forth) of the animals. Variations in basal hormone levels due to sex, circadian rhythm, or the estrus cycle altered the LH plasma level in etherization (Turpen et al., 1976). Age may also be an important factor. The transient rise observed in young male rats cannot be elicited in aged animals (Riegle and Meites, 1976a), probably as a consequence of decreased hypothalamus-pituitary responsiveness.

Other stimuli may induce a rapid fall in plasma gonadotropin levels. In ovariectomized rats pretreated with estrogen and progesterone to stabilize the hormonal background, the stress of a novel environment (Baldwin, Colombo, and Sawyer, 1974) or combined ether-surgery and a novel environment depressed plasma LH levels (Colombo and Sawyer, 1975), and spreading depression prevented the effect. Small but significant decreases in LH and FSH levels were observed 15 minutes after the combined stress of bleeding and restraint (Libertun and McCann, 1976). Döhler et al. (1977) found a slight transient rise in serum FSH 15 minutes after exposing rats to disturbance stress, while the serum LH level showed only slight fluctuations.

In humans, both surgery under general anesthesia and gastroscopy were followed by a rise in serum LH level, but FSH failed to change (Sowers et al., 1977). A strenuous running exercise of short duration caused a significant rise in plasma LH (Kuoppasalmi et al., 1976), in contrast to an exercise of long duration causing no change (Dessypris, Kuoppasalmi, and Adlercreutz, 1976).

The evidence presently available about the response of gonadotropins is best summarized in the opinion of McCann et al. (1973) that gonadotrophins often show a biphasic response: frequently there is an acute discharge of the hormones followed by a fall below the normal levels.

2.6. Vasopressin Secretion in Stress

It has been known for more than 25 years that vasopressin is involved in the control of blood osmolarity, volume, and pressure and is influenced by a number of factors, (for a recent review see Robertson, 1977). Until recently it was widely accepted that any form of nonspecific stress is an effective stimulus of vasopressin secretion, and it was debatable whether or not vasopressin might be the natural hypothalamic factor mediating the release of corticotropin. High concentrations of vasopressin have been found in the portal plasma sampled under severe surgical stress in the monkey (Zimmermann et al., 1973) and the rat (Oliver, Mical, and Porter, 1977). In the rat, vasopressin level in the portal plasma significantly dropped after acute removal of the neural lobe, but still remained at a much higher level than in the peripheral blood (Oliver et al. 1977. This shows (1) that vasopressin is secreted from the stalk–median eminence and (2) that vasopressin originating from the neural lobe can reach the portal vessels, at least under the conditions of their acute cannulation. Moreover, vasopressin can reach the anterior pituitary in high concentration and might influence its secretory functions. Vasopressin has also been detected in the anterior lobe of the pituitary, and its amount varied in parallel with the activity of the pituitary-adrenal system, i.e., increased after adrenalectomy and decreased in corticoid treatment (Chateau, Burlet, and Boulange, 1977).

In spite of this, it is clear that vasopressin is not identical with the ACTH-releasing substance that can be extracted from the stalk–median eminence or the neural lobe. CRF activity was observed in the ME and the hypothalamus of Brattleboro rats genetically lacking vasopressin (Krieger, Liotta, and Brownstein, 1977a), and such rats are capable of increasing ACTH and glucocorticoid secretion in response to a variety of stressors (McCann et al., 1966; Arimura et al., 1967). CRF activity can be demonstrated in bioassay systems nonresponsive to vasopressin

(Yasuda and Greer, 1976a). CRF and vasopressin release can be dissociated in vitro by pharmacological means (Jones, Hillhouse, and Burden, 1976), and vasopressin and CRF-like activity of hypothalamic extracts can be separated by biochemical techniques (Saffran and Schally, 1977a,b) or by immunoneutralization (Lutz-Bucher, Koch, and Mialhe, 1977).

With recent advances in the radioimmunoassay of plasma vasopressin, it became feasible to reevaluate the role of vasopressin release in the hormonal response to stress. It became apparent that, provided they do not change blood pressure or osmolality, none of the stressors employed—light ether anesthesia, water immersion, pain (Brennan, Shelton, and Robertson, 1975), or acceleration stress (Keil and Severs, 1977)—had any detectable effect on vasopressin levels, although they elevated plasma corticosterone levels (Brennan et al., 1975). In rats dehydrated for elevated vasopressin levels, ether inhalation and acceleration stress induced a rapid reduction rather than the expected rise in the level of vasopressin (Keil and Severs, 1977). However, in severe stress with changes in the pressure, volume, or osmolality of blood, vasopressin may be released (secondarily) and have a role on its own.

3. HORMONAL CHANGES DURING THE STAGE OF RESISTANCE

The concepts of adaptation of the organism and adaptation of the hormonal response(s) to stress are to be clearly separated. In principle the development of resistance to any given stressor may or may not be accompanied by a sustained hormonal response such as adrenocortical hypersecretion. ''Adaptation'' of the hormonal response might be regarded also as a return to normal or to the pre-stress state.

Early morphological observations during prolonged stress of adrenal hypertrophy with restored ascorbic acid and lipid content, were interpreted as signs of sustained adrenal hyperfunction. This was accompanied by indirect signs of decreased secretion of other pituitary hormones, and it is suggested that during the stage of resistance there would be a shift in pituitary functions, predominantly corticotropin being secreted at the expense of the other hormones. At the same time doubts arose about a sustained adrenal hyperfunction during the stage of resistance: the thymus regained its weight; blood lymphocyte and eosinophil granulocyte counts returned to normal.

3.1. Corticotropin in Chronic Stress

The hypothalamus-pituitary-adrenal system does not seem to "adapt" easily to repeated stress over limited time. Ether, tourniquet, or "broken leg" stresses repeated at 90-minute intervals up to three times, or ether stress once daily for three days, resulted in no decrease in either plasma ACTH or corticosterone response (Cook et al., 1974). On a longer time scale, repeated or chronic exposure to various stressors often, but not invariably, results in a gradual diminution of the adrenocortical response, usually measured in the rat as changes of plasma corticosterone. When compared to the response seen after the first or initial exposure, there is a marked reduction (sometimes to pre-stress levels) of the plasma corticosteroid level in the stage of resistance. The stressors studied were: daily injection of formaldehyde (Vecsei, 1962; Stark et al., 1965, 1968; Mikulaj et al., 1973), administration of insulin (Kraicer and Logothetopoulos, 1963), bacterial endotoxins (Stark et al., 1968), immobilization (Mikulaj et al., 1973; Riegle, 1973; Kawakami, Seto, and Kimura, 1972), traumatization in the Noble-Collip drum (Mikulaj et al., 1973), forced swimming (Frenkl et al., 1968, 1969), heat (Strosser et al., 1974), cold (Daniels-Severs et al., 1973), chronic environmental stress elicited by alternating audiogenic stimulation, and flashing lights and motion stimuli (Buckley, 1973).

It became apparent from these studies that various lengths of time were required for the "adaptation" of the adrenocortical response to the various stressors. The response to handling or injections of moderate doses of formaldehyde or bacterial endotoxin is reduced within two weeks, whereas with trauma in the Noble-Collip drum or immobilization it took six weeks for the inhibition to appear. An interesting aspect is that "adapted" animals appear to secrete corticosterone at a lesser rate and for a shorter period that nonadapted ones. In some experiments, rats adapted to one kind of stressor showed a substantial elevation of plasma corticosterone level upon administration of another (Stark et al., 1968; Daniels-Severs et al., 1973; Sakellaris and Vernikos-Danellis, 1975).

There are, however, well documented examples of chronic or repeated stressors producing the same plasma corticosterone response as did the first exposure. When a single powerful electrical shock, which caused an approximately threefold rise of plasma corticosterone level, was administered daily for 30 days, the response to the last exposure was the same as that to the first (Stark et al., 1968). Similar observations were made with the chronic stressor of crowding rats. Although crowding elicited no adrenal hypertrophy, elevated adrenal and plasma corticosterone levels were measured over one to eight weeks (Daniels-Severs et al., 1973).

From the evidence available the following general conclusions might be derived: *First,* persistent adrenal hypertrophy is often, but not invariably, associated with a return toward normal of corticoid blood levels. *Second,* the reduction of the adrenal response cannot be due to an exhaustion of the pituitary or the adrenals, since injection of corticotropin or introduction of another stressor quickly raised plasma hormone levels. In other words the "adaptation" of the adrenal response has considerable stimulus specificity and probably takes place in the hypothalamic circuits or somewhere along the afferent pathways. *Third,* the "adaptation" cannot be due solely to inhibition of ACTH release by the negative feedback action because such an inhibition would be relatively unselective and affect to a similar degree various stressful stimuli. It appears that chronic stress causes an increased drive in the central control of corticotropin secretion which compensates for or overrides the glucocorticoid feedback (Dallman and Jones, 1973; Sakellaris and Vernikos-Danellis, 1975).

The varying time course of adaptation to various stimuli, and the apparent lack of "adaptation" of the hormonal response to at least two nonspecific stressors support the idea that the response to nonspecific stress is stereotypic only in the limited sense of being invariably accompanied by an acute activation of the pituitary-adrenal system. However, when mechanisms or pathways are considered, or the very existence or the speed of adaptation, there are various response patterns, probably specific to the type of stimulus. This is one more reason to consider the apparently nonspecific acute hormonal response as a specific expression of a more general mechanism, depending on the hypothalamic neural circuits that control the endocrine system by decoding various peripheral inputs for the final "decision" on whether the organism exposed to stress ought or ought not to increase its corticotropin and glucocorticoid secretion.

3.2. Prolactin, Somatotropin, Gonadotropin, and Thyrotropin Secretion in Chronic Stress

In contrast to what is known of the response of the pituitary-adrenal system to chronic stress, there is very little reliable information on the response patterns of other pituitary hormones. Although decreases in body weight, reproductive function, and endocrine gland weights are charactistic consequences of severe chronic stress, this change is not necessarily caused via diminution of pituitary hormone secretion; for changes in weight of peripheral endocrine organs are poor indicators of endocrine function, especially since direct neural influences were demonstrated in adrenal, ovarian, and testicular weight changes.

Indirect evidence led Selye (1950) to suggest that during chronic stress a shift in anterior pituitary function occurs, so that hypersecretion of one hormone, namely corticotropin, would be accompanied by decreased secretion of other hormones by the same gland. Since then it has become evident that the various pituitary hormones are synthetized by separate cells—although LH and FSH, on the one hand, and corticotropin, melanotropins, and lipotropin, on the other, are produced in the same cells—and that there is no compulsive inverse relationship between the secretion of the various hormones. Numerous acute stressors are capable of simultaneously activating the release of three or more other pituitary hormones. Some recent morphological findings also seem to contradict the "shift theory." Using a signaled unpredictable footshock regimen Bassett, and Cairncross, (1976) have shown by an ultrastructural study of the adenohypophysis that the initial *hyperactivity* in response to stress affected all the tropic cell types, and that adrenal function as well as cellular morphology showed a gradual return to normal after 10–20 days.

Direct chemical or immunochemical hormone measurements during chronic stress are scarce. Using a complex chronic stress protocol, it has been shown (Nagy et al., 1971) that no change occurs during adaptation in somatotropin and prolactin content of the anterior pituitary. Simultaneous measurements of hormone levels in blood plasma or serum are available only in two situations. In starvation, which is a rather special stressor, Chowers, Einat, and Feldman (1969) found evidence for a sustained release of corticotropin, whereas Campbell et al. (1977) found decreased serum levels of somatotropin, prolactin, thyrotropin, LH, and FSH. Using TRH and LHRH injections, they obtained evidence that the depression of hormone levels by starvation was primarily due to reduced hypothalamic hormone secretion rather than the inability of the pituitary to secrete its hormones. The possible shift in adenohypophyseal activity was also studied by Taché et al. (1976) using chronic intermittent immobilization. Female rats were immobilized for 8 hours daily up to 15 days, and blood was sampled only at the end of the immobilization sessions. This treatment depressed the weight of the body, the pituitary, and the ovary but not of the thyroid, while the adrenals were hypertrophied. An increase of plasma corticosterone, and a clear-cut decrease of somatotropin and LH was maintained throughout the study period, while changes in FSH, thyrotropin, and prolactin were either biphasic or very slight. After injection of TRH + LHRH, significant rises of LH, FSH, prolactin, and thyrotropin occurred. Since in the case of corticotropin release it is known that hormone level returns to normal between the restraint sessions (Mikulaj et al., 1973), whereas Riegle and Meites (1976b) found sustained high levels of prolactin *between* sessions of intermittent immobilization while at the *end* of the twentieth session there was still a decrease, it appears that during intermittent stress the hormone levels measured during or immediately after the last stress exposure do not reflect what happens during much of the stress period. One cannot know, therefore, whether in the above-mentioned experiments normal basal secretion was maintained and the pituitary responded with the same response pattern to the first and the fifteenth immobilization sessions, or whether there was a sustained shift due to repetition of tropic hormone secretions in either direction.

From the fragmentary data available, one may conclude that there is only partial support as yet for the shift theory of Selye, and that more information is needed about the secretory profiles of the various pituitary hormones in a number of chronic stressful situations before a comprehensive picture can be drawn. It seems probable, however, that if a shift is proved to exist in chronic severe stress, it will be primarily a *shift in the secretion of hypothalamic hypophyseotrophic hormones* rather than a primary hypophyseal shift.

4. SITES OF PRODUCTION AND RELEASE OF HYPOPHYSIOTROPIC SUBSTANCES

Although the expression "hypophysiotrophic hormones" might be adequate for summarizing certain neurohumoral substances under a general title, and with a certain concept in mind, the term is now only of didactical value in view of the very different kinds of mechanisms and substances, partly known, partly unknown, that are involved. Some of these substances have been identified chemically; the existence of others can be inferred indirectly from their action on the anterior pituitary. The chemically identified substances are summarized in Table 12.1. The other releasing or release-inhibiting hormones—among them CRF, the main factor mediating stress mechanisms—are still unknown. The chemical identification of this CRF was thought to have been successful (Schally, Lipscomb, and Guillemin, 1962; Schally and Bowers, 1964); however, the control of its activity did not substantiate this claim (Saffran and Schally, 1977a,b).

One of the main difficulties in the identification of these neurohormones is a certain lack of specificity. It turned out that various kinds of neurohormones (or transmitters), in most cases peptides, may be responsible for a given hypophysiotropic effect. Even the identified releasing or release-inhibiting hormones can also influence, albeit to a lesser degree, the release of the other pituitary hormones. Hence, hypophysiotropic effects, and among them those occurring during stress, can no longer be considered as the result of the release or inhibition of release of a single hypothalamic mediator.

An analysis of the central mechanisms involved in stress has to be based, therefore, upon a thorough study of the action mechanisms and of the sites of synthesis and/or release of these neurohumors. This has become relatively simple with the chemically identified neurohumors, especially if radioimmunoassay and immunocytochemical methods for their localization are already available. Unfortunately, this is not the case with the most important putative neurohumor, CRF. Also, the identification of

Table 12.1 Structures of Peptides

TRH	(Pyro)Glu His Pro(NH$_2$)
Oxytocin	CyS-Tyr-Phe-Glu(NH$_2$)-Asp(NH$_2$)-CyS-Pro-Lys-Gly(NH$_2$)
	1 2 3 4 5 6 7 8 9
Vasopressin	CyS-Tyr-Ile-Glu(NH$_2$)-Asp(NH$_2$)-CyS-Pro-Leu-Gly(NH$_2$)
LH-RH	(Pyro)Glu-His-Trp-Ser-Tyr-Gly-Leu-Pro-Gly(NH$_2$)
Somatostatin	Ala-Gly-CyS-Lys-Asn-Phe-Phe-Trp-Lys-Thr-Phe-Thr-Ser-CyS
Enkephalins	Tyr-Gly-Gly-Phe-Met-OH
	Tyr-Gly-Gly-Phe-Leu-OH
Angiotensin II	Asp-Arg-Val-Tyr-Ile-His-Pro-Phe-OH
	1 2 3 4 5 6 7 8
Substance P	Arg-Pro-Lys-Pro-Gln-Gln-Phe-Phe-Gly-Leu-Met(NH$_2$)
Neurotensin	Glu-Leu-Tyr-Glu-Asn-Lys-Pro-Arg-Arg-Pro-Tyr-Ileu-Leu-OH

certain neurohumors raised unexpected new difficulties: it was soon realized that most of the "hypothalamic" neurohumors occur in many intracentral and extracentral sites. Among the intracentral sites that they are present in, there are many (spinal cord, lower brainstem, cerebellum, and so on) from which there is no way (apart from that over complex neuronal chains) to reach the hypophysis. It is also unlikely that their synthesis in other neural structures would mean that they are to reach the pituitary over the systemic circulation; their significance is mainly local, subserving synaptic transmission or modulation.

The major new message coming through from studies based upon immunocytochemistry, is the understanding—in contrast to the very generally held traditional opinion (see a summary of the earlier literature in Szentágothai et al., 1962, 1965, 1968)—that not all the perikarya synthesizing hypophysiotropic hormones are localized in the hypothalamus. Unfortunately, while it is relatively easy to detect, by aid of immunocytochemical methods, hypothalamic neurohumors in the nerve terminals at the surface zone of the median eminence and of the pituitary stalk (including some other zones of massed nerve terminals, for example in the vascular organ of the lamina terminalis), this is not so easy in the case of the perikarya. Also, the specificity of the methods appears to be much less satisfactory if applied to perikarya. At any rate the number of cells containing the neurohumors, and identified immunochemically with sufficient specificity, is far smaller than what would be required by the number of terminals. This might be due to the presence of a precursor only in the perikarya, while the complete neurohumor might be available only in the axon terminals. Also, much appears to depend on the nature of the antisera (Hoffman, 1977; Hofmann et al., 1977, 1978a,b). Particular difficulties arise from substantial species differences.

4.1. Chemically Identified Neurohumors

We shall not enter into a discussion, in any depth, of the chemical nature of the peptidic neurohormones (and/or mediators), or into that of their mode of action on the membrane receptor level. The reader is referred for this whole complex body of relatively new knowledge to the excellent survey by Cooper, Bloom, and Roth (1978). It might be worthwhile, though, to include Table 12.1, to have a comprehensive list of the known neurohumors. Only a minority of them have been so far reliably shown to have a direct role in hypothalamic mechanisms. In the following paragraph only those will be dealt with, the role of which is reasonably well documented.

4.1.1 Luteinizing Hormone-Releasing Hormone (LH-RH). According to location of the perikarya, two fields of LH-RH cells can be distinguished: LH-RH field I and field II (Hoffman, 1977; Hoffman et al., 1977, 1978a). Field I includes the intrah;ypothalamic LH-RH cells, localized mainly in the arcuate and in the dorsal premamillary nuclei. Field II includes the medial preoptic, interstitial nucleus of the stria terminalis, and to some extent cells located in the nucleus of the diagonal tract. In the rodent field II is dominant, while in the dog, in the monkey, and in man, fields I and II seem to be of equal importance (Hoffman, 1977). Apart from these two fields, LH-RH cells have also been described in other territories of the brain (Barry, Dubois, and Poulain, 1973; Silverman, 1976; Barry, 1977; Hoffman, 1977; Hoffman et al., 1978b).

LH-RH fibers and axon terminals are found in abundance in the median eminence and in the vascular organ of the lamina terminalis (OVLT), (Barry et al., 1973; Leonardelli, Barry, and Dubois, 1973; Kordon et al., 1974; King et al., 1974; Baker, Dermody, and Reel, 1974; Sétáló et al., 1975a,b, 1976a,b; Barry and Carette, 1975; Barry and Dubois, 1976; Silverman, 1976; Barry, 1977, 1978; Hoffman, 1977; Hoffman et al., 1978a,b). The highest content in LH-RH is being found in the same regions by radioimmunoassay methods (Palkovits, et al., 1974; Wheaton, Krulich, and McKann, 1975; Kizer, Palkovits, and Brownstein, 1976). From field II the axons of the LH-RH cells can be traced toward the OVL and to the rear toward the median eminence (Barry, 1977, 1978; Barry and Carette, 1975; Palkovits et al., 1978). Most of the latter have to traverse the arcuate nucleus, where they are joined by the axons originating from the cells of field I. In the rat the majority of LH-RH fibers originate from the preoptic region, as also shown by the virtual disappearance of LH-RH fibers and terminals after anterior or complete deafferentation of the medial-basal hypothalamus (Barry et al., 1973; Weiner et al., 1975, Sétáló et al., 1975a,b, 1976b), under which circumstances the LH-RH content of the median eminence is reduced by 75–85% (Weiner et al., 1975; Brownstein et al., 1976a; Palkovits, Brownstein, and Kizer, 1976b). It must be mentioned, though, that the number of LH-RH fibers is considerable behind the region of detachment of the pituitary stalk from the median eminence (Barry et al., 1973; Baker et al., 1974; Kordon et al., 1974; Sétáló et al., 1975b), as well as in various regions of the diencephalon and mesencephalon (Barry and Carette, 1975; Barry and Dubois, 1976; Sétáló, 1976; Silverman, 1976; Barry, 1977, 1978).

4.1.2. Thyrotropin-Releasing Hormone (TRH).

The presence of TRH has been observed in almost all parts of the CNS with radioimmunoassay methods (Winokur and Utiger, 1974; Jackson and Reichlin, 1974a,b; Oliver et al., 1974) and immunocytochemistry (Hökfelt et al., 1975b, 1976). The localization of cell bodies, however, by immunocytochemical methods remained unsuccessful. As regards tissue concentration in TRH, the medial eminence exceeds all other regions of the brain by two orders of magnitude (Brownstein et al., 1974). The TRH content of the median eminence seems to be largely of extrahypothalamic origin because complete de-afferentation of the medial-basal hypothalamus causes a loss of 80% of its original TRH content, while that of other brain regions remained unchanged (Brownstein et al., 1975b).

4.1.3. Growth Hormone–Release Inhibiting Hormone (Somatostatin).

The concentration of somatostatin in the CNS is higher by an order of magnitude than that of any other releasing hormone (Brownstein et al., 1975a; Palkovits et al., 1976a; Epelbaum et al., 1977). It can be found in all parts of the CNS, but also in other, nonneural tissues (gastric, enteric mucosa, pancreas (Hökfelt et al., 1975a). Its concentration also is at its maximum in the median eminence.

By aid of immunohistological methods somatostatin-containing perikarya could be detected in many parts of the CNS (Hökfelt et al., 1974, 1975a; Sétáló et al., 1975c; Baker and Yu, 1976). Only a small part of the cells are localized in the medial-basal hypothalamus, where they occur mainly in anterior and periventricular location, but scattered cells can also be found in the dorsomedial nucleus and inserted into the median forebrain bundle (Hökfelt et al., 1975a; Elde and Parsons, 1975; Alpert et al., 1976; Bennett-Clarke, 1977). In the surface zone of the median eminence and of the proximal stalk, numerous axon terminals containing somatostatin can be detected (Hökfelt et al., 1974; Sétáló et al., 1975c; King et al., 1975). They appear to enter this region from the anterior direction because in anterior and total de-afferentation of the medial-basal hypothalamus the concentration of somatostatin in the median eminence drops by 76–84% (Brownstein et al., 1977).

4.1.4. Oxytocin. Oxytocin can be demonstrated immunocytochemically both in perikarya and in axons and their terminals (Vandesande and Dierickx, 1975; Vandesande, Dierickx, and De Mey, 1975a,b; Dierickx, Vandesande, and De Mey, 1976; Buijs et al., 1978). The cells are located in the magnocellular hypothalamic nuclei (paraventricular, supraoptic, magnocellular, accessory). It occurs and is transported together with a carrier protein (neurophysin I) mainly via the supraoptico-hypophyseal tract in the interior stratum of the median eminence into the neurohypophysis. Its concentration is highest in the neural lobe, followed by the median eminence, and subsequently by the nuclei of its synthesis.

4.1.5. Vasopressin. Vasopressin is synthesized in the same nuclei as oxytocin but in different cells (Vandesande et al., 1975a,b; Vandesande and Dierickx, 1975; Silverman and Zimmerman, 1975; Zimmerman, 1976; Dierickx et al., 1976; Zimmerman et al., 1977). Perikarya containing vasopressin were also found in the suprachiasmatic nucleus (Vandesande et al., 1975b; Zimmerman, 1976). The course of vasopressin-containing axons is the same as of oxytocin-conveying axons, but they also terminate in the palizade zone of the stalk–median eminence (Zimmerman et al., 1977). Vasopressin-containing fibers also occur at other sites of the CNS (Buijs et al., 1978). Its carrier protein (neurophysin II) is not identical with that of oxytocin. The results of radioimmunoassay in tissue samples and of immunocytochemistry for vasopressin run parallel in the neurohypophysis, the median eminence, and the hypothalamus.

4.2. Unidentified Hypothalamic Neurohumors

Only those will be enumerated in the following paragraphs that have a known significant role in the stress mechanisms.

4.2.1. Corticotropin-Releasing Factor (CRF). In the absence of an unequivocal chemical identification, neither radioimmunoassay nor immunocytochemical observations are available on this substance. Using bioassay methods, CRF-like activity has been shown to exist in all hypothalamic nuclei and in the median eminence (Vernikos-Danellis, 1964, 1965; Lang et al., 1976; Krieger et al., 1977a). The highest activity is present in the median eminence.

There is no immunocytochemical technique available that would help us to decide whether CRF activity in the medial-basal hypothalamus is localized in perikarya or nerve terminals. Some observations argue in favor of intrahypothalamic localization of CRF cell bodies (Yasuda and Greer, 1976b; Krieger et al., 1977a). Others, in contrast, claim that CRF cells are situated outside the medial-basal hypothalamus and the high CRF activity found there is due to the CRF stored in nerve terminals. CRF activity in stalk–median eminence extracts from rats with complete or antero-lateral surgical isolation of the medial-basal hypothalamus, was at least ten times less than that in the controls (Makara et al., in press/[no #]c). Electrical stimulation in the rat tuber cinereum and various stressful stimuli induced a rise in the plasma corticosterone level. However, seven to ten days after complete or antero-lateral isolation of the medial-basal hypothalamus, neither the electrical stimulation (Makara, Stark, and Palkovits, 1978) nor various stressful stimuli (Makara et al., 1969, 1970, in press/b; Palkovits, Makara, and Stark, 1976c) elicited significant increments of plasma corticosterone. These data suggest that the majority of CRF enters the medial-basal hypothalamus from outside and runs toward the neurohemal regions of the stalk–median eminence.

4.2.2. Prolactin-Inhibiting Factor (PIF).   There are numerous data suggesting that dopamine might inhibit prolactin release; it has even been assumed that PIF is identical with dopamine (see Meites et al., 1972; MacLeod, 1976). However, this identification rests, for the time being, on shaky grounds. The dopamine in the stalk–median eminence is undoubtedly synthesized by nerve cells located predominantly in the arcuate and periventricular nuclei (Dahlström and Fuxe, 1964; Fuxe, 1965; Fuxe and Hökfelt, 1966; Björklund et al., 1970, 1973). Numerous dopaminergic axons are present in the median eminence adjacent to the portal blood vessels. Dopamine is secreted into portal blood in significant quantities during pregnancy as well as during the day of estrus, during early diestrus, and least on the day of proestrus, supporting the important role of dopamine in the regulation of anterior pituitary function (Ben-Jonathan et al., 1977).

4.2.3. Growth Hormone-Releasing Factor (GRF).   GRF has recently been chemically purified (Redding and Schally, 1977), but radioimmuno- or immunocytochemical techniques are not yet available. Bioassay studies point to the existence in the medial-basal hypothalam;us of a substance that releases growth hormone from the pituitary (Krulich et al., 1971, 1977).

4.2.4. Factors of Putative Significance: Enkephalins, Endorphins, Substance P, Neurotensins, α-MSH. Various other peptides may have some role in influencing (or modulating) the release of hypothalamic neurohormones, and may be involved in the mechanisms of responses to stress.

The undecapeptide Substance P (Table 12.1) is widely distributed in the CNS, as demonstrated immunocytochemically (Hökfelt et al., 1975c; Cuello and Kanazawa, 1978), and by radioimmunoassay (Brownstein et al., 1976b). A dense plexus of Substance P immunoreactive nerve terminals in the median eminence was presented by Hökfelt et al. (1978).

β-Lipotropin consisting of 91 amino acids contains several smaller biologically active peptides: β-MSH, ACTH, β-lipotropin, methionine-enkephalin, and endorphins (α, β, γ). In the brain the highest concentration was found in the hypothalamus (Krieger et al., 1977b), where β-lipotropin perikarya (in the arcuate nucleus) and axons (in the arcuate, dorsomedial, and paraventricular nuclei and the external layer of the median eminence) could be demonstrated by the immunoperoxydase technique (Zimmerman, Liotta, and Krieger, 1978).

The chemically identified endorphins can be regarded as fragments of β-lipotropin. Relatively high concentrations were found in the hypothalamus (Guillemin et al., 1977; Krieger et al., 1977b). β-endorphin-containing axons in the hypothalamus were demonstrated with the aid of immunofluorescence techniques (Guillemin et al., 1977; Rossier et al., 1977).

α-Melanocyte stimulating hormone (α-MSH) was shown in the CNS in the same distribution as β-lipotropin (Oliver and Porter, 1978; Dubé et al., 1978).

Enkephalins (methionin- and leucin-enkephalin (see Table 12.1)) are widely but unevenly distributed in the CNS (Simantov et al., 1976; Yang, Hong, and Costa, 1977; Hong et al., 1977; Kobayashi et al., 1978). Axons containing enkephalins do occur in the median eminence and various regions of the hypothalamus (Elde et al., 1976; Simantov, Kuhar, and Uhl, 1977; Hökfelt et al., 1977).

The high concentration in the hypothalamus of tridecapeptide neurotensin (see Table 12.1) was demonstrated recently (Uhl and Snyder, 1976; Uhl, Kuhar, and Snyder, 1977; Kobayashi, Brown, and Vale, 1977).

In spite of the increasing number of observations related to the high concentrations of neural peptides in the median eminence and hypothalamus, it would still be premature to try to fit the data into any coherent hypothesis.

5. A REASSESSMENT OF ENDOCRINE HYPOTHALAMIC ANGIOARCHITECTONICS

The still-very-much-alive concept of two basic mechanisms, a neurogenic and a systematic one, in stress, makes it all the more important to try to bring the huge new body of information on endocrine hypothalamic mechanisms into line with its angioarchitectonics, which, after all, was the main lead from which our whole understanding of the hypothalamo-hypophyseal relationship originated.

The basic principle of pituitary blood supply as described in the classical studies of Harris and Green (1947, 1948, 1949, 1951) is still generally accepted as valid, the essence of this being that anterior pituitary tissue is supplied from the so-called *pituitary portal vessels* which arise from the primary arteriolar plexus on the surface of the median eminence and pituitary stalk. A system of specific metaarteriolar loops penetrates through the tissue of the stalk–median eminence almost to the lower wall of the third ventricle. The primary arteriolar plexus of the stalk–median eminence is fed by three hypophyseal arteries in the rat (two in man), and its drainage was assumed largely if not exclusively over the portal vessels that break up into a second capillary bed in the tissue of the anterior lobe. The metaarterioles (or some may be true capillaries) of the primary plexus and of the median eminence loops are covered throughout with fenestrated endothelium (Figure 12.2), which fits well with the observation that this region of the capillary bed of the CNS lacks the usual blood-brain barrier (Wislocki and King, 1936; Duke and Smith, 1974). A dense system of nerve terminals has been observed immediately adjoining the vessels of the primary plexus of the median eminence and of the specific loops (see Palkovits and Záborszky, in press). These structural features are well in accord with the concept of hypothalamic neurohumor being taken up into the blood, draining toward the anterior pituitary tissue by way of the portal vessels. There can hardly be any doubt about the validity of the general concept; it is likely to remain the main basis of all understanding of hypothalamo-pituitary mechanisms. However, as was pointed out long ago (Szentágothai et al., 1962), there were some inconsistencies among then-apparently-minor structural features, which could become crucial if the general idea were schematized and cut down to a

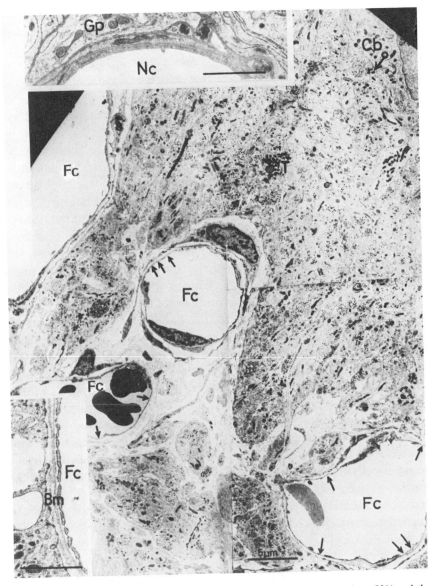

Figure 12.2. Fenestrated capillaries (Fc) in the zone between the arcuate nucleus (NA) and the median eminence. Arrows point to fenestrated endothelium. In the upper left inset are details from a nonfenestrated capillary (Nc) from the middle of the NA; in the right upper corner, axo-somatic synapse (ringed arrow) characteristic of the NA. *Abbr.:* Bm = basal membrane; Cb = cell body; Gp = glial process; T = tanycyte process.

simplistic dogmatic description, as is often done in the neuroendo-crinological literature. These inconsistencies in the classical concept may be of minor significance for the general functional principle of hypothalamo-pituitary interrelations; however, in the intricacies of any specific functional mechanism like that integrating the response of the organism to stress, and particularly in the interpretation of the results of modern and highly sophisticated experimental approaches, the considera-tion of all details may become important.

Our recent studies, using more advanced injection procedures for the identification of the position within the entire vascular circuit of any small vessel (Ambach and Palkovits, 1974), made it possible to straighten out earlier observed inconsistencies between the classical concept and all structural features, and to put them together into a picture of satisfactory coherence (Ambach, Palkovits, and Szentágothai, 1966). The main data can be summed up briefly as follows:

(a) The hypophyseal arteries supply not only the median eminence and the tissue of the anterior pituitary, but also the arcuate nucleus and a considerable part of the retrochiasmatic area of the hypothalamus (Figure 12.3). The vascular bed of the medial basal hypothalamus forms an intimately interconnected system of metaarterioles and capillaries, which is separated from the vascular bed of the remaining part of the hypothalamus. Three main circuits can, nevertheless, be distinguished in this ensemble (Ambach et al., 1976): (1) The *classical portal circuit* consists of hypophyseal arteries, primary plexus, specific stalk–median eminence loops, pituitary portal veins, anterior lobe sinusoids, and ven-ous drainage of the anterior lobe; the specific median eminence capillary loops are not the only roots of the portal veins, which receive some of the blood directly from the primary metaarteriolar plexus on the surface of the median eminence. (2) The *subependymal metaarteriolar plexus*, which receives its input, in part, directly from penetrating branchlets of the hypophyseal arteries and partially from the special median capillary loops of the median eminence, is localized immediately beneath the bottom of the third ventricle; although this plexus has some outlet toward smaller tuberal veins, its main drainage is secured around the lateral edges of the infundibular recess of the third ventricle toward the capillary network of the arcuate nucleus. (3) The *arcuate nucleus circuit* receives its arterial supply from two sources, direct penetrating branches of the hypophyseal arteries and branches of the subependymal (meta)arteriolar plexus curving around the lateral edges of the infundibular recess; the venous drainage of

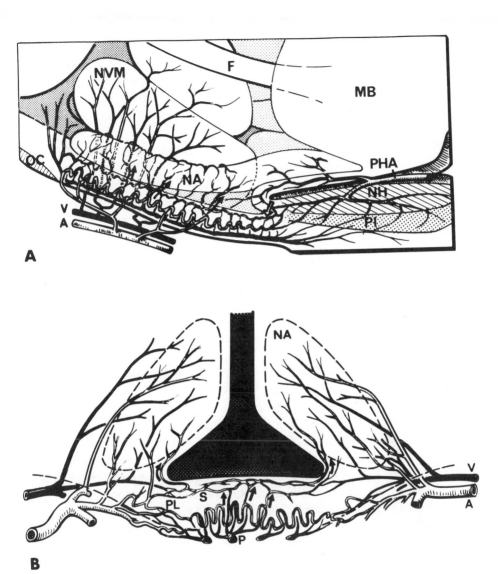

Figure 12.3. Schematic illustration of blood vessels in the stalk–median eminence and arcuate nucleus (a = sagittal, and b = frontal views). Directions of blood flow from the primary plexus (Pl) and metarteriolar loops in the median eminence to the subependymal plexus (S) and capillaries supplying the arcuate nucleus (NA) are indicated by arrows. Portal veins (p) originating from the primary plexus and metarteriolar loops are directed to the distal lobe of the pituitary gland. Some of these vessels are connected with those of the posterior pituitary artery (PHA) at the caudal end of the pituitary stalk (⟹). *Abbr.*: NH = posterior lobe; Pl = intermediate lobe; NVM = ventromedial nucleus; MB = mamillary body; OC = optic chiasm; A = internal carotid artery; V = basilar vein; AHA = anterior pituitary artery; MHA = middle pituitary artery.

309

this circuit is ensured over a separate row of tuberal veins starting from the retrochiasmatic area and continuing until the premamillary region. There is very little, other than collateral capillary connectivity, between this entire vascular bed and that of the remaining part of the hypothalamus, especially of the ventromedial nucleus, supplied by the tuberal arteries (Ambach and Palkovits, 1977).

(b) The complexity and unity of the vascular bed supplying not only the median eminence, pituitary stalk, and the entire pituitary, but additionally large parts of the medial basal hypothalamus, arcuate nucleus, and retrochiasmatic area, call for a certain reevaluation of the classical concepts about the hypothalamo-hypophyseal vascular relation. Instead of an unequivocal unidirectional blood flow from the hypophyseal arteries → primary plexus → special vascular loops → pituitary portal vessels, another direction of flow has to be considered, viz.: hypophyseal arteries → primary plexus → special vascular loops → subependymal plexus → arcuate nucleus, etc. This means that a possibility hinted at briefly by Szentágothai et al. (1962, ed., pp. 94–95; 1968 ed., pp. 87–92) is no longer a vague possibility but has now become a real mechanism, which cannot be neglected. If part of the blood passing the median eminence and becoming enriched in the neurohumors present in abundance (see section 4 of this chapter) passes over the capillary bed of the arcuate nucleus and the retrochiasmatic region, a repercussion (in fact, a [short] feedback action) of these neurohumors upon the neural structures of these regions becomes almost a necessity. This feedback may become especially important in the interpretation of the fundamental "hypophysiotrophic area effect" of Halász, Pupp, and Uhlarik (1962), which in the extreme case might mean that the effect is due, not to the neurohormones being secreted by cell bodies in the region defined by the hypophysiotrophic area, but to the drainage of blood from the median eminence toward the same hypothalamic territory (see also Sétáló et al., 1976a,b). It is obvious that various kinds of short feedback mechanisms potentially involved in the stress mechanism cannot be interpreted correctly without taking account of these circumstances. In fact, the anatomical situation illustrated in Figure 12.3 would suggest the possibility of a backflow to the medial-basal hypothalamus of blood having passed parts of both lobes of the pituitary. Scanning electron microscopic studies (Page and Bergland, 1977; Bergland and Page, 1978), hormone measurements in the portal blood of intact and median eminence–transected animals (Oliver et al., 1977), and determination of the labeled ACTH-fragment in the CNS after intrapituitary or intrasellar injections (Mezey et al., 1978), all serve as evidence for the existence of a significant backflow from the pituitary gland to the CNS.

(c) Since the main arterial supply of the neurohypophysis comes from the posterior hypophyseal artery, which contributes considerably to the posterior primary plexus and to a number of capillary loops in the postinfundibular part of the pituitary stalk and particularly on its dorsal surface with connection to the intermediate lobe, similar considerations as expounded above in (b) may arise in connection with the role of the neurohypophyseal hormones.

(d) All these considerations suffer from one common weakness, lack of knowledge about the exact distribution of fenestrated capillaries in the hypothalamo-pituitary vascular bed and/or of local variations of permeability (blood-brain barrier) in this entire region. But even so, the angioarchitectonics of this region cannot be omitted from consideration whenever any mechanism is speculated on.

6. A NEW LOOK AT THE NEURAL APPARATUS OF THE ENDOCRINE HYPOTHALAMUS

Earlier notions about the participation of neural structures in adrenocorticotropic mechanisms, as reflected in Figure 12.1, were based on the assumption that CRF is synthetized in the medial-basal hypothalamus, i.e., chiefly in the arcuate nucleus and possibly in the retrochiasmatic area and/or the anterior periventricular nucleus. This assumption appeared then to be fully in accord (1) with the anatomical observation of axons originating in the arcuate nucleus and terminating in the surface zone of the median eminence (Szentágothai et al., 1962, Fig. 49,; Szentágothai, 1964); (2) with the original interpretation of the observations by Halász et al. (1962) on the "hypophysiotrophic area" in the basal hypothalamus; and finally (3) with the observation that responses to various types of stress were preserved after neural de-afferentation or isolation of the basal hypothalamus from the remaining part of the CNS, while an intact connection remained between the basal hypothalamus and the pituitary (Halász and Pupp, 1965; Halász et al., 1967; Feldman et al., 1968; Voloschin, Joseph, and Knigge, 1968; Makara et al., 1970). What remained for demonstrating a purely neural feedback was to find a pathway connecting receptors from the periphery with the medial-basal hypothalamus. The solution suggested in Figure 12.1 was based on some highly indirect evidence of a crossed neural connection from assumed adrenal cortical capsular receptors to the ventromedial nucleus (Halász and Szentágothai, 1959). Some of the subsequent reinvestigations failed to substantiate the original effect; however, the existence of a crossed purely neural relation was later shown to exist by more advanced experimental techniques (Gerendai et al., 1974). A more recent, careful study by Dallman, Engeland, and McBride (1977) suggests the possibility of a purely neural reflex mechanism involved in compensatory adrenal hypertrophy, a concept that might explain many inconsistencies in the whole body of experimental results.

Although the basic principle of the concept illustrated in Figure 12.1 may still be valid, confidence in such a solution—which we now recognize to be simplistic—was shattered by the following developments: (1) As mentioned above in paragraph 4.2.1, most of the CRF may not be produced in the basal hypothalamus at all; it may even be of extrahypothalamic origin (Makara et al., 1978, in press/b,c). Hence, in a purely neural feedback the afferent pathway from the periphery has to reach this extrahypothalamic site of the CRF-producing cells. Until this site has been identified, it is of little use to speculate about the neuronal mechanism translating neural information about local stressful stimuli (for example tissue damage) into an increase of CRF release. (2) The possible need to shift the interpretation of the "hypophysiotrophic area" (see section 5) from assuming it to be the site of synthesis of the hypothalamic neurohumors toward that of the brain region, instigated by blood passing through the stalk–median eminence, where most neurohumors are delivered by the (free) nerve endings, would remove the medial-basal hypothalamus and its immediate environment from being the main candidate for the neural region upon which the humoral feedback by the corticoids (or any other chemical signal) could be exercised. The site of translation of the humoral signals into neural signals could be anywhere—particularly, of course, in the dendrites and perikarya of the hypophyseotrophic neurons. (3) The involvement (or possible involvement) in responses to stress of numerous other neurohumoral mechanisms, as discussed in section 2 of this chapter, shows that the mechanisms of mobilizing the defense of the body against harmful influences cannot be reduced to a "single-track" mechanism of mobilizing the release of CRF. We have to look, therefore, for some more general neural framework of pathways, connections in very different parts of the CNS, and involving various kinds of specific neuron systems, and/or mediation mechanisms that might satisfy these demands.

In spite of these doubts, the structural facts, upon which the earlier concepts were based, are too well founded and documented to be now discarded. Even if the cells producing CRF were not localized in the medial-basal hypothalamus, the majority of the free nerve terminals in the surface zone of the median eminence and the proximal part of the stalk have their origin in the MBH (Réthelyi and Halász, 1970). Any neural mechanism to be proposed for explanation of the involvement of the hypothalamus and of neural mechanisms in responses to stress has to take this into account; it must even start from the basic structural facts known about the magnocellular and the parvicellular neurosecretory systems. This was done recently by Palkovits (1977), who considered three possibilities by which extrahypothalamic pathways may interact in the MBH or in the median eminence: (1) extrahypothalamic pathways may terminate synaptically on the perikarya of the parvicellular system; (2) they may terminate by means of axo-axonic synapses upon the nerve endings of the parvicellular neuron system; and finally (3) they may terminate separately among the nerve terminals of the median eminence. From these three possibilities, numbers (1) and (3) have, so far, been shown to exist anatomically (van Cuc, Láránth, and Palkovits, in press).

In the following sections we shall summarize very briefly some more recent evidence about the pathways involved in mediating surgical stress (6.1) and some more general information about the neural structure of the basal hypothalamus (6.2).

6.1. Pathways of Extrahypothalamic Origin Involved in the Hormonal Response to Stress

The introduction by Halász and Pupp (1965) of the stereotaxic technique of hypothalamic de-afferentation and isolation has given rise to considerable optimism concerning a quick solution of all problems related to the neural pathways and mechanisms involved in conveying information to the hypothalamus about tissue damage, and about changes in the adrenal in consequence of the former. This optimism appeared justified, for some time, following the first studies by Halász et al. (1967) on corticotropin secretion after total or partial de-afferentation. While the consequences of total de-afferentation of the MBH, and the maintenance of a certain basal level in ACTH, remained uncontested, the interpretation of this as a proof that CRF-producing cells were localized in the MBH was not generally acceptable (Makara et al., 1978, in press/b,c). The results of partial de-afferentation remained equivocal, probably largely because of the lack of sufficient histological control in uninterrupted section series. Systematic studies on the point of entrance into the hypothalamus of the neural pathways conveying information about stress (Palkovits et al., 1976c) indicates that this is a rather circumscribed territory in the so-called lateral retrochiasmatic area (RCAL) in the rat (Figure 12.4). This is a small window on the medial border of the medial forebrain bundle (MFB), through which the pathways involved in conveying stress signals enter the hypothalamus radiating through and below the anterior hypothalamic nucleus (Figure 12.5). The relatively anterior location of this window in the caudal levels between the posterior edge of the optic chiasma and the anterior border of the median eminence explains that this region may have been completely destroyed or left partially intact both in anterior and, similarly, in lateral de-afferentations, thus giving rise to the controversial results. A complete destruction of this window in the RCAL is the only condition, in addition to complete isolation of the MBH, that abolishes any response to surgical (Palkovits et al., 1976c) and ether stress (Makara et al., in press/c). The anatomical reality is shown by degeneration of terminal fibers in the MBH after lesions in the RCAL (Figure 12.6).

Since this apparently crucial territory can be considered as a window to the MFB, a considerable number of fiber tracts both ascending and descending in this bundle can be considered as possible contributors to the stress pathways. Additionally, however, there are four other pathways, not otherwise belonging to the MFB, that enter the hypothalamus through the same window (Figure 12.4): these are the supraoptico-hypophyseal tract, the direct amydalohypothalamic tract, the supraoptic decussation, and an anatomically unidentified CRF-tract suggested by physiological evidence (Makara et al., 1978, in press/a,b,c). Palkovits (1977) has discussed *in extenso* the possible significance in ACTH release of these several pathways, so that it might suffice to summarize very briefly the meager—and for the time being rather inconclusive—evidence about the relative significance of the known pathways entering the hypothalamus through the RCAL: (1) Descending fibers of the MFB, partially also from the whole rostral territory of the limbic system, may be involved in ACTH release by inhibitory mechanisms. However, this inhibition is probably largely exercised by the hippocampus (Endröczi et al. 1959; Knigge, 1961; Knigge and Hays, 1963; Mandell et al. 1963). (2) The vasopressin-containing fibers from the paraventricular and supraoptic nuclei (supraoptico-hypophyseal tract), entering the hypothalamus through the same window, may be involved indirectly, as discussed already in part 2.6 of this chapter. (3) A direct amygdalo-hypothalamic

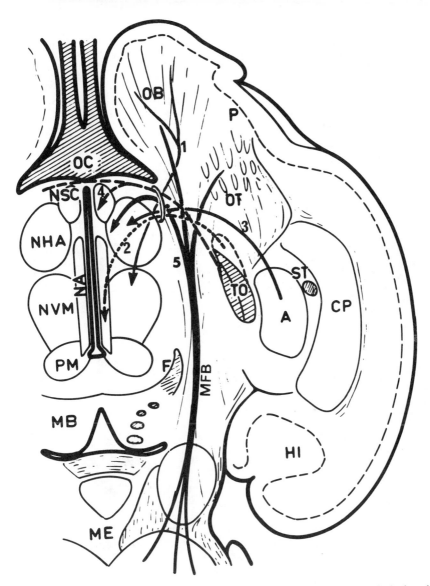

Figure 12.4. Illustration of pathways entering the medial-basal hypothalamus through the lateral retrochiasmatic area. Horizontal section at the level of the medial forebrain bundle (MFB). 1 = descending fibers of the MFB from the rostral limbic areas, 2 = supraoptico-hypophyseal tract, 3 = ventral amygdalofugal pathway, 4 = supraoptic decussations, and 5 = ascending fibers in the MFB. *Abbr.*: OB = olfactory bulb; P = pyriform cortex; OC = optic chiasm ; NSC = suprachiasmatic nucleus; OT = olfactory tubercle; NHA = anterior hypothalamic nucleus; NVM = ventromedial hypothalamic nucleus; NA = arcuate nucleus; TO = optic tract; A = amygdala; ST = stria terminalis; CP = caudate putamen; F = fornix; PM = premamillary nuclei; MB = mamillary body; HI = hippocampus; ME = mesencephalon.

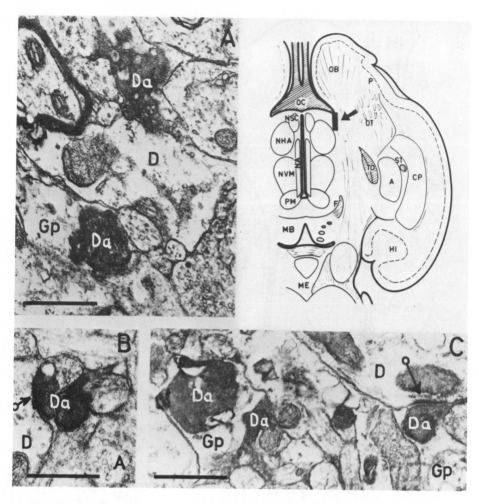

Figure 12.5. Degenerated nerve terminals in the arcuate nucleus (*A* and *C*) and ventromedial nucleus (*B*) two days after parasagittal transection (→) of the lateral retrochiasmatic area (Palkovits, Makara, Léránth, and van Cuc, unpublished. Some axons established synaptic contact (ringed arrows) with dendritic profiles. Bar scale: 1 µm. *Abbr.*: D = dendrite; Da = degenerated nerve terminals; Gp = glial process; A = intact nerve terminals. (Abbr. on drawing: see Figure 12.4).

pathway was first mentioned by Krieg (1932), but no other later anatomical confirmations (Szentágothai et al., 1962; Leonard and Scott, 1971) or more direct physiological observations on a possible participation of the amygdalar complex in stress-induced ACTH release (see Palkovits, 1977), were able to clarify the role of the direct amygdalo-hypothalamic

ions between the ventromedial and arcuate nucleus and
ence. This "quasi-segmental" organization of internal
ld have already been *guessed* from early Golgi pictures
al., 1962, Fig. 36), especially from the fact that in-
terminal arborizations always seemed to expand in the
e also Fig. 2 in Szentágothai, 1969). The apparent dis-
n the two architectural principles is resolved easily when
gi information, gained from horizontally oriented section
ered.

lar" Organization Principle of the Hypothalamus

e of using transverse (coronal or frontal) section series in
as been found to present a great disadvantage for gaining
overall connectivity organization in any original part of
it the spinal cord, the medulla, the lower brainstem, or
ll see, the hypothalamus. A recent Golgi study of the rat
Palkovits and van Cuc, in press) based mainly on horizon-
s revealed that a large part of the transversally oriented
the hypothalamus from the medial forebrain bundle are
pers (Figure 12.6B) of this bundle, appearing not at ran-
r numbers at certain sites. The lateral retrochiasmatic area
agraph 6.1 is one of such major concentration of fibers
y; however, here the majority are not collaterals, but the
es. It is not quite clear whether some of the transversal
s, which leave the hypothalamus and upon entering the
n bundle arborize into an ascending and a descending
scription as well as the figures of the Golgi material by
al. (1962) might certainly be interpreted in this way,
pect of the Golgi architecture was not pursued at that time.
ugh much sparser, longitudinal fiber system can be recog-
ntal Golgi sections (Figure 12.6), running immediately
dyma of the third ventricle; this is the periventricular
has a similar relation to the hypothalamic nuclei as the
n bundle. The individual collaterals entering the hypo-
tend to arborize there in the transversal (coronal) plane
bushy terminal arbors confined to relatively small
ntágothai et al., 1962; Szentágothai, 1969), so that it often
se terminals were directed to a single cell by forming

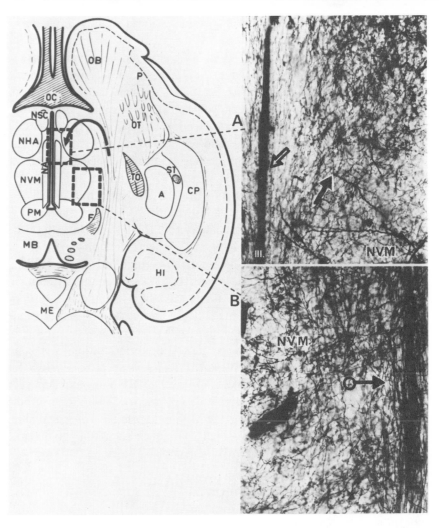

Figure 12.6. Neuronal networks of the hypothalamus. A = anterior hypothalamic, B = middle
hypothalamic levels as indicated on the horizontal drawing of rat forebrain. Golgi impregnation
technique. Axons and collaterals are indicated by arrows: = retrochiasmatic area, NVM = ventromedial nucleus, = periventricular fiber system, = medial forebrain bundle, III = third ventricle.
Other abbreviations as on Figure 12.4.

pathway. (4) The composition of the supraoptic decussation and the
courses and origins of its elements are far from being sufficiently clarified
(Minderhoud, 1967), but cannot be discarded from a possible role in
stress mechanisms. (5) Undoubtedly the most important pathways re-

sponsible for conveying to the hypothalamus neural signals about stressful stimuli are the ascending systems of the MFB. An interruption of the MFB below the level of the RCAL significantly reduces the response to stress by peripheral tissue damage (Feldman, Conforti, and Chowers, 1971). From the various specific ascending systems the noradrenergic pathway (Ungerstedt, 1971; Sachs, Jonsson, and Fuxe, 1973; Björklund et al., 1973) may be of crucial importance for two reasons: (i) it enters the hypothalamus mainly through the said window (Palkovits et al., 1977a); and (ii) its fibers terminate in the surface zone of the median eminence (Björklund et al., 1973; Palkovits et al., 1977b). However, this does not mean in itself that it has to have a direct role in stress mechanisms. There is even less evidence for other ascending aminergic systems (adrenaline, dopamine, serotonin). Most unfortunately, the final common path of the neural chain, the CRF neurons, have still eluded detection.

The most reasonable view of the ascending neural limb of a combined neural-humoral functional chain, connecting tissue damage with an increased release of ACTH, is the assumption of a nonspecific sensory pathway crossing in the level of the spinal cord and being relayed in the lower brainstem (reticular formation) to various specific ascending mechanisms (noradrenergic, cholinergic) or possibly chains. These, in turn, would be conveyed through the MFB and its specific window for stress pathways in the RCAL, eventually to the CRF neurons. This very general concept does not solve the crucial problem of the CRF neurons; however, until direct immunohistochemical evidence becomes available, hypothalamic nuclei like ventromedial, arcuate, or anterior hypothalamic nuclei, even cells located in the MFB, cannot be discarded a priori.

6.2. Intrahypothalamic Connectivity

From the general considerations discussed in sections 1 and 2, it became apparent that the mobilization of the defense of the organism, far from being a monolithic and generalized mechanism, is a highly differentiated complex of numerous interconnected mechanisms involving in one way or another almost the whole endocrine hypothalamus and its related hormonal mechanisms. If so, it would be hopeless to try to separate or to sort out from the ensemble of the hypothalamo-hypophyseal complex any single center or particular neural mechanism that would be responsible for stress mechanisms. On the contrary, what we would have to expect would be an intricate internal connectivity system of the hypothalamus. At-

tempts at understanding the hypothalamu
been made in earlier syntheses (Szentágot
results were rudimentary, owing to the ra
though the technical possibilities have
mainly through the introduction of more
niques, especially on the level of the ele
more advanced experimental procedur
methods of anterograde and retrograde
our understanding of intrahypothalamic
The following account is based mainly
and Makara (1979), taking advantage
both the intact and the chronically iso
avoid misinterpretation by interrupting
running through it), and of degeneratio
as visible under the electron microsco

Besides yielding evidence for the te
of fibers arising from the ventromedia
terior hypothalamic area, the observ
(1979) indicated a very large interr
hypothalamus. The rich intranuclear
nucleus was to be expected after the
ágothai et al. (1962), but the abunda
the preoptic area, suprachiasmatic r
cleus, and the premamillary region,
interconnections between the arcuate
by earlier studies (Halász et al., 197
also be substantiated. Additionally,
fibers to the anterior periventricular
this is not quite certain (for technic
area (Makara, Harris, and Spyer,

As can already be judged from t
ity appears to be built on two seem
quasi-segmental organization, and
along the antero-posterior axis of
organization principle, mainly of
complex, was assumed explicit
local dopaminergic neuron system
well as the recent degeneration
would seem to indicate that this a

all local
the medi
connecti
(Szentág
trahypotl
coronal p
crepancy
some rece
series, is

6.3. The

The usual
Golgi stud
insight int
the neurax
even, as w
hypothalar
tal section
fibers ente
collaterals
dom but in
discussed i
turning med
fibers them
fibers are a
medial fore
branch. The
Szentágotha
although this
A similar, al
nized in hor
below the e
system, whic
medial foreb
thalamic nuc
and may sh
spaces (see S
looks as if t

baskets around their cell bodies. (Recent studies, on Golgi-stained axonal arborizations by reembedding them and analyzing them by electronmicroscopy in thin section series, do not support such subjective impressions given by the Golgi picture.)

If this aspect of Golgi architecture were combined with the degeneration results discussed in paragraph 6.2, the hypothalamus might be viewed in a similar way, as was first done for the lower brainstem reticular formation by Scheibel and Scheibel (1958), and as more recently has become widely used for the spinal cord (see a general discussion and survey of the earlier literature in Szentágothai and Arbib, 1974). Figure

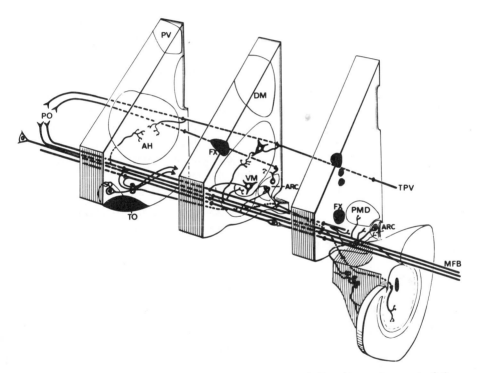

Figure 12.7. Simplified stereodiagram illustrating the "modular" architectural concept of the hypothalamus. The flat coronally oriented slabs cut out from various regions of the left half of the hypothalamus represent the building blocks, discussed in detail in the text. Especially, the interconnections between the arcuate nucleus (ARC), the ventromedial nucleus (VM), and the median eminence are arrayed within the blocks, while the connections between "blocks" and with afferents (and/or efferents) are conveyed by the medial forebrain bundle (MFB) and the periventricular tract (TPV). Capillary loops are indicated, for the sake of simplicity, only in the lower part of the stalk. *Abbr.*: PO = preoptic region; PV = paraventricular nucleus; AH = anterior hypothalamic nucleus; TO = optic tract; FX = fornix; DM = dorsomedial nucleus; PMD = dorsal premamillary nucleus.

12.7 tries to illustrate this architectural principle quite diagrammatically, and, as a very preliminary synthesis, as it could be applied to the hypothalamus. In this view the nuclear substance (''grey matter'') of the hypothalamus could be visualized as being built of quasi-repetitive transversal disclike building blocks, connected among themselves and with afferent (and perhaps also efferent) pathways by the medial forebrain bundle and the periventricular fiber system (corresponding to the ''white matter'' of the spinal cord). The connection of each ''building block'' with the median eminence would then be essentially ''segmental,'' with the difference that, owing to the elongation of the median eminence into the pituitary stalk, many of the descending fibers from both the arcuate and the ventromedial nucleus become ''pulled'' in the caudal direction.

Such a view might seem rather unorthodox and even perhaps provocative for the time being; however, it might explain the great complexity of neuroendocrine regulatory mechanisms. A neural machine of this kind might be able to work like a ''computer,'' receiving all information of the prevailing ''external'' circumstances (including tissue damage or toxic influence), of the momentary functional state of the endocrine systems, and of the whole internal ''tuning'' of the CNS (comprising ongoing higher, i.e., psychic, functions and the traces of earlier experience), and to elaborate a complex function pattern adapted to the total ensemble. Although we would still be very far from understanding the working of such a mechanism, we would have to expect that, for example, under circumstances of stress, most of the various hypothalamo-hypophyseal mechanisms would be mobilized in one way or another.

7. CONCLUDING REMARKS

Considering the various aspects of the neuroendocrine mechanisms involved in the response to stress leads to a radically different picture from the classical concepts of a more or less uniform mechanism centered around an increased release by the pathway of ACTH. Strangely, the identity, site, and mechanism of elaboration of CRF are more obscure than most other aspects of the wide array of changes elicited by the various kinds of stress imposed upon the organism. Whether this obscurity is due primarily to the unknown chemical identity of CRF, and all controversial data will suddenly fall into a clear picture when this information becomes available, or whether other reasons are the decisive ones, remains for clarification by future studies.

References

Ajika, K., Kalra, S. P., Fawcett, C. P., Krulich, L., and McCann, S. M. The effects of stress and nembutal on plasma levels of gonadotropin and prolactin in ovariectomized rats. *Endocrinology 90:* 707–715, 1972.

Alpert, L. C., Brawer, J. R., Patel, Y. C., and Reichlin, S. Somatostatinergic neurons in anterior hypothalamus: Immunohistochemical localization. *Endocrinology 98:* 255–258, 1976.

Ambach, G., and Palkovits, M. Blood supply of the rat hypothalamus. I. Nucleus supraopticus. *Acta morph. Acad. Sci. Hung. 22:* 291–310, 1974.

Ambach, G., and Palkovits, M. Blood supply of the rat hypothalamus. V. The medial hypothalamus (nucleus ventromedialis, nucleus dorsomedialis, nucleus perifornicalis). *Acta morph. Acad. Sci. Hung. 25:* 259–278, 1977.

Ambach, G., Palkovits, M., and Szentágothai, J. Blood supply of the rat hypothalamus. IV. Retrochiasmatic area, median eminence, arcuate nucleus. *Acta morph. Acad. Sci. Hung. 24:* 93–118, 1976.

Arimura, A., Saito, T. M., Bowers, C. Y., and Schally, A. V. Pituitary-adrenal activation in rats with hereditary hypothalamic diabetes insipidus. *Acta Endocrinologica 54:* 155–165, 1967.

Arimura, A., Smith, W. D., and Schally, A. V. Blockade of the stress-induced decrease in blood GH by anti-somatostatin serum in rat. *Endocrinology 98:* 540, 1976.

Baker, B. L., Dermody, W. C., and Reel, J. R. Localization of luteinizing hormone-releasing hormone in the mammalian hypothalamus. *Am. J. Anat. 139:* 129–134, 1974.

Baker, B. L., and Yu, Y. Distribution of growth hormone–release-inhibiting hormone (somatostatin) in the rat brain as observed with immunohistochemistry. *Anat. Rec. 186:* 343–356, 1976.

Baldwin, D. M., Colombo, J. A., and Sawyer, C. H. Plasma prolactin, LH, and corticosterone in rats exposed to a novel environment. *Am. J. Physiol. 226:* 1366–1369, 1974.

Barry, J. Immunofluorescence study of LRF neurons in man. *Cell Tiss. Res. 181:* 1–14, 1977.

Barry, J. Septo-epithalamo-habenular LRF-reactive neurons in monkeys. *Brain Res. 151:* 183–187, 1978.

Barry, J., and Carette, B. Immunofluorescence study of LRF neurons in primates. *Cell Tiss. Res. 164:* 163–178, 1975.

Barry, J., and Dubois, M. P. Immunoreactive neurosecretory pathways in mammals. *Acta Anat. (Basel) 94:* 497–503, 1976.

Barry, J., Dubois, M. P., and Poulain, P. LRF producing cells of the mammalian hypothalamus. *Z. Zellforsch. 146:* 351–366, 1973.

Ben-Jonathan, N., Oliver, C., Weiner, H. J., Mical, R. S., and Porter, J. C. Dopamine in hypophysial portal plasma of the rat during the estrous cycle and throughout pregnancy. *Endocrinology 100:* 452–458, 1977.

Bennett-Clarke, C. A. Immunocytochemical localization of LHRH and SRIF in the rat CNS. *Anat. Rec. 187:* 536, 1977.

Bergland, R. M., and Page, R. B. Can the pituitary secrete directly to the brain? (Affirmative anatomical evidence) *Endocrinology 102:* 1325–1338, 1978.

Björklund, A., Falck, B., Hromek, F., Owman, C., and West, K. A. Identification and terminal distribution of the tubero-hypophyseal monoamine fibre system in the rat by means of stereotaxic and microspectrofluorimetric techniques. *Brain Res. 17:* 1–23, 1970.

Björklund, A., Moore, R. Y., Nobin, A., and Stenevi, U. The organization of tubero-hypophyseal and reticulo-infundibular catecholamine neuron systems in the rat brain. *Brain Res. 51:* 171–191, 1973.

Bodoky, M., and Réthelyi, M. Dendritic arborization and axon trajectory of neurons in the hypothalamic arcuate nucleus of the rat. *Exp. Brain Res. 28:* 543–555, 1977.

Brennan, T. C., Shelton, R. L., and Robertson, G. L. Cited by Robertson. *Clin. Res. 23:* 234A, 1975.

Brownstein, M. J., Arimura, A., Fernandez-Durango, R., Schally, A. V., Palkovits, M., and Kizer, J. S. The effect of hypothalamic deafferentation on somatostatin-like activity in the rat brain. *Endocrinology 100:* 246–249, 1977.

Brownstein, M., Arimura, A., Sato, H., Schally, A. V., and Kizer, J. S. The regional distribution of somatostatin in the rat brain. *Endocrinology 96:* 1456–1461, 1975b.

Brownstein, M., Arimura, A., Schally, A. V., Palkovits, M., and Kizer, J. S. The effect of surgical isolation of the hypothalamus on its luteinizing hormone–releasing hormone content. *Endocrinology 98:* 662–665, 1976a.

Brownstein, M. J., Mroz, E. A., Kizer, J. S., Palkovits, M., and Leeman, S. E. Regional distribution of Substance P in the brain of the rat. *Brain Res. 116:* 299–305, 1976b.

Brownstein, M. J., Palkovits, M., Saavedra, J. M., Bassiri, R. M., and Utiger, R. D. Thyrotropin-releasing hormone in specific nuclei of the brain. *Science 185;* 267–269, 1974.

Brownstein, M., Utiger, R. D., Palkovits, M., and Kizer, J. S. Effect of hypothalamic deafferentation on thyrotropin releasing hormone levels in rat brain. *Proc. Nat. Acad. Sci. USA 72:* 4177–4179, 1975a.

Buckley, J. P. Biochemical and physiological effects of intermittent neurogenic stress. In Nemeth, S. (ed.), *Hormones, Metabolism and Stress. Recent Progress and Perspectives.* Bratislava: Publishing House of the Slovak Academy of Sciences, 1973, pp. 165–177.

Buijs, R. M., Swaab, D. F., Dogterom, J., and van Leeuwen, F. W. Intra- and extrahypothalamic vasopressin and oxytocin pathways in the rat. *Cell Tiss. Res. 186:* 423–433, 1978.

Campbell, G. A., Kurcz, M., Marshall, S., and Meites, J. Effects of starvation in rats on serum levels of follicle stimulating hormone, luteinizing hormone, thyrotropin, growth hormone and prolactin response to LH-releasing hormone and thyrotropin releasing hormone. *Endocrinology 100:* 580–587, 1977.

Chateau, A., Burlet, M., and Boulange, M. Identification of a hypothalamic infundibular system and its relationship with pituitary adrenal function. (Abstr. No. 376.) *XXVII Congress of the IUPS, Paris, 1977.*

Chowers, I., Einat, R., and Feldman, S. Effects of starvation on levels of corticotrophin releasing factor, corticotrophin and plasma corticosterone in rats. *Acta Endocr. 61:* 687–694, 1969.

Collu, R., Jequier, J.-C., Letarte, J., Leboeuf, G., and Ducharme, J. R. Effect of stress and hypothalamic deafferentation on the secretion of growth hormone in the rat. *Neuroendocrinology 11:* 183–190, 1973.

Colombo, J. A., and Sawyer, C. H. Effects of spreading depression on stress-induced changes in plasma prolactin and LH. *Proc. Soc. Exp. Biol. Med. 150:* 211–214, 1975.

Cook, D. M., Allen, J. P., Greer, M. A., and Allen, C. F. Lack of adaptation of ACTH secretion to sequential ether, tourniquet or leg-break stress. *Endocr. Res. Comm. 1:* 347–357, 1974.

Cooper, J. R., Bloom, F. E., and Roth, R. H. *The Biochemical Basis of Neuropharmacology,* third ed. New York: Oxford University Press, 1978.

Cuc, H. van, Léránth, Cs., and Palkovits, M. Light and electron microscopic studies on the medial forebrain bundle in rat. Degenerated nerve elements in the medial hypothalamic nuclei following surgical transections of the medial forebrain bundle. *Brain Res. Bull,* in press.

Cuello, A. C., and Kanazawa, I. The distribution of Substance P immunoreactive fibers in the rat nervous system. *J. Comp. Neurol. 178:* 129–156, 1978.

Dahlström, A., and Fuxe, K. Evidence for the existence of monoamine-containing neurons in the central nervous system. I. Demonstration of monoamines in the cell bodies of brain stem neurons. *Acta Physiol. Scand. 62,* Suppl. 232: 1–55, 1964.

Dallman, M. F., Engeland, W. C., and McBride, M. H. The neural regulation of compensatory adrenal growth. In Krieger, D. T., and Ganong, W. F. (eds.), *ACTH and Related Peptides: Structure, Regulation and Action. Ann. N.Y. Acad. Sci. 297:* 373–392, 1977.

Dallman, M. F., and Jones, M. T. Corticosteroid feedback control of ACTH secretion: Effect of stress-induced corticosterone secretion on subsequent stress responses in the rat. *Endocrinology 92:* 1367–1375, 1973.

Daniels-Severs, A., Goodwin, A., Keil, L. C., and Vernikos-Danellis, J. Effect of chronic crowding and cold on the pituitary-adrenal system: Responsiveness to an acute stimulus during chronic stress. *Pharmacology 9:* 348–356, 1973.

Davidson, J. M., and Feldman, S. Effects of extrahypothalamic dexamethasone implants on the pituitary-adrenal system. *Acta Endocrinol. 55:* 240–245, 1967.

Dessypris, A., Kuoppasalmi, K., and Adlercreutz, H. Plasma cortisol, testosterone, androstenedione and luteinizing hormone (LH) in a non-competitive marathon run. *J. Steroid Biochem. 7:* 33–37, 1976.

Dewhurst, K. E., El Kabir, D. J., Harris, G. W., and Mandelbrote, B. M. A review of the effect of stress on the activity of the central nervous-pituitary-thyroid axis in animals and man. *Confin. Neurol. 30:* 161–196, 1968.

Dierickx, K., Vandesande, F., and DeMey, J. Identification, in the external region of the rat median eminence, of separate neurophysin-vasopressin and neurophysin-oxytocin containing nerve fibers. *Cell Tiss. Res. 168:* 141–151, 1976.

Döhler, K-D., Gärtner, K., Mühlen, A., von Zur, and Döhler, U. Activation of anterior pituitary, thyroid and adrenal gland in rats after disturbance stress. *Acta Endocr. 86:* 489–497, 1977.

Dubé, D., Lissitzky, J. C., Leclerc, R., and Pelletier, G. Localization of α-melanocyte-stimulating hormone in rat brain and pituitary. *Endocrinology 102:* 1283–1291, 1978.

Ducommun, P., Sakiz, E., and Guillemin, R. Lability of plasma TSH levels in the rat in response to nonspecific exteroceptive stimuli. *Proc. Soc. Exp. Biol. 121:* 921–923, 1966.

Duke, J. E., and Smith, G. C. The blood-brain barrier in the hypothalamohypophyseal complex. *J. Anat. (Lond.) 118:* 395–396, 1974.

Dunn, J. D., Arimura, A., and Scheving, L. E. Effects of stress on circadian periodicity in serum LH and prolactin concentration. *Endocrinology 90:* 29–33, 1972.

Dunn, J. D., Schindler, W. J., Hutchins, M. D., Scheving, L. E., and Turpen, C. Daily variation in rat growth hormone concentration and the effect of stress on periodicity. *Neuroendocrinology 13:* 69–78, 1973/74.

Dupont, A., Bastarache, A., Endröczi, E., and Fortier, C. Effect of hippocampal stimulation on the plasma thyrotropin (TSH) and corticosterone responses to acute cold exposure in the rat. *Canad. J. Physiol. Pharmacol. 50:* 364–367, 1972.

Elde, R., Hökfelt, T., Johansson, O., and Terenius, L. Immunohistochemical studies using antibodies to leucine-enkephalin: Initial observations of the nervous system of the rat. *Neurosci. 1:* 349–351, 1976.

Elde, R. P., and Parsons, J. A. Immunocytochemical localization of somatostatin in cell bodies of the rat hypothalamus. *Am. J. Anat. 144:* 541–548, 1975.

Engeland, W. C., Shinsako, J., Winget, C. M., Vernikos-Danellis, J., and Dallman, M. F. Circadian patterns of stress-induced ACTH secretion are modified by corticosterone responses. *Endocrinology 100:* 138–147, 1977.

Enjalbert, A., Priam, M., and Kordon, C. Evidence in favor of the existence of a dopamine-free prolactin-inhibitory factor (PIF) in rat hypothalamic extracts. *Europ. J. Pharmacol. 41:* 243–244, 1977.

Endröczi, E., Lissák, K., Bohus, B., and Kovács, S. The inhibitory influence of archiocortical structures on pituitary-adrenal function. *Acta physiol. Acad. Sci. Hung. 16:* 17–25, 1959.

Epelbaum, J., Brazeau, P., Tsang, D., Brawer, J., and Martin, J. B. Subcellular distribution of radioimmunoassayable somatostatin in rat brain. *Brain Res. 126:* 309–323, 1977.

Euker, J. E., Meites, J., and Riegle, G. D. Effects of acute stress on serum LH and prolactin in intact, castrate and dexamethasone-treated male rats. *Endocrinology 96:* 85–92, 1975.

Feldman, S., Conforti, N., and Chowers, I. The role of the medial forebrain bundle in mediating adrenocortical responses to neurogenic stimuli. *J. Endocr. (Lond.) 51:* 745–749, 1971.

Feldman, S., Conforti, N., Chowers, I., and Davidson, J. M. Differential effects of hypothalamic deafferentation on responses to different stresses. *Israel J. Med. Sci. 4:* 908–910, 1968.

Fenske, M., and Wuttke, W. Development of stress-induced pituitary prolactin and TSH release in male rats. *Acta Endocr. 85:* 729–735, 1977.

Fortier, C. Dual control of adrenocorticotrophin release. *Endocrinology 49:* 782–788, 1951.

Fortier, C. Nervous control of ACTH secretion. In Harris, G. W., and Donovan, B. T. (eds.), *The Pituitary Gland,* Vol. 2: *Anterior Pituitary.* London: Butterworths, 1966, pp. 195–234.

Frenkl, R., Csalay, L., and Csákváry, G. A study of the stress reaction elicited by muscular exertion in trained and untrained man and rats. *Acta physiol. Acad. Sci. Hung. 36:* 365–370, 1969.

Frenkl, R., Csalay, L., Csákváry, G., and Zelles, T. Effect of muscular exertion on the reaction of the pituitary-adrenocortical axis in trained and untrained rats. *Acta physiol. Acad. Sci. Hung. 33:* 435–438, 1968.

Frohman, L. A., Horton, E. S., and Lebovitz, H. E. Growth hormone releasing action of a *Pseudomonas* endotoxin (Piromen). *Metabolism 16:* 57–67, 1967.

Fuxe, K. Evidence for the existence of monoamine neurons in the central nervous system. IV. The distributions of monoamine nerve terminals in the central nervous system. *Acta Physiol. Scand. 64,* Suppl. 247: 39–85, 1965.

Fuxe, K., and Hökfelt, T. Further evidence for the existence of tuberoinfundibular dopamine neurons. *Acta Physiol. Scand. 66:* 245–246, 1966.

Gerendai, I., Kiss, J., Molnár, J., and Halász, B. Further data on the existence of a neural pathway from the adrenal gland to the hypothalamus. *Cell Tiss. Res. 153:* 559–564, 1974.

Green, J. D. The histology of the hypophysial stalk and median eminence in man, with special reference to blood vessels, nerve fibers and a peculiar neurovascular zone in this region. *Anat. Rec. 100:* 273–296, 1948.

Green, J. D. The comparative anatomy of the hypophysis with special reference to its blood supply and innervation. *Am. J. Anat. 88:* 225–311, 1951.

Green, J. D., and Harris, G. W. Observations of the hypophysioportal vessels of the living rat. *J. Physiol. (Lond.) 108:* 359–361, 1949.

Guillemin, R., Ling, N., Lazarus, L., Burgus, R., Minick, S., Bloom, F., Nicoll, R., Siggins, G., and Segal, D. The endorphins, novel peptides of brain and hypophysial origin, with opiate-like activity: Biochemical and biologic studies. *Ann. N.Y. Acad. Sci. 297:* 131–157, 1977.

Halász, B., Köves, K., Réthelyi, M., Bodoky, M., and Koritsánszky, S. Recent data on neuronal connections between nervous structures involved in the control of the adenohypophysis. In Stumpf, W. E., and Grant, L. D. (eds.), *Anatomical Neuroendocrinology.* Basel-München-Paris-London-New York-Sydney: S. Karger, 1975, pp. 9–14.

Halász, B., and Pupp, L. Hormone secretion of the anterior pituitary gland after physical interruption of all nervous pathways to the hypophysiotrophic area. *Endocrinology 77:* 553–562, 1965.

Halász, B., Pupp, L., and Uhlarik, S. Hypophysiotrophic area in the hypothalamus. *J. Endocr. (Lond.) 25:* 147–154, 1962.

Halász, B., Slusher, M., and Gorski, R. A. Adrenocorticotrophic hormone secretion in rats after partial or total deafferentation of the medial basal hypothalamus. *Neuroendocrinology 2:* 43–55, 1967.

Halász, B., and Szentágothai, J. Histologischer Beweis einer nervösen Signalübermittlung von der Nebennierenrinde zum Hypothalamus. *Z. Zellforsch. 50:* 297–306, 1959.

Harris, A. R. C., Christianson, D., Smith, M. S., Fang, S.-L., Braverman, L. E., and Vagenakis, A. G. The physiological role of thyrotropin-releasing hormone in the regulation of thyroid-stimulating hormone and prolactin secretion in the rat. *J. Clin. Invest. 61:* 441–448, 1978.

Harris, G. W. The blood vessels of the rabbits pituitary gland and the significance of the pars and zona tuberalis. *J. Anat. (Lond.) 81:* 343–351, 1947.

Hodges, J. R., and Jones, M. T. The effect of injected corticosterone on the release of adrenocorticotrophic hormone in rats exposed to acute stress. *J. Physiol. (Lond.) 167:* 30-37, 1963.

Hoffman, G. E. Immunogenecity of gonadotropin releasing factors in mammalian neurons. *Anat. Rec. 187:* 606, 1977.

Hoffman, G. E., Joseph, S. A., and Knigge, K. M. Evidence for two different fields of gonadotropin releasing factor (GnRF) neurons in mouse and rat brain. *Endocrinology 100,* Suppl. 18: 65, 1977.

Hoffman, G. E., Knigge, K. M., Moynihan, J. A., Melnyk, V., and Arimura, A. Neuronal fields containing luteinizing hormone releasing hormone (LHRH) in mouse brain. *Neuroscience 3:* 219-231, 1978a.

Hoffman, G. E., Melnyk, V., Hayes, T., Bennett-Clarke, C., and Fowler, E. Immunocytology of LHRH neurons. In Scott, D. E., Kozlowski, G. P., and Weindl, A. (eds.), *Brain-Endocrine Interaction. III. Neural Hormones and Reproduction.* Basel: Karger, 1978b, pp. 67-82.

Hökfelt, T., Efendić, S., Hellerström, C., Johansson, O., Luft, R., and Arimura, A. Cellular localization of somatostatin in endocrine-like cells and neurons of the rat with special reference to the A1 cells of the pancreatic islets and to the hypothalamus. *Acta Endocrin. (KBH.) 200,* Suppl.: 1-41, 1975a.

Hökfelt, T., Efencić, S., Johansson, O., Luft, R., and Arimura, A. Immunohistochemical localization of somatostatin (growth hormone-release inhibiting factor) in the guinea pig brain. *Brain Res. 80:* 165-169, 1974.

Höfelt, T., Elde, R., Johansson, O., Terenius, L., and Stein, L. The distribution of enkephalin immunoreactive cell bodies in the rat central nervous system. *Neurosci. Lett. 5:* 25-31, 1977.

Hökfelt, T., Fuxe, K., Johansson, O., Jeffcoate, S., and White, N. Distribution of thyrotropin-releasing hormone (TRH) in the central nervous system as revealed with immunocytochemistry. *Eur. J. Pharmacol. 34:* 389-392, 1975b.

Hökfelt, T., Fuxe, K., Johansson, O., Jeffcoate, S., and White, N. Thyrotropin releasing hormone (TRH)-containing nerve terminals in certain brain stem nuclei and in the spinal cord. *Neurosci. Lett. 1:* 133-139, 1976.

Hökfelt, T., Kellerth, J. O., Milsson, G., and Pernow, B. Substance P: Localization in the central nervous system and in some primary sensory neurons. *Science 190:* 889-890, 1975c.

Hökfelt, T., Pernow, B., Nilsson, G., Wetterberg, L., Goldstein, M., and Jeffcoate, S. L. Dense plexus of Substance P immunoreactive nerve terminals in eminentia medialis of the primate hypothalamus. *Proc. Nat. Acad. Sci. USA 75:* 1013-1015, 1978.

Hong, J. S., Yang, H.-Y., Fratta, W., and Costa, E. Determination of methionine enkephalin in discrete regions of rat brain. *Brain Res. 134:* 383-386, 1977.

Hunter, W. M., and Greenwood, F. C. Studies on the secretion of human pituitary growth hormone. *Brit. Med. J. 5386:* 804, 1964.

Jackson, I. M., and Reichlin, S. Thyrotropin releasing hormone (TRH) distribution in the brain, blood and urine of the rat. *Life Sci. 14:* 2259-2266, 1974a.

Jackson, I. M. D., and Reichlin, S. Thyrotropin releasing hormone (TRH): Distribution in hypothalamic and extrahypothalamic brain tissues of mammalian and submammalian chordates. *Endocrinology 95:* 854-862, 1974b.

Jones, M. T., and Hillhouse, E. W. Structure-activity relationship and the mode of action of corticosteroid feedback on the secretion of corticotrophin-releasing factor. *J. Steroid Biochem. 7:* 1189–1202, 1976.

Jones, M. T., Hillhouse, E. W., and Burden, J. L. Secretion of corticotropin-releasing hormone *in vitro*. In Martini, L., and Ganong, W. F. (eds.), *Frontiers of Neuroendocrinology*, Vol. 4. New York: Raven Press, 1976.

Kawakami, M., Seto, K., and Kimura, F. Influence of repeated immobilization stress upon the circadian rhythmicity of adrenocorticoid biosynthesis. *Neuroendocrinology 9:* 207–214, 1972.

Keil, L. C., and Severs, W. B. Reduction in plasma vasopressin levels of dehydrated rats following acute stress. *Endocrinology 100:* 30–38, 1977.

Kendall, J. W., Tang, L., and Cook, D. M. Sites of feedback control in the pituitary-adrenocortical system. In Stumpf, W. E., and Grant, L. D. (eds.), *Anatomical Neuroendocrinology*. Basel: Karger, 1975, pp. 276–283.

King, J. C., Gerall, A. A., Fishback, J. B., Elkind, K. E., and Arimura, A. Growth hormone–release inhibiting hormone (GH–RIH) pathway of the rat hypothalamus revealed by the unlabeled antibody peroxidase-antiperoxidase method. *Cell Tiss. Res. 160:* 423–430, 1975.

King, J. C., Parsons, J. A., Erlandsen, S. L., and Williams, T. A. Luteinizing hormone-releasing hormone (LH-RH) pathway of the rat hypothalamus revealed by the unlabeled antibody peroxidase-antiperoxidase method. *Cell Tiss. Res. 153:* 211–217, 1974.

Kizer, J. S., Palkovits, M., and Brownstein, M. J. Releasing factors in the circumventricular organs of the rat brain. *Endocrinology 98:* 311–317, 1976.

Knigge, K. M. Adrenocortical response to stress in rats with lesions in hippocampus or amygdala. *Proc. Soc. Exp. Biol. Med. 108:* 18–21, 1961.

Knigge, K. M., and Hays, M.: Evidence of inhibitive role of hippocampus in neural regulation of ACTH release. *Proc. Soc. Exp. Biol. Med. 114:* 67–69, 1963.

Kobayashi, R. M., Brown, M., and Vale, W. Regional distribution of neurotensin and somatostatin in rat brain. *Brain Res. 126:* 584–588, 1977.

Kobayashi, R. M., Palkovits, M., Miller, R. J., Chang, K.-J., and Cuatrecasas, P. Distribution of enkephalin in the brain is unaltered by hypophysectomy. *Life Sci. 22:* 527–530, 1978.

Koch, Y., Goldhaber, G., Fireman, I., Zor, U., Shani, J., and Tal, E. Suppression of prolactin and thyrotropin secretion in the rat by antiserum to thyrotropin-releasing hormone. *Endocrinology 100:* 1476–1478, 1977.

Kohler, P. O., O'Malley, B. W., Rayford, P. L., Lipsett, M. B., and Odell, W. D. Effect of pyrogen on blood levels of pituitary trophic hormones. Observations on the usefulness of the growth hormone response in the detection of pituitary disease. *J. Clin. Endocr. 27:* 219–226, 1967.

Kordon, C., Kerdelhué, B., Pattou, E., and Jutisz, M.: Immunocytochemical localization of LHRH in axons and nerve terminals of the rat median eminence. *Proc. Soc. Exp. Biol. Med. 147:* 122–127, 1974.

Kraicer, J., and Logothetopoulos, J. Adrenal cortical response to insulin-induced hypoglycaemia in the rat. I. Adaptation to repeated daily injections of protamine zinc insulin. *Acta Endocrin. (Kbh.) 44:* 259–271, 1963.

Krieg, W. S. The hypothalamus of the albino rat. *J. Comp. Neurol. 55:* 19–89, 1932.

Krieger, D. T., Kiotta, A., and Brownstein, M. J. Corticotropin releasing factor distribution in normal and Brattleboro rat brain, and effect of deafferentation, hypophysectomy and steroid treatment in normal animals. *Endocrinology 100:* 227–237, 1977a.

Krieger, D. T., Liotta, A., Suda, T., Palkovits, M., and Brownstein, M. J. Presence of immunoassayable β-lipotropin in bovine brain and spinal cord: Lack of concordance with ACTH concentrations. *Biochem. Biophys. Res. Commun. 76:* 930–936, 1977b.

Krulich, L., Hefco, E., and Aschenbrenner, J. E. Mechanism of the effects of hypothalamic deafferentation in prolactin secretion in the rat. *Endocrinology 96:* 107–118, 1975.

Krulich, L., Hefco, E., Illner, P., and Read, C. B. The effects of acute stress on the secretion of LH, FSH, prolactin and GH in the normal male rat, with comments on their statistical evaluation. *Neuroendocrinology 16:* 292–311, 1974.

Krulich, L., Quijada, M., and Illner, P. Localization of prolactin-inhibiting hormone (PIF), prolactin-releasing factor (PRF), growth hormone releasing factor (GRF), and GIF activities in the hypothalamus of the rat. (Abstr. 82.) *Program 53rd Meeting Endocrine Soc.,* 1971.

Krulich, L., Quijada, M., Wheaton, J. E., Illner, P., and McCann, S. M. Localization of hypophysiotrophic neurohormones by assay of sections from various brain areas. *Fed. Proc. 36:* 1953–1959, 1977.

Kuoppasalmi, K., Näveri, H., Rehunen, S., Harköknen, M., and Adlercreutz, H. Effect of strenous anaerobic running exercise on plasma growth hormone, cortisol, luteinizing hormone, testosterone, adrostenedione, estrone and estradiol. *J. Steroid Biochem. 7:* 823–829, 1976.

Lang, R. E., Voight, K.-H., Fehm, H. L., and Pfeiffer, E. F. Localization of croticotropin-releasing activity in the rat hypothalamus. *Neurosci. Lett. 2:* 19–20, 1976.

Leonard, C. M., and Scott, J. W. Origin and distribution of the amygdalofugal pathways in the rat: An experimental-neuroanatomical study. *J. Comp. Neurol. 141:* 313–330, 1971.

Leonardelli, J., Barry, J., and Dubois, M.-P. Mise en évidence par immunofluoroscence d'un constituant immunologiquement apparenté au LH–RF dans l'hypothalamus et l'éminence mediane chez les Mammifères. *C.R. Acad. Sci. [D] (Paris) 276:* 2043–2046, 1973.

Libertun, C., and McCann, S. M. The possible role of histamine in the control of prolactin and gonadotropin release. *Neuroendocrinology 20:* 110–120, 1976.

Lutz-Bucher, B., Koch, B., and Mialhe, C. Comparative *in vitro* studies on corticotropin releasing activity of vasopressin and hypothalamic median eminence extract. *Neuroendocrinology 23:* 181–192, 1977.

Lymangrover, J. R., and Brodish, A. Tissue-CRF: An extrahypothalamic corticotrophin releasing factor (CRF) in the peripheral blood of stressed rats. *Neuroendocinology 12:* 225–235, 1973.

MacLeod, R. M. Regulation of prolactin secretion. In Martini, L., Ganong, W. F. (eds.), *Frontiers in Neuroendocrinology,* Vol. 4. New York: Raven Press, 1976, pp. 169–194.

Makara, G. B., Harris, M. C., and Spyer, K. M. Identification and distribution of tubero-infundibular neurones. *Brain Res. 40:* 283–290, 1972.

Makara, G. B., and Hodács, L. Rostral projections from the hypothalamic arcuate nucleus. *Brain Res. 84:* 23–29, 1975.

Makara, G. B., Stark, E., and Mészáros, T. Corticotrophin release induced by *E. coli* endotoxin after removal of the medial hypothalamus. *Endocrinology 88:* 412–414, 1971.

Makara, G. B., Stark, E., and Palkovits, M. Afferent pathways of stressful stimuli: Corticotrophin release after hypothalamic deafferentation. *J. Endocrin. 47:* 411–416, 1970.

Makara, G. B., Stark, E., and Palkovits, M. ACTH release after tuberal electrical stimulation in rats with various cuts around the medial basal hypothalamus. *Neuroendocrinology, 27:* 109–118, 1978.

Makara, G. B., Stark, E., and Palkovits, M. Reevaluation of the pituitary-adrenal response to ether in rats with various cuts around the medial basal hypothalamus. *Neuroendocrinology,* in press/b.

Makara, G. B., Stark, E., Palkovits, M., Révész, T., and Mihály, K. Afferent pathways of stressful stimuli: Corticotrophin release after partial deafferentation of the medial basal hypothalamus. *J. Endocr. 44:* 187–193, 1969.

Makara, G. B., Stark, E., Rappay, G., Karteszi, M., and Palkovits, M. Changes in ACTH releasing factor (CRF) of the stalk–median eminence in rats with various cuts around the medial basal hypothalamus. *J. Endocr.,* in press/c.

Mandell, A. J., Chapman, L. F., Rand, R. W., and Walter, R. D. Plasma corticosteroids: Changes in concentration after stimulation of hippocampus and amygdala. *Science 139:* 1212, 1963.

Mannistö, P. T., Saarinen, A., and Ranta, T. Anesthetics and thyrotropin secretion in the rat. *Endocrinology 99:* 875–880, 1976.

Martin, J. B. Plasma growth hormone (GH) response to hypothalamic or extrahypothalamic electrical stimulation. *Endocrinology 91:* 107–115, 1972.

Martin, J. B. Brain regulation of growth hormone secretion. In Martini, L., and Ganong, W. F. (eds.), *Frontiers in Neuroendocrinology,* Vol. 4. New York: Raven Press, 1976, p. 129.

McCann, S. M., Ajika, K., Fawcett, C. P., Hefco, E., Illner, P., Negro-Vilar, A., Orias, R., Watson, J. T., and Krulich, L. Hypothalamic control of the adenohypophyseal response to stress by releasing and inhibitory neurohormones. In Németh, S. (ed.), *Hormones, Metabolism and Stress. Recent Progress and Perspectives.* Bratislava: Publishing House of the Slovak Academy of Sciences, 1973, pp. 67–78.

McCann, S. M., Antunes-Rodriguez, J., Naller, R., and Valtiny, H. Pituitary-adrenal function in the absence of vasopressin. *Endocrinology 79:* 1058–1064, 1966.

Meites, J., Lu, K. H., Wuttke, W., Welsch, C. W., Nagasawa, H., and Quadri, S. K. Recent studies on functions and control of prolactin secretion in rats. *Recent Progr. Horm. Res. 28:* 471–516, 1972.

Meyer, V., and Knobil, E. Growth hormone secretion in the unanesthetized Rhesus monkey in response to noxious stimuli. *Endocrinology 80:* 163–171, 1967.

Mezey, É., Palkovits, M., de Kloet, E. R., Verhoef, J., and de Wied, D. Evidence for pituitary-brain transport of a behaviorally potent ACTH analog. *Life Sci. 22:* 831–838, 1978.

Mikulaj, L., Mitro, A., Murgaš, K., and Dobraková, M. Adrenocortical activity during and after stress with respect to adaptation. In Németh, S. (ed.), *Hormones, Metabolism and Stress. Recent Progress and Perspectives.* Bratislava: Publishing House of the Slovak Academy of Sciences, 1973, pp. 115–128.

Minderhoud, J. M. Observations on the supraoptic decussations in the albino rat. *J. Comp. Neurol. 129:* 297–312, 1967.

Mitchell, J. A., Hutchins, M., Schindler, W. J., and Critchlow, V. Increases in plasma growth hormone concentration and naso-anal length in rats following isolation of the medial basal hypothalamus. *Neuroendocrinology 12:* 161–173, 1973.

Morishige, W. K., and Rotchild, I. A paradoxical inhibiting effect of ether on prolactin release in the rat: Comparison with effect of ether on LH and FSH. *Neuroendocrinology 16:* 95–107, 1974.

Muller, E. E. Nervous control of growth hormone secretion. *Neuroendocrinology 11:* 338–369, 1973.

Nagy, I., Do, N. T., Maderspach, K., and Kurcz, M. Pituitary somatotropin and prolactin content after repeated stress effect. (Abstr.) *Acta physiol. Acad. Sci. Hung. 39:* 209, 1971.

Nagy, I., Kurcz, M., Halmy, L., Mosonyi, L., Baranyai, P., and Kiss, Cs. Effect of stress, drugs, and hypothalamic extract on anterior pituitary somatotropin content in the rat. *Acta physiol. Acad. Sci. Hung. 38:* 357–370, 1970a.

Nagy, I., Kurcz, M., Kiss, Cs., Baranyai, P., Mosonyi, L., and Halmi, L. The effect of suckling, stress and drugs on pituitary prolactin content in the rat. *Acta physiol. Acad. Sci. Hung. 38:* 371–380, 1970b.

Neill, J. D. Effect of stress on serum prolactin and luteinizing hormone levels during the estrous cycle of the rat. *Endocrinology 87:* 1192–1197, 1970.

Oliver, C., Eskay, N. L., Ben-Jonathan, N., and Porter, J. C. Distribution and concentration of TRH in the rat brain. *Endocrinology 95:* 540–546, 1974.

Oliver, C., Mical, R. S., and Porter, J. C. Hypothalamic-pituitary vasculature: Evidence for retrograde blood flow in the pituitary stalk. *Endocrinology 101:* 598–604, 1977.

Oliver, C., and Porter, J. C. Distribution and characterization of α-melanocyte-stimulating hormone in the rat brain. *Endocrinology 102:* 697–705, 1978.

Page, R. B., and Bergland, R. M. The neurohypophyseal capillary bed. I. Anatomy and arterial supply. *Am. J. Anat. 148:* 345–358, 1977.

Palkovits, M. Neural pathways involved in ACTH regulation. In Krieger, D. T., and Ganong, W. F. (eds.), *ACTH and Related Peptides, Structure, Regulation and Action. Ann. N.Y. Acad. Sci. 297:* 455–476, 1977.

Palkovits, M., Arimura, A., Brownstein, M., Schally, A. V., and Saavedra, J. M. Luteinizing hormone–releasing hormone (LH–RH) content of the hypothalamic nuclei in rat. *Endocrinology 96:* 554–558, 1974.

Palkovits, M., Brownstein, M., Arimura, A., Sato, H., Schally, A. V., and Kizer, J. S. Somatostatin content of the hypothalamic ventromedial and arcuate nuclei and the circumventricular organs in the rat. *Brain Res. 109:* 430–434, 1976a.

Palkovits, M., Brownstein, M., and Kizer, J. S. Effect of total hypothalamic deafferentation on releasing hormone and neurotransmitter concentrations of the mediobasal hypothalamus in rat. In Endröczi, E. (ed.), *International Symposium on Cellular and Molecular Bases of Neuroendocrine Processes.* Budapest: Academic Press, 1976b, pp. 575–599.

Palkovits, M., and Cuc, H. van. Axons, axoncollaterals and neuronal network in the rat hypothalamus. A Golgi study. *Brain Res. Bull.,* in press.

Palkovits, M., Fekete, M., Makara, G. B., and Herman, J. P. Total and partial hypothalamic deafferentation for topographical identification of catecholaminergic innervations of certain preoptic and hypothalamic nuclei. *Brain Res. 127:* 127–136, 1977a.

Palkovits, M., Léránth, Cs., Záborszky, L., and Brownstein, M. J. Electron microscopic evidence of direct neuronal connections from the lower brain stem to the median eminence. *Brain Res. 136:* 339–344, 1977b.

Palkovits, M., Makara, G. B., and Stark, E. Hypothalamic region and pathways responsible for adrenocortical response to surgical stress in rats. *Neuroendocrinology 21:* 280–288, 1976c.

Palkovits, M., Mezey, É., Ambach, G., and Kivovics, P. Neural and vascular connections between the organum vasculosum laminae terminalis and preoptic nuclei. In Scott, D. E., Kozlowski, G. P., and Weindl, A. (eds.), *Brain-Endocrine Interaction. III. Neural Hormones and Reproduction.* Basel: Karger, 1978, pp. 302–313. 313.

Palkovits, M., and Záborszky, L. Neural connections of the hypothalamus. In Morgane, P. J., and Panksepp, J. (eds.), *Handbook of the Hypothalamus,* Chapter 16. New York: M. Dekker, in press.

Pollard, I., Bassett, J. R., and Cairncross, K. D. Plasma glucocorticoid elevation and ultrastructural changes in the adenohypophysis of the male rat, following prolonged exposure to stress. *Neuroendocrinology 21:* 312–330, 1976.

Redding, T. W., and Schally, A. V. The purification of a growth hormone–releasing factor from porcine hypothalamic tissue. *Endocrinology 100:* A350, 1977.

Réthelyi, M., and Halász, B. Origin of the nerve endings in the surface zone of the median eminence of the rat hypothalamus. *Exp. Brain Res. 11:* 145–158, 1970.

Rice, R. W., and Critchlow, V. Extrahypothalamic control of stress-induced inhibition of growth hormone secretion in the rat. *Endocrinology 99:* 970–976, 1976.

Riegle, G. D. Chronic stress effects on adrenocortical responsiveness in young and aged rats. *Neuroendocrinology 11:* 1–10, 1973.

Riegle, G. D., and Meites, J. Effects of aging on LH and prolactin after LHRH, L-dopa, methyl-dopa and stress in male rats. *Proc. Soc. Exp. Biol. Med. 151:* 507–511, 1976a.

Riegle, G. D., and Meites, J. The effect of stress on serum prolactin in the female rat. *Proc. Soc. Exp. Biol. Med. 152:* 441, 1976b.

Robertson, G. L. The regulation of vasopressin function in health and disease. *Recent Progr. Hormone Res. 33:* 333–374, 1977.

Rossier, J., Vargo, T. M., Minick, S., Ling, N. Bloom, F. E., and Guillemin, R. Regional dissociation of β-endorphin and enkephalin contents in rat brain and pituitary. *Proc. Nat. Acad. Sci. USA 74:* 5162–5165, 1977.

Roth, J., Glick, S. M., Yalow, R. S., and Berson, S. A. Secretion of growth hormone: Physiologic and experimental modification. *Metabolism 12:* 577–579, 1963.

Sachs, C., Jonsson, G., and Fuxe, K. Mapping of central noradrenaline pathways with 6-hydroxy-DOPA. *Brain Res. 63:* 249–261, 1973.

Saffran, M., and Schally, A. V. Corticotropin-releasing factor: Isolation and chemical properties. *Ann. N.Y. Acad. Sci. 297:* 395–404, 1977a.

Saffran, M., and Schally, A. V.: The status of the corticotropin releasing factor (CRF). *Neuroendocrinology 24:* 359–375, 1977b.

Sakellaris, P. C., and Vernikos-Danellis, J. Increased rate of response of the pituitary-adrenal system in rats adapted to chronic stress. *Endocrinology 97:* 597–602, 1975.

Sayers, A., and Sayers, M. A. Regulation of pituitary adrenocorticotrophic activity during the response of the rat to acute stress. *Endocrinology 40:* 265–273, 1947.

Schalch, D. S. The influence of physical stress and exercise on growth hormone and insulin secretion in man. *J. Lab. Clin. Med. 69:* 256–269, 1967.

Schalch, D. S., and Reichlin, S. Plasma growth hormone concentration in the rat determined by radioimmunoassay. Influence of sex, pregnancy, lactation, anesthesia, hypophysectomy and extrasellar pituitary transplants. *Endocrinology 79:* 275–280, 1966.

Schally, A. V., and Bowers, C. Y. Corticotropin-releasing factor and other hypothalamic peptides. *Metabolism 13:* 1190–1205, 1964.

Schally, A. V., Lipscomb, H. S., and Guillemin, R. Isolation and amino acid sequence of α_2-corticotropin-releasing factor (α_2-CRF) from hog pituitary glands. *Endocrinology 71:* 164–173, 1962.

Scheibel, M. E., and Scheibel, A. B. Structural substrates for integrative patterns in the brain stem reticular core. In Jasper, H. H., Proctor, L. D., Knighton, R. S., Noshay, W. C., and Costello, R. T. (eds.), *Reticular Formation of the Brain.* Boston, Toronto: Little, Brown and Co., 1958, pp. 33–68.

Selye, H. A syndrome produced by diverse nocuous agents. *Nature 138:* 32, 1936.

Selye, H. The general adaptation syndrome and the diseases of adaptation. *J. Clin. Endocr. 6:* 117–230, 1946.

Selye, H. *Stress. The Physiology and Pathology of Exposure to Systemic Stress.* Montreal: Acta Inc., 1950.

Selye, H., and Heuser, G. *Fifth Annual Report on Stress,* Montreal: Acta Inc., 1956.

Sétáló, G. Anatomy, using new histologic techniques. In *Endocrinology,* Vol. 1. Amsterdam: Excerpta Medica, 100–104, 1976.

Sétáló, G., Vigh, S., Hagino, N., and Flerkó, B. Immunohistological observations on the "hypophysiotrophic area" of the hypothalamus. *Acta morph. Acad. Sci. Hung. 24:* 79–91, 1976a.

Sétáló, G., Vigh, S., Schally, A. V., Arimura, A., and Flerkó, B. Immunohistological investigations on the LH-RH-synthetizing neuron system of the rat. In Endröczy, E. (ed.), *Cellular and Molecular Bases of Neuroendocrine Processes.* Budapest: Akadémiai Kiadó, 1975a, pp. 77–88.

Sétáló, G., Vigh, S., Schally, A. V., Arimura, A., and Flerkó, B. LH–RH containing neural elements in the rat hypothalamus. *Endocrinology 96:* 135–142, 1975b.

Sétáló, G., Vigh, S., Schally, A. V., Arimura, A., and Flerkö, B. GH-RIH-containing neural elements in the rat hypothalamus. *Brain Res. 90:* 352–356, 1975c.

Sétáló, G., Vigh, S., Schally, A. V., Arimura, A., and Flerkó, B. Immunohistological study of the origin of LH–RH containing nerve fibres of the rat hypothalamus. *Brain Res. 103:* 597–602, 1976b.

Silverman, A. J. Distribution of luteinizing hormone–releasing hormone (LHRH) in the guinea pig brain. *Endocrinology 99:* 30–41, 1976.

Silverman, A. J., and Zimmerman, E. A. Ultrastructural immunocytochemical localization of neurophysin and vasopressin in the median eminence and posterior pituitary of the guinea pig. *Cell Tiss. Res. 159:* 291–301, 1975.

Simantov, R., Kuhar, M. J., Pasternak, G. W., and Snyder, S. H. The regional distribution of a morphine-like factor enkephalin in monkey brain. *Brain Res. 106:* 189–197, 1976.

Simantov, R., Kuhar, M. J., Uhl, G. R., and Snyder, S. H. Opioid peptide enkephalin: Immunohistochemical mapping in the rat central nervous system. *Proc. Nat. Acad. Sci. USA 74:* 2167–2171, 1977.

Smelik, P. G. Relation between blood level of corticoids and their inhibiting effect on the hypophyseal stress response. *Proc. Soc. Exp. Biol. Med. 113:* 616–619, 1963.

Smelik, P. G., Gaarenstroom, J. H., Konynendyk, W., and de Wied, D. Evaluation of the role of the posterior lobe of the hypophysis in the reflex secretion of corticotrophin. *Acta Physiol. Pharmacol. Neerl. 11:* 295, 1962.

Sowers, J. R., Raj, R. P., Hershman, J. M., Carlson, H. E., and McCallum, R. W. The effect of stressful diagnostic studies and surgery on anterior pituitary hormone release in man. *Acta Endocrinol. (Kbh.) 86:* 25, 1977.

Stark, E., and Fachet, J. Effect of blood corticosteroid levels on ACTH release caused by stress. *Acta med. Acad. Sci. Hung. 9:* 366–370, 1963.

Stark, E., Fachet, J., Makara, G. B., and Mihály, K. An attempt to explain differences in the hypophyseal-adrenocortical response to repeated stressful stimuli by their dependence on differences in pathways. *Acta med. Acad. Sci. Hung. 25:* 251–260, 1968.

Stark, E., Fachet, J., and Mihály, K. Untersuchung der Nebennierenrindenfunktion nach Wiederholung eines aspezifischen Reizes. *Endokrinologie 49:* 29–35, 1965.

Stark, E., Makara, G. B., Marton, J., and Palkovits, M. ACTH release in rats after removal of the medial hypothalamus. *Neuroendocrinology 13:* 224–233, 1973/74.

Strosser, M. T., Bucher, B., Briaud, B., Lutz, B., Koch, B., and Mialhe, C. Effet de la chaleur sur la secretion de l'hormone de croissance et sur l'activité du cortex surrénalien du rat. *J. Physiol. (Paris) 68:* 181–191 (1974.

Szentágothai, J. The parvicellular neurosecretory system. *Progr. Brain Res. 5:* 135–146, 1964.

Szentágothai, J. The synaptic architecture of the hypothalamo-hypophyseal neuron system. *Acta Neurol. Belg. 69:* 453–468, 1969.

Szentágothai, J., and Arbib, M. A. Conceptual models of neural organization. *Neurosciences Research Program Bulletin, 12:* 305–510, 1974.

Szentágothai, J., Flerkó, B., Mess, B., and Halász, B. *Hypothalamic Control of the Anterior Pituitary,* 1st ed. Budapest: Publishing House of the Hungarian Academy of Sciences, 1962.

Szentágothai, J., Flerkó, B., Mess, B., and Halász, B. *Hypothalamic Control of the Anterior Pituitary,* 2nd ed. Budapest: Publishing House of the Hungarian Academy of Sciences, 1965.

Szentágothai, J., Flerkó, B., Mess, B., and Halász, B. *Hypothalamic Control of the Anterior Pituitary,* 3rd ed. Budapest: Publishing House of the Hungarian Academy of Sciences, 1968.

Taché, Y., du Ruisseau, P., Taché, J., Selye, H., and Collu, R. Shift in adenohypophyseal activity during chronic intermittent immobilization of rats. *Neuroendocrinology 22:* 325–336, 1976.

Takeuchi, A., Kajihara, A., and Suzuki, M. Effect of acute exposure to cold on the levels of corticosterone and pituitary hormones in plasma collected from free conscious cannulated rats. *Endocrinol. Japon. 24:* 109–114, 1977.

Terry, L. C., Willoughby, J. O., Brazeau, P., Martin, J. B., and Patel, Y. Antiserum to somatostatin prevents stress-induced inhibition of growth hormone secretion in the rat. *Science 192:* 565–567, 1976.

Turpen, C., Johnson, D. C., and Dunn, J. D. Stress-induced gonadotropin and prolactin secretory patterns. *Neuroendocrinology 20:* 339–351, 1976.

Uhl, G. R., Kuhar, M. J., and Snyder, J. H. Neurotensin: Immunohistochemical localization in rat central nervous system. *Proc. Nat. Acad. Sci. USA 74:* 4059–4063, 1977.

Uhl, G. R., and Snyder, S. H. Regional and subcellular distributions of brain neurotensin. *Life Sci. 19:* 1827–1832, 1976.

Ungerstedt, U. Stereotaxic mapping of the monoamine pathways in the rat brain. *Acta Physiol. Scand. 82,* Suppl. 367: 1–48, 1971.

Vandesande, F., and Dierickx, K. Identification of the vasopressin producing and of the oxytocin producing neurons in the hypothalamic magnocellular nerusecretory system of the rat. *Cell Tiss. Res. 164:* 153–162, 1975.

Vandesande, F., Dierickx, K., and DeMey, J. Identification of the vasopressin-neurophysin II and the oxytocin-neurophysin I producing neurons in the bovine hypothalamus. *Cell Tiss. Res. 156:* 189–200, 1975a.

Vandesande, F., Dierickx, K., and DeMey, J. Identification of vasopressin-neurophysin neurons of the rat suprachiasmatic nuclei. *Cell Tiss. Res. 156:* 377–380, 1975b.

Vecsei, P. Verhalten des Corticosterongehaltes im peripheren Blut weisser Ratten nach Formolbehandlung. *Endokrinologie 42:* 154–157, 1962.

Vernikos-Danellis, J. Estimation of corticotropin-releasing activity of rat hypothalamus and neurohypophysis before and after stress. *Endocrinology 75:* 514–520, 1964.

Vernikos-Danellis, J. Effect of stress, adrenalectomy, hypophysectomy and hydrocortisone onthe corticotropin-releasing activity of rat median eminence. *Endocrinology 76:* 122–126, 1965.

Voloschin, L., Joseph, S. A., and Knigge, K. M. Endocrine function in male rats following complete and partial isolations of the hypothalamo-pituitary unit. *Neuroendocrinology 3:* 387–397, 1968.

Wakabayashi, H., Arimura, A., and Schally, V. Effect of pentobarbital and ether stress on serum prolactin levels in rats. *Proc. Soc. Exp. Biol. Med. 137:* 1181–1193, 1971.

Weiner, R. I., Pattou, E., Kerdelhué, B., and Kordon, C. Differential effects of hypothalamic deafferentation upon luteinizing hormone–releasing hormone in the median eminence and organum vasculosum of the laminae terminalis. *Endocrinology 97:* 1597–1600, 1975.

Wheaton, J. E., Krulich, L., and McCann, S. M. Localization of luteinizing hormone–releasing hormone in the preoptic area and hypothalamus of the rat using radioimmunoassay. *Endocrinology 97:* 30–38, 1975.

Winokur, A., and Utiger, R. D. Thyrotropin-releasing hormone: Regional distribution in rat brain. *Science 185:* 265–267, 1974.

Wislocki, G. B., and King, L. S. The permeability of the hypophysis and hypothalamus to vital dyes; with a study of the hypophysial vascular supply. *Am. J. Anat. 58:* 421–472, 1936.

Yang, H.-Y., Hong, J. S., and Costa, E. Regional distribution of leu and met-enkephalin in rat brain. *Neuropharmacology 16:* 303–307, 1977.

Yasuda, N., and Greer, M. A. Studies on the corticotrophin releasing activity of vasopressin using ACTH secretion by cultured rat adenohypophyseal cells. *Endocrinology 98:* 936–942, 1976a.

Yasuda, N., and Greer, M. A. Rat hypothalamic corticotropin-releasing factor (CRF) content remains constant despite marked acute or chronic changes in ACTH secretion. *Neuroendocrinology 22:* 48–56, 1976b.

Yates, F. E., Leeman, S. E., Glenister, D. W., and Dallman, M. F. Interaction between plasma corticosterone concentration and adrenocorticotropin-releasing stimuli in the rat: Evidence for the reset of an endocrine feedback control. *Endocrinology 69:* 67–80, 1961.

Yates, F. E., and Maran, J. W. *Handbook of Physiology,* Section 7: Endocrinology, Vol. 4. Washington, D.C.: Am. Physiol. Soc., 1974, p. 367.

Záborszky, L., and Makara, G. B. Intrahypothalamic connections: An electron microscopic study in the rat. *Exp. Brain Res., 34:* 201–215, 1979.

Zimmerman, E. A. Localization of hypothalamic hormones by immunocytochemical techniques. In Martini, L., and Ganong, W. F. (eds.), *Frontiers in Neuroendocrinology.* New York: Raven Press, 1976, pp. 25–62.

Zimmerman, E. A., Carmel, P. W., Husain, M. K., Ferin, M., Tannenbaum, M., Frantz, A. G., and Robinson, A. G. Vasopressin and neurophysin: High concentrations in monkey hypophyseal portal blood. *Science 182:* 925–927, 1973.

Zimmerman, E. A., Liotta, A., and Krieger, D. T. β-Lipotropin brain: Localization in hypothalamic neurons by immunoperoxydase technique. *Cell Tiss. Res. 186:* 393–398, 1978.

Zimmerman, E. A., Stillman, M. A., Recht, L. D., Antunes, J. L., and Carmel, P. W. Vasopressin and corticotropin-releasing factor: An axonal pathway to portal capillaries in the zona externa of the median eminence containing vasopressin and its interaction with adrenal corticoids. In Krieger, D. T., and Ganong, W. F. (eds.), *ACTH and Related Peptides: Structure, Regulation and Action. Ann. N.Y. Acad. Sci. 297:* 405–419, 1977.

Epilogue

At first it might seem useless to select a few subjects a year for special discussion because a volume so constructed obviously could not give a satisfactory, complete overview of our field; besides, I have already written an encyclopedic treatise, based on 7,500 scientific articles, that covers all fields of stress research. Yet comprehensiveness has its limitations. A comprehensive approach is necessarily very sketchy, and subject to the selection of the editor and the interpretation of each individual author.

The present volume is an attempt to cover stress research in the detail and variety it requires, and yet to avoid the gigantic and insuperable task of editing and publishing that such an undertaking seemingly would entail. It was thought that if a yearly volume were offered which included only the best authors dealing with the most timely topics in the stress field, the effort behind it would have been well worthwhile.

In any case, this is only part of the program we have set for our International Institute of Stress (IIS), which is devoted to the furtherance of research on stress, and to the dissemination of knowledge already existing but not easily accessible to those who devote their time to highly specific, individual problems. In order to accomplish these aims, we have created the largest stress library and documentation service; it contains 150,000 entries, which are now available to everybody interested in any particular problem related to stress. We are also in the process of organizing an international network of affiliated stress institutes and stress teaching centers, which will be able to use the supportive work of our center, its documentation service, its teaching facilities and its lecturers.

A great deal is known about the various aspects of stress in medicine, biochemistry, psychology, law, daily life, and so on, and the knowledge is still growing. However, as more data accumulate, the work of correlating relevant findings becomes more difficult, and in themselves isolated facts are of virtually no value. Undoubtedly, the most important accomplishment of an institute such as ours would be the construction of a code of behavior acceptable to everybody irrespective of race, religion, traditions or any other specific factor. Just as drugs, surgery and other orthodox procedures afford protection from physical hazards, such a code would be a protective guide helping us to navigate among the many difficulties of life without being in contradiction with, or dependent upon, our lasting belief in the authority of any ''infallible'' leading spirit. Let us now consider the basic tenets of such a philosophy of life or code of behavior, which we have attempted to deduce from current knowledge of stress.

THE PRINCIPLE OF ALTRUISTIC EGOISM

From laboratory and clinical work on stress we have tried to arrive at a code of ethics founded, not on the traditions of our society, inspiration or blind faith in the infallibility of the teachings of any particular prophet, religious leader or man-made political doctrine, but on the scientifically verifiable laws of Nature that govern the body's reactions in maintaining homeostasis and living in satisfying equilibrium with its surroundings.

When you meet a helpless drunk who showers you with insults but is obviously quite unable to do you any harm, nothing happens if you go past and ignore him. However, if you respond by fighting or even only preparing to fight, the consequences may be tragic. You discharge adrenalines that increase blood pressure and pulse rate, while your whole nervous system becomes alarmed and tense in anticipation of combat. If you happen to be a coronary candidate, the result may be a fatal heart accident. In this case, who would be the murderer? The drunk will not have touched you. This is biologic suicide! Death will have been caused by choosing the wrong reaction. If, on the other hand, the man who showers you with insults is a homicidal maniac with a dagger in his hand, evidently determined to kill you, you must take an aggressive attitude. You must try to disarm him, even at the calculated risk of injury to yourself from the physical accompaniments of the alarm reaction in preparation for a fight. Contrary to common opinion, Nature, as usually interpreted, does always know best, since on both the cellular and the interpersonal level we do not always recognize what is and what is not worth fighting for. Both somatic and intellectual adaptive reactions are based on laws of Nature, and both must be combined for optimal efficiency.

Like all the lower animals, man has to fight and work for some goal that he considers worthwhile and satisfying. He must use his innate capacities to enjoy the eustress of fulfillment. Only through effort, often aggressive, egoistic effort, can he maintain his fitness and assure the security of his homeostatic equilibrium with the surrounding society and the inanimate world. To achieve this, his activities must earn lasting results; the fruits of his work must be cumulative and must provide a capital gain to meet future needs. To succeed, we have to accept the scientifically established fact that man has an inescapable, natural urge to work egoistically for things that can be stored to strengthen his homeostasis in unpredictable situations with which life may face him. These are not instincts we should combat or be ashamed of. We can do nothing about having been built to work, and to work primarily for our own good. Organs that are not used (muscles, bones, even the brain) undergo inactivity atrophy. There is no example in Nature of a creature guided exclusively by altruism and the desire to protect others. In fact, a code of universal altruism would be highly immoral, since it would expect others to look out for us more than for themselves.

The command "Love the neighbor as thyself" is full of wisdom, but, as originally expressed, it is incompatible with biologic laws; no one ought to develop an inferiority complex if he cannot love all his fellow men on command. Neither should he feel guilty because he works for a capital that can be safely stored to ensure his future homeostasis. Hoarding is a vitally important biologic instinct that we share with all animals, such as ants, bees, squirrels and beavers.

We must learn to live by a code of ethics that accepts, as morally correct, egoism and working to hoard personal capital. The "philosophy of altruistic egoism" advocates the creation of feelings of accomplishment and security through the inspiration in others of love, goodwill and gratitude for what we have done or are likely to do in the future. We must be useful and necessary to others. As explained in *Stress without Distress* (page iii), the basic concepts and guidelines are:

1. *Find your own natural stress level and run toward what you accept as your own goal.* People differ with regard to the amount and kind of work they consider worth doing to meet the exigencies of daily life and to

assure their future security and happiness. In this respect, all of us are influenced by hereditary predispositions and the traditions of our society. Only through planned self-analysis can we establish what we really want. Granted, this is difficult and takes much time, but too many people suffer all their lives because they are too conservative to risk a radical change and break with tradition.

2. *Practice altruistic egoism.* The selfish hoarding of the goodwill, respect, esteem, support and love of our neighbor is the most efficient way to give vent to our pent-up energy while creating enjoyable, beautiful or useful things.

3. *Earn thy neighbor's love.* This motto, unlike the command to love, is compatible with man's natural structure, and, although it is based on altruistic egoism, it could hardly be attacked as unethical. Who would blame anyone who wants to assure his own homeostasis and happiness by accumulating the treasure of other people's benevolence and gratitude toward him? This gives him self-esteem and at the same time makes him quite secure, for nobody wants to attack and destroy those upon whom he depends.

Man is a social being. If you have earned your neighbor's love, you will never be alone, and he who desires safety must avoid remaining alone in the midst of our overcrowded society. You must try to trust at least some people, despite their apparent untrustworthiness, or you will have no friends, no support.

These three main principles are derived from observations on the basic mechanisms that maintain homeostasis in cells, organs, people and entire societies, and that help them to face the stressors encountered in their constant fight for survival, security and happiness. In some people they have developed naturally during evolution, without the need for scientific proof. But evolution has not yet reached its final completion; it is still in progress. Meanwhile, we can best use these guidelines by conscious understanding and voluntary control.

In view of the advances made in our knowledge of the role played by chemical compounds (adrenal and pituitary hormones, endorphins, 5-HT, psychotropic drugs) and nervous processes, it is by studying this field that we can see the greatest future for the further development of a code of behavior based on biologic laws. But this will take a great deal of time; meanwhile we can make excellent use of a philosophy of life based on the scientific principles already established.

Let me close by expressing the hope that this yearly *Guide to Stress Research* will help support one of the most important of our activities, namely the correlation of detail and its dissemination and teaching. Thus it could act as a cement unifying the many efforts that are now being made to use the stress concept as a guide to a better understanding among people, a cement that keeps the most dissimilar facets of stress research together.

H.S.

Index